# ECHOCARDIOGRAPHY

## Practical Pocket Guide

*for Intensivists and Emergency Medicine Physicians*

A Quick Learning Initiative

## Declaration

# ECHOCARDIOGRAPHY

## Practical Pocket Guide

## *for Intensivists and Emergency Medicine Physicians*

## A Quick Learning Initiative

*Editors*

**Puneet Khanna**
MD
Additional Professor
Department of Anesthesiology, Pain Medicine and Critical Care
All India Institute of Medical Sciences
New Delhi, India

**Gourav Mittal**
DM (Critical Care Medicine)
Associate Consultant
Department of Medical Intensive Care Unit
Max Super Specialty Hospital
Noida, Uttar Pradesh, India

JAYPEE

JAYPEE BROTHERS MEDICAL PUBLISHERS
*The Health Sciences Publisher*
New Delhi | London

JAYPEE **Jaypee Brothers Medical Publishers (P) Ltd**

**Headquarters**
EMCA House
23/23-B, Ansari Road, Daryaganj
New Delhi - 110 002, India
Landline: +91-11-23272143, +91-11-23272703
+91-11-23282021, +91-11-23245672
E-mail: jaypee@jaypeebrothers.com

**Corporate Office**
4838/24, Ansari Road, Daryaganj
New Delhi - 110 002, India
Phone: +91-11-43574357
Fax: +91-11-43574314
E-mail: jaypee@jaypeebrothers.com

**Overseas Office**
J.P. Medical Ltd
83 Victoria Street, London
SW1H 0HW (UK)
Phone: +44 20 3170 8910
E-mail: info@jpmedpub.com

**EU GPSR** Authorised Representative
Logos Europe, 9 rue Nicolas Poussin
17000, La Rochelle, France
Phone: +33 (0) 6 67 93 73 78
E-mail: contact@logoseurope.eu

Website: www.jaypeebrothers.com
Website: www.jaypeedigital.com



**Inquiries for bulk sales may be solicited at:** jaypee@jaypeebrothers.com

***Echocardiography: Practical Pocket Guide for Intensivists and Emergency Medicine Physicians—A Quick Learning Initiative***

*First Edition:* 2025
*Reprint:* **2026**
ISBN: 978-93-5696-968-1
*Printed at: Samrat Offset Pvt. Ltd.*

## Dedication

*To the teachers and residents in anesthesiology and critical care*
*for their endeavor to dissipate and acquire knowledge,*
*My parents for their blessings,*
*My daughter Ziva for her patience and tolerance*
*shown to loss of many precious moments and finally to*
*my wife Ishita for her understanding and encouragement*

**Puneet Khanna**

*To my late father, whose enduring inspiration continues to light my path*
*To my mother, the unwavering pillar of my strength and support*
*To my nephew Aarav and niece Anaika, whose love and joy enrich my life everyday*
*And to all the patients and Residents in Critical Care Medicine at AIIMS, who placed their trust in me—this book is dedicated to you, with heartfelt gratitude and love.*

**Gourav Mittal**

# Contributors

**Ajay Singh** MD
Assistant Professor
Department of Anesthesia and Intensive Care
Post Graduate Institute of Medical Education and Research
Chandigarh, India

**Amit Kumar Malviya** MD
Assistant Professor
Department of Anesthesiology, Pain Medicine and Critical Care
All India Institute of Medical Sciences
New Delhi, India

**Anant Vikram Pachisia** MBBS MD FNB
Consultant
Department of Critical Care Medicine
Medanta—The Medicity
Gurugram, Haryana, India

**Aravindhan Manoharan** MD DM
Senior Resident
Division of Pediatric Pulmonology and Intensive Care
Department of Pediatrics
MIOT International Hospital
Chennai, Tamil Nadu, India

**Arshdeep Singh** MBBS MD
Senior Resident
Division of Cardiac Anesthesia and Intensive Care
Department of Anesthesia and Intensive Care
Post Graduate Institute of Medical Education and Research
Chandigarh, India

**Avneet Singh**
MBBS MD DM (Cardiac Anesthesia) FTEE
Assistant Professor
Division of Cardiac Anesthesia
Department of Anesthesia and Intensive Care
Government Medical College and Hospital
Chandigarh, India

**Balaji Rajaraman**
MD IDCCM EDIC DM (Critical Care Medicine)
Consultant
Department of Critical Care Services
Apollo Main Hospitals
Chennai, Tamil Nadu, India

**Bhavana Kayarat** MD
Senior Resident (Academic)
Department of Anesthesiology, Pain Medicine and Critical Care
All India Institute of Medical Sciences
New Delhi, India

**Gourav Mittal** DM (Critical Care Medicine)
Associate Consultant
Department of Medical Intensive Care Unit
Max Super Specialty Hospital
Noida, Uttar Pradesh, India

**Gyaninder Pal Singh** MD DM
Professor
Department Neuroanesthesiology and Neurocritical Care
All India Institute of Medical Sciences
New Delhi, India

**Kandaswamy N**
MD DNB (Anesthesiology) DM (Critical Care Medicine) EDIC
Assistant Professor
Department of Anesthesiology and Critical Care
Jawaharlal Institute of Postgraduate Medical Education and Research (JIPMER)
Puducherry, India

**Kapil Dev Soni** MD (Anesthesiology)
Professor Critical and Intensive Care
JPN Apex Trauma Centre
All India Institute of Medical Sciences
New Delhi, India

**Kiran Jangra** MD DM (Neurasthenia)
Additional Professor
Division of Neuroanesthesiology
and Neurocritical Care
Postgraduate Institute of Medical Education
and Research (PGIMER)
Chandigarh, India

**Kulbhushan Saini**
MD (Anesthesia) DM (Cardiac Anesthesia)
Associate Professor
Department of Anesthesia and Intensive Care
Postgraduate Institute of Medical Education and
Research (PGIMER)
Chandigarh, India

**Meera Rajeev** MD
DM Trainee (Cardiac Surgical Intensive Care)
Department of Cardiothoracic and Vascular
Surgery
All India Institute of Medical Sciences
New Delhi, India

**Mohd. Luqman** MD DM
Assistant Professor
Department of Anesthesiology, Pain Medicine
and Critical Care
All India Institute of Medical Sciences
Bathinda, Punjab, India

**Mukkelli Vinay Gandhi** MD DM
Senior Resident
Department of Anesthesiology, Pain Medicine
and Critical Care
All India Institute of Medical Sciences
New Delhi, India

**Nitin Rai** MD DM (Critical Care Medicine)
HOD, Department of Critical Care Medicine
Health City Vistaar Superspecialty Hospital
Lucknow, Uttar Pradesh, India

**Puneet Khanna** MD
Additional Professor, Department of
Anesthesiology, Pain Medicine and Critical Care
All India Institute of Medical Sciences
New Delhi, India

**Rakesh Lodha** MD
Professor, Department of Pediatrics
All India Institute of Medical Sciences
New Delhi, India

**Rakupathy S** MD DM (Critical Care) IDCCM
Senior Resident
Department of Anesthesiology, Pain Medicine
and Critical Care
All India Institute of Medical Sciences
New Delhi, India

**Richa Saroa** MD
Professor
Department of Anesthesia and Intensive Care
Government College and Hospital
Chandigarh, India

**Sanjeev Palta** MD
HOD
Department of Anesthesiology, Pain Medicine
and Critical Care
Government College and Hospital
Chandigarh, India

**Sarvesh Pal Singh** MD DM FIACTA FTEE
Additional Professor of Intensive Care for CTVS
Cardiothoracic and Vascular Surgery
All India Institute of Medical Sciences
New Delhi, India

**Shrikanth Srinivasan** MD DNB FNB EDIC FICCM
Chairman
Manipal Institute of Critical Care Medicine
Manipal Hospitals
New Delhi, India

**Srikant Behera**
MD PDCC DM (Critical Care Medicine)
Assistant Professor
Department of General Medicine
All India Institute of Medical Sciences
Bhubaneswar, Odisha, India

**Velmurugan Selvam** MD DM
Associate Professor
Department of Critical Care
Sri Ramachandra Medical College
Chennai, Tamil Nadu, India

**Vinay Kumar** MD
Assistant Professor
Department of Anesthesiology, Pain medicine
and Critical Care
Government Institute of Medical Sciences
Greater Noida, Uttar Pradesh, India

# Preface

Two-dimensional echocardiography plays a pivotal role, particularly in distinguishing various types of shock, guiding the use of vasopressors and fluid resuscitation, and facilitating goal-directed management of cardiac issues. The ability to perform echocardiographic assessments at the bedside empowers clinicians to make informed, real-time decisions, which are often critical for saving lives.

However, mastering echocardiography and ultrasound in the intensive care unit (ICU) poses challenges due to the steep-learning curve. Typically, the first point of contact for critically ill patients is a newly joined resident or a physician in the early stages of their training. These residents, while eager to learn, face heavy workloads and long hours rotating through various specialties, leaving little time to study complex materials. Watching videos or reading dense textbooks on ultrasound and echocardiography often feels impractical amidst the relentless demands of the ICU.

For intensivists, the challenge is even greater. Unlike cardiologists, who undergo structured and specialized training in cardiovascular medicine, intensivists must develop expertise across multiple systems—cardiovascular, respiratory, renal, and neurological—each with its own diagnostic and therapeutic complexities. Understanding the interplay of these systems in critically ill patients adds another layer of difficulty to acquiring in-depth knowledge of specialized procedures such as echocardiography.

While an abundance of literature exists on this subject, much of it is too dense and theoretical for those who need actionable, practical knowledge. The overwhelming volume of material can discourage residents, who are already fatigued from long-duty hours and frequent rotations. Even when residents manage to read these materials, the content often remains theoretical, with limited immediate applicability at the bedside. This gap between theoretical knowledge and practical application can lead to uncertainty, reliance on more experienced colleagues, or worse—turning to unreliable sources such as Internet searches during critical moments. Such scenarios compromise patient care and safety.

In the ICU, where every second counts, delays in diagnosis or treatment can have dire consequences. The goal of any intensivist is to deliver rapid, efficient, and accurate care. Without proper training and support, however, residents may struggle to confidently and competently use ultrasound for patient assessments, undermining the goal of a *Swift ICU, Safe ICU*. A truly safe ICU ensures that all medical staff, regardless of experience, are equipped with the necessary knowledge and tools to act decisively.

**The Need for Practical, Accessible Knowledge**

To address these challenges, we have developed a practical, easy-to-use guide specifically designed for intensivists and ICU residents. The cornerstone of this guide is simplicity and usability—providing residents with quick access to essential information without overwhelming them with unnecessary details or lengthy texts. The goal is to create a resource that is immediately applicable at the bedside.

Our book focuses on concise, targeted content, emphasizing the practical aspects of ultrasound and echocardiography in the ICU. It includes algorithms, normal values, essential concepts, and step-by-step guides, all of which can be quickly referenced during busy shifts. The information is deliberately crisp and direct, enabling residents to grasp key concepts in a short amount of time.

What sets our book apart from other publications is its focus on providing practical knowledge that is directly applicable to the day-to-day work of Intensivists and ICU Residents. While many books and resources focus on theoretical concepts, our guide aims to bridge the gap between theory and practice. By distilling complex medical concepts into easily digestible, actionable steps, our book empowers residents to make informed, confident decisions at the bedside. Moreover, the inclusion of interdisciplinary knowledge, such as how ultrasound integrates with other monitoring modalities and treatment strategies in the ICU, provides a holistic approach to patient care. The integration of various diagnostic tools—ultrasound, echocardiography, hemodynamic monitoring, and ventilatory support—helps intensivists form a complete picture of a patient's condition, allowing for timely interventions and more personalized care plans.

Through our unique knowledge cards and accompanying multimedia resources, we hope to empower healthcare professionals to provide swift, accurate, and safe care to critically ill patients. Our book is more than just a guide; it is a tool for improving patient care, enhancing medical education, and ultimately ensuring that every ICU remains a safe, effective, and responsive environment.

**Puneet Khanna**
**Gourav Mittal**

# Acknowledgments

We are thankful to Shri Jitendar P Vij (Group Chairman), Mr Ankit Vij (Managing Director), Mr MS Mani (Group President), Dr Neeraj Chaudhary—Associate Director (Publishing), Ms Pooja Bhandari [Director—Production (Books and Journals)], Ms Nikita Chauhan (Publishing Manager), Ms Ruby Sharma (Business Manager), and Mr Prashant Mahajan (Development Editor) of M/s Jaypee Brothers Medical Publishers (P) Ltd., New Delhi, India, for giving the go-ahead at the very beginning and helping us in every way possible to bring out this book.

We would like to thank Bhawna Kayrat for proofreading.

# Contents

# Video Contents

**Kindly refer to the all videos by scanning the QR code**

CHAPTER 1

# Indications of TTE and TEE in ICU. What is the need to go beyond POCUS to Critical Care Echocardiography? How is Critical Care Echocardiography Different from Cardiologist Echocardiography?

*Mukkelli Vinay Gandhi, Puneet Khanna*

## INTRODUCTION

*Echocardiography in the intensive care unit (ICU) serves multiple crucial purposes:* Assessing cardiac function, diagnosing abnormalities, guiding therapy, evaluating responses to treatment, and monitoring. Critical care echocardiography (CCE) provides a more thorough assessment, which is essential for effectively managing critically ill patients. It differs from cardiologist echocardiography in its focus on real-time decision-making and procedural guidance in the ICU. Critical care physicians require specialized training encompassing fundamental skills, interpretation abilities, and seamless integration into clinical practice. Adherence to guidelines and updated knowledge empowers caregivers to provide high-quality care.

## INDICATIONS OF TTE AND TEE IN INTENSIVE CARE UNIT[1-5]

- Evaluating the mechanisms of circulatory failure
- To titrate pharmacological or mechanical circulatory support
- Evaluation of cardiac causes of respiratory failure
- Etiology evaluation of systemic embolism
- Categorization of pulmonary embolism
- Evaluation of cardiac trauma
- Evaluation of complications after cardiac procedures/cardiothoracic surgery
- Evaluation of etiology of cardiac arrest
- Assessment of regional wall motion abnormalities (RWMA) and complications of acute coronary syndrome (ACS)
- Classification of aortic dissection
- Diagnosis of infective endocarditis, pericarditis, and cardiac tamponade
- Placement and monitoring of mechanical circulatory devices
- Assessment of valvular pathology, diastolic dysfunction, and pulmonary hypertension

## INDICATIONS OF CRITICAL CARE TRANSESOPHAGEAL ECHOCARDIOGRAPHY[6-9]

Transesophageal echocardiography (TEE) offers higher-resolution assessment when transthoracic echocardiography is not sufficient.

- Inadequate TTE windows for assessment of hemodynamic instability and shock.
- Diagnosis and assessment of intracardiac shunt lesions.
- Evaluation of etiology of cardiac arrest, i.e., aortic dissection, pulmonary embolism, cardiac tamponade, etc.
- Procedural guidance and monitoring of mechanical circulatory devices (MCDs).

- Assessment of cardiac trauma, i.e., traumatic valvular abnormalities, aortic injuries, and etiologies of shock.
- To identify right ventricular (RV) failure and intracardiac shunting in respiratory failure.
- Assessment of valvular pathologies, diagnosis of endocarditis, prosthetic valvular function, intracardiac thrombus, and atrial myxomas.
- Difficult TTE windows, i.e., obesity, subcutaneous emphysema, and thoracic drains and dressing.
- Evaluation of complications after cardiac procedures/cardiothoracic surgery.

**What is the need to go beyond the cardiac point of care ultrasound (POCUS) to CCE?[10-13]**

Cardiac POCUS utilizes a focused imaging protocol to identify specific conditions or to enable rapid follow-up assessments, whereas CCE uses extensive protocols and diagnoses conditions relevant to critical care. It often incorporates Doppler assessments and evaluations beyond standard transthoracic echocardiography.

In critically ill patients, Echocardiography measurements are interpreted cautiously, these are affected by rapidly changing physiological states due to fluid resuscitation, vasoactive agents, and changes in intrathoracic pressure. Cardiac output is traditionally determined by heart rate, contractility, preload, and afterload. However, practical scenarios also consider left and right heart function, systemic vascular resistance, ventricular interdependence, and venous return for a comprehensive understanding of circulatory failure. CCE examines these parameters using Doppler, providing insights into cardiac output and ventricular filling pressures.

Mixed (cardiogenic and noncardiogenic) shock was frequently encountered in ICU patients, accurate discernment is critical. Intensivists skilled in CCE use metrics such as stroke volume and left ventricular outflow tract velocity time integral (LVOT VTI) to accurately determine the shock profile, irrespective of the underlying cause or existing cardiomyopathy.

In critically ill patients, missing significant valvular dysfunction, such as severe aortic regurgitation in those with an intra-aortic balloon pump, can be dangerous. CCE utilizing continuous wave Doppler is crucial for determining the severity of regurgitations.

Right ventricular function evaluation is crucial in patients with ARDS, receiving mechanical ventilation with high positive end-expiratory pressure (PEEP). CCE evaluation of RV function with variable PEEP may help in selecting the most appropriate ventilator settings and optimizing heart-lung interactions.

Critical care echocardiography involves the dynamic assessment of cardiac function, interpreting changes based on rapidly evolving physiological conditions. This enables the implementation of therapeutic interventions, potentially aiding in the early stabilization of the patient.

## HOW IS CCE DIFFERENT FROM CARDIOLOGIST ECHOCARDIOGRAPHY (TABLES 1 AND 2)?[10]

### Cardiologist Echocardiography

Using advanced techniques, comprehensive evaluations are performed once per admission or when there is a change in clinical status. The evaluation thoroughly addresses all findings, whether related to the referral question or incidental, with standard practice incorporating comparisons to prior studies. All findings, both primary and incidental, are mandatorily recorded in detailed imaging. Images are archived on picture archiving

**TABLE 1:** How is CCE different from cardiologist echocardiography.

| | *Cardiac POCUS* | *CCE* |
|---|---|---|
| Definition | Utilizes specific imaging protocols based upon suspicion of a specific disease | Focused on obtaining specific findings relevant to the care of the critically ill (e.g., volume status, and CO) |
| Frequency | Usually once | More frequently |
| Quantification | Quantification is optional | Requires quantification |
| Indication | Clinical suspicion | Medical necessity |
| Time required | Rapid assessment (5–10 minutes) | Depends on indication |
| Training duration | Training requires weeks to months | Requires months |
| Utility | • Assessment of LV and RV function, LV wall thickness, LA size, pericardial effusion, IVC size, and variability<br>• Evaluation of findings associated with cardiac tamponade, pulmonary embolism, HFrEF, and HFpEF | • Evaluation of functional anatomy<br>• Of heart chambers<br>• *Evaluation of:* Valvular, pericardial, and great vessels pathologies (IVC, SVC, and aorta)<br>• Guidance and monitoring of devices (CVCs and TPIs)<br>• Evaluation of adult congenital heart diseases<br>• Classification and management of shock<br>• Assessment of volume status<br>• Assessment of cardiovascular emergencies (AMI, RWMA, CHD, and CHF)<br>• Cardiac trauma<br>• Evaluation of cardiac causes of respiratory failure<br>• Etiologic evaluation of cardiac arrest |

(AMI: acute myocardial infarction; CCE: critical care echocardiography; CHD: coronary heart disease; CO: cardiac output; CVCs: central venous catheters; HFrEF: heart failure with reduced ejection fraction; HFpEF: heart failure with preserved ejection fraction; IVC: inferior vena cava; LA: left atrium; LV: left ventricle; POCUS: point of care ultrasound; RV: right ventricular; RWMA: regional wall motion abnormalities; SVC: superior vena cava; TPIS: transjugular intrahepatic portosystemic shunt)

and communication systems (PACS), accompanied by a formal report.

The echocardiography machines used for CCE often differ from those used for cardiologist echocardiography. Most radiologic equipment in the ICU features 2D, color, and spectral Doppler capabilities but may have limited options for image modification. In contrast, standard echocardiography equipment features comprehensive and modifiable controls, multiple transducers, and durability.

In CCE, patient positioning is frequently constrained; patients are often intubated, and their ventilation mode can affect dynamics. Patients are usually supine, and pacer/defibrillator pads may obstruct access, requiring infection precautions. Conversely, cardiologist echocardiography is optimized with the patient in the left lateral position, often with a bed cutout for apical imaging, typically for nonportable exams.

Critical care echocardiography involves a basic assessment of valves, filling pressures,

**TABLE 2:** Comparison between critical care echocardiography and comprehensive echo.

| | *CCE* | *Comprehensive echo* |
|---|---|---|
| Diagnostic expectations | Focused on a collection of specific views/findings pertinent to the care of the critically ill (e.g., cardiac output and fluid-responsive) | Comprehensive, all findings, quantification; increasingly use advanced techniques |
| Application frequency | On admission or change in clinical status, potentially frequently | Once (per admission, change in clinical status) |
| Interpretation of findings | Primary and incidental findings recorded in views | All findings, primary and incidental recorded in comprehensive imaging |
| Quantification | Typically | Mandatory |
| Indication | Medical necessity | Medical necessity |
| Documentation | Images archived, formal report | Images archived on PACS, formal report |
| Teaching required | Advanced (years) | Advanced (years) |

(CCE: critical care echocardiography; PACS: picture archiving and communication systems)

and cardiac output, and may include chamber quantification. Standard echocardiography, on the other hand, entails meticulous comprehensive measurements of all standard areas, increasingly incorporating advanced quantification techniques, three-dimensional (3D) imaging, and strain analysis.

The scanning protocol and interpretation in CCE focus on findings pertinent to the clinical situation, often including evaluations of other organs. Standard echocardiography; however, provides a comprehensive evaluation of the heart alone.

In CCE, all views and at least basic techniques are used to evaluate clinical diagnoses. In contrast, standard echocardiography requires the use of all views and techniques, with advanced valvular quantification, strain, and 3D imaging becoming standard practices.

## TRAINING AND EXPERTISE REQUIRED FOR CRITICAL CARE ECHOCARDIOGRAPHY[14-19]

An expert roundtable on echocardiography in the ICU produced an international consensus statement on training standards for advanced CCE in 2014.

They recognized general CCE and advanced CCE as separate entities, for Advanced CCE requires separate special training and additional competence.

Various specialty societies have emphasized the need for circular training of health care professionals, and WINFOCUS emphasized the training requirements for cardiac POCUS in critical care.

In 2020, the American Society of Echocardiography provided recommendations for echocardiography laboratories involved in cardiac POCUS and CCE training. CCE training curriculum requires ≥2–3 months of training, the trainee should do a minimum of 150 CCE scans with image review and interpretation, under the supervision of a National Board of Echocardiography (NBE)-certified physician.

Trainees should develop competencies in evaluating the anatomy and physiological function of the heart, as well as pathologies related to valvular, pericardial, and great vessels. They should also be proficient in the placement and monitoring of devices and foreign bodies and the diagnosis and management of adult congenital heart diseases, shock, acute cardiovascular presentations, trauma, respiratory failure, and cardiac arrest. Additionally, trainees should acquire technical skills and knowledge in the physics of ultrasonography, Doppler techniques, and image optimization. These are just a few examples of the CCE components in which trainees should become proficient.

## EDUCATION GUIDELINE[14-19]

Critical care echocardiography has become an essential tool in the management of critically ill patients. The education guidelines for CCE are designed to ensure that healthcare professionals acquire the necessary knowledge, skills, and competencies to effectively utilize this technology.

Core competencies and curriculum.

*The guidelines emphasize the importance of developing core competencies in several areas:*

- *Anatomy and physiological function:* Understanding the structural and functional aspects of the heart is fundamental. Trainees must be able to assess cardiac chambers, valves, and pericardium accurately.
- *Pathological conditions:* Competence in identifying and managing conditions, such as valvular disease, pericardial pathologies, and great vessel abnormalities is crucial.
- *Technical skills:* Proficiency in the technical aspects of echocardiography, including the physics of ultrasound, Doppler techniques, and image optimization, is necessary.
- *Clinical applications:* Training should cover the use of CCE in various clinical scenarios, including shock, acute cardiovascular presentations, trauma, respiratory failure, and cardiac arrest.

### Training Methods

The guidelines recommend a combination of theoretical knowledge and practical experience:

- *Didactic learning:* Trainees should undergo formal education through lectures, seminars, and self-study materials. This foundational knowledge is crucial for understanding the principles of echocardiography.
- *Hands-on training:* Supervised practice with real patients is essential. Trainees should perform a minimum number of echocardiographic examinations to achieve proficiency.
- *Simulation:* The use of simulation-based training can enhance learning, particularly in complex or rare cases where real-life practice opportunities may be limited.

### Assessment and Certification

Assessment methods include both formative and summative evaluations:

- *Formative assessments:* Continuous feedback during training helps identify areas for improvement. This can include direct observation, logbooks, and reflective practice.
- *Summative assessments:* Formal examinations, including written tests and practical evaluations, are used to certify competence. Successful completion of these assessments is often required for credentialing in CCE.

### Challenges and Recommendations

Implementing these guidelines presents several challenges:

### *Resource Limitations*

Access to training resources, including qualified instructors and advanced equipment, can be limited in some settings.

### *Standardization*

Ensuring consistent training quality across different institutions and regions is challenging. The development of universal standards and regular updates to the guidelines are recommended to address this.

## CONCLUSION

The education guidelines for CCE provide a comprehensive framework for training healthcare professionals in this vital skill. By adhering to these guidelines, training programs can ensure that trainees develop the necessary competencies to effectively use CCE in clinical practice. Continued efforts to address implementation challenges and update the guidelines in response to technological and clinical advancements will be essential for maintaining high standards of care.

## REFERENCES

1. Barman B, Parihar A, Kohli N, Agarwal A, Dwivedi D, Kumari G. Impact of bedside combined cardiopulmonary ultrasound on etiological diagnosis and treatment of acute respiratory failure in critically ill patients. Indian J Crit Care Med. 2020;24(11):1062-70.
2. Soliman-Aboumarie H, Pastore MC, Galiatsou E, Gargani L, Pugliese NR, Mandoli GE, et al. Echocardiography in the intensive care unit: an essential tool for diagnosis, monitoring and guiding clinical decision-making. Imaging. 2021;14(1):1-15.
3. Peng X, Luo T, Yao L, Kessner R, Wu W, Bonavina L, et al. Ultrasonography in the intensive care unit: a bibliometrics analysis. J Thorac Dis. 2024;16(1):623-31.
4. Volpicelli G, Mayo P, Rovida S. Focus on ultrasound in intensive care. Intensive Care Med. 2020;46(6):1258-60.
5. Guevarra K, Greenstein Y. Ultrasonography in the Critical Care Unit. Curr Cardiol Rep. 2020;22(11):145.
6. Prager R, Bowdridge J, Pratte M, Cheng J, McInnes MD, Arntfield R. Indications, clinical impact, and complications of critical care transesophageal echocardiography: a scoping review. J Intensive Care Med. 2023;38(3):245-72.
7. Andrade H, Carroll J, Tomkiewicz E, Jackson E. Hemodialysis catheter–associated right atrial thrombus diagnosed via point of care transesophageal echocardiogram. POCUS J. 2024;9(1):25-8.
8. Teran F, West FM, Jelic T, Taylor L, Jafry ZM, Burns KM, et al. Resuscitative transesophageal echocardiography in emergency departments in the United States and Canada: a cross-sectional survey. Am J Emerg Med. 2024;76:164-72.
9. Grotberg JC, McDonald RK, Co IN. point-of-care echocardiography in the difficult-to-image patient in the ICU: a narrative review. Crit Care Explor. 2024;6(1):e1035.
10. Kirkpatrick JN, Grimm R, Johri AM, Kimura BJ, Kort S, Labovitz AJ, et al. Recommendations for Echocardiography Laboratories Participating in Cardiac Point of Care Cardiac Ultrasound (POCUS) and Critical Care Echocardiography Training: Report from the American Society of Echocardiography. J Am Soc Echocardiogr. 2020;33(4):409-22.e4.
11. Kimura BJ. Point-of-care cardiac ultrasound techniques in the physical examination: better at the bedside. Heart. 2017;103(13):987-94.
12. Salinas P, Dieiev V. Critical care echocardiography: assessing left and right ventricular function in the intensive care unit. Semin Ultrasound CT MRI. 2024;45(1):58-73.
13. Orde S, Slama M, Hilton A, Yastrebov K, McLean A. Pearls and pitfalls in comprehensive critical care echocardiography. Crit Care. 2017;21(1):279.
14. Vieillard-Baron A, Mayo P, Vignon P, Cholley B, Slama M, Pinsky MR, et al. International consensus statement on

training standards for advanced critical care echocardiography. Intensive Care Med. 2014;40(5):654-66.

15. Cecconi M, De Backer D, Antonelli M, Beale R, Bakker J, Hofer C, et al. Consensus on circulatory shock and hemodynamic monitoring. Task force of the European Society of Intensive Care Medicine. Intensive Care Med. 2014;40(12):1795-815.
16. Millington SJ, Arntfield RT, Guo RJ, Koenig S, Kory P, Noble V, et al. The Assessment of Competency in Thoracic Sonography (ACTS) scale: validation of a tool for point-of-care ultrasound. Crit Ultrasound J. 2017;9(1):25.
17. Millington SJ, Hewak M, Arntfield RT, Beaulieu Y, Hibbert B, Koenig S, et al. Outcomes from extensive training in critical care echocardiography: identifying the optimal number of practice studies required to achieve competency. J Crit Care. 2017;40:99-102.
18. Price S, Via G, Sloth E, Guarracino F, Breitkreutz R, Catena E, et al. Echocardiography practice, training and accreditation in the intensive care: document for the World Interactive Network Focused on Critical Ultrasound (WINFOCUS). Cardiovasc Ultrasound. 2008;6(1):49.
19. Gaudet J, Waechter J, McLaughlin K, Ferland A, Godinez T, Bands C, et al. Focused critical care echocardiography: development and evaluation of an image acquisition assessment tool. Crit Care Med. 2016;44(6):e329-35.

CHAPTER 2

# Physics in Echocardiography

*Bhavana Kayarat, Puneet Khanna*

## INTRODUCTION

Echocardiography is the primary noninvasive imaging modality that provides us with qualitative and quantitative information about cardiac anatomy. A brief pulse of the ultrasound wave is propagated through the cardiac structures, which is subsequently reflected. The ultrasound transducer records the duration of time delay with each returning reflection. This permits us to precisely calculate the location of the cardiac structures to create an image map of the heart. A basic understanding of the fundamental physical principles of cardiac ultrasound is therefore necessary. In this section, we will discuss the physical principles of ultrasound wave mechanics, its propagation through tissues, along with applications of Doppler echocardiography.

## SOUND WAVE: GENERAL PHYSICAL PRINCIPLES

Sound travels through a medium in the form of a propagating wave, typically represented graphically as a sine wave **(Fig. 1)**. Typically, ultrasound used in medical practice employs

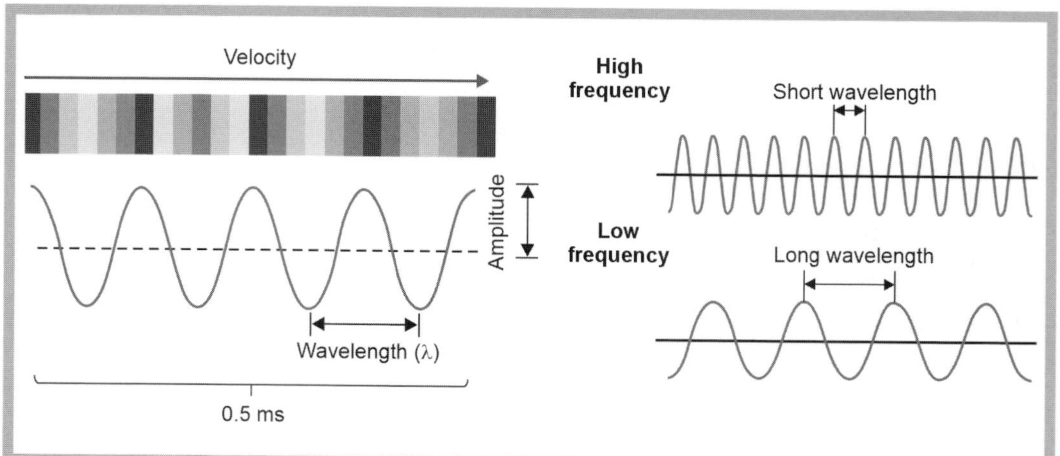


**Fig. 1:** Sound wave. Vibrations from the transducer cause cycles of compression and rarefaction in the adjacent tissue. The ultrasound wave is characterized by amplitude, frequency, wavelength, and propagation velocity.

*Source:* Adapted from In: Perino A (Ed). A Practical Approach to Transesophageal Echocardiography, 3rd edition. Philadelphia: Lippincott Williams & Wilkins; 2014.

sound waves at frequencies ranging from 1 to 20 MHz.

- *Amplitude (A)* represents the maximum compression of particles above the baseline and is measured in decibels (dB). Changes in amplitude are what create the grayscale images seen in two-dimensional (2D) echocardiography.
- *Intensity (I)* indicates the amount of sound energy within a specific area of tissue and is measured as watts per square centimeter (watts/cm$^2$). It is calculated using the formula: Intensity (I) = Power (watts)/beam area (cm$^2$). Intensity is directly proportional to the square of the ultrasound wave's amplitude. Higher amplitude results in greater intensity, which increases the risk of tissue injury.

The distance the wave travels through one cycle is called *wavelength (λ)*. It is the distance between one peak of the wave to the next peak. The number of waves that pass in a given unit of time is referred to as the frequency of the *wave (f)*. The product of wavelength (λ) and frequency (f) gives us the propagation velocity of the wave. Since the propagation velocity of sound waves in human cardiac tissues is a constant (i.e., 1,540 m/s); we can say that the wavelength is related inversely to the frequency.

## INTERACTION OF ULTRASOUND WAVES WITH TISSUES

### Acoustic Impedance

Acoustic impedance refers to the resistance a medium offers to the propagation of sound. It is the product of the velocity of the sound and the density of the medium it passes through. When sound traverses a homogeneous medium, it follows a linear path. However, when the sound wave encounters an interface; i.e., when it passes between two tissues with two different densities (acoustic impedances), a part of the sound beam gets reflected back to the source. The extent to which this reflection occurs is determined by the disparity in their acoustic impedances. A greater difference in acoustic impedance between the two tissues results in a higher proportion of the ultrasound wave being reflected. The magnitude of the reflected beam received by the transducer is contingent upon the angle between the ultrasound beam and the tissue interface. Optimal reflection, or the maximum return of the reflected ultrasound, is achieved when the angle of incidence is 90° (perpendicular) to the interface.

### Scattering

Scattering refers to the phenomenon where ultrasound waves encounter irregularly shaped or small structures (e.g., red blood cells) and this results in the reflection of waves in multiple directions. These scattered reflections are considerably weaker compared to specular reflections **(Fig. 2)**.

### Attenuation

Attenuation refers to the reduction in the strength of the ultrasound wave as it traverses through various tissues. This decrease in signal strength occurs primarily due to the absorption of ultrasound energy, which is converted to heat. Attenuation is influenced by both frequency and wavelength. Additionally, attenuation is also affected by acoustic impedance. Air exhibits very high acoustic impedance. This explains the attenuation of signal we observe when imaging through lung tissue, especially appreciated in cases of emphysema. Conversely, the presence of fluid in the pleural space enhances ultrasound imaging.

## GENERATION OF ULTRASOUND BEAM

### Piezoelectric Effect

Ultrasound is produced through the piezoelectric effect. When an electric charge is applied to a piezoelectric crystal, the dipoles within the crystal realign with the electric field, resulting in distortion and vibration of the crystal. These vibrations generate ultrasonic waves that propagate into the body. The ultrasound transducer also functions as a receiver; the reflected ultrasonic waves cause slight movements in the crystal's dipoles, inducing an electric field. This electric field is detected by electrodes, subsequently amplified, and processed for display by the ultrasound machine.

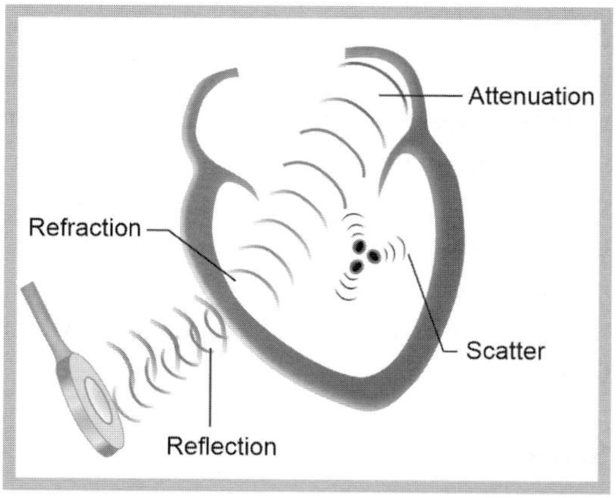


**Fig. 2:** Interaction of ultrasound waves and tissues.
*Source:* Adapted from In: Perino A (Ed). A Practical Approach to Transesophageal Echocardiography, 3rd edition. Philadelphia: Lippincott Williams & Wilkins; 2014.

### Transducers

The structure of a transducer includes the following **(Figs. 3A to C)**:

- Acoustic insulation
- Backing layer
- Piezoelectric crystals
- Matching layer
- Acoustic lens

The *acoustic insulation* in the transducer ensures that no other sound waves interfere

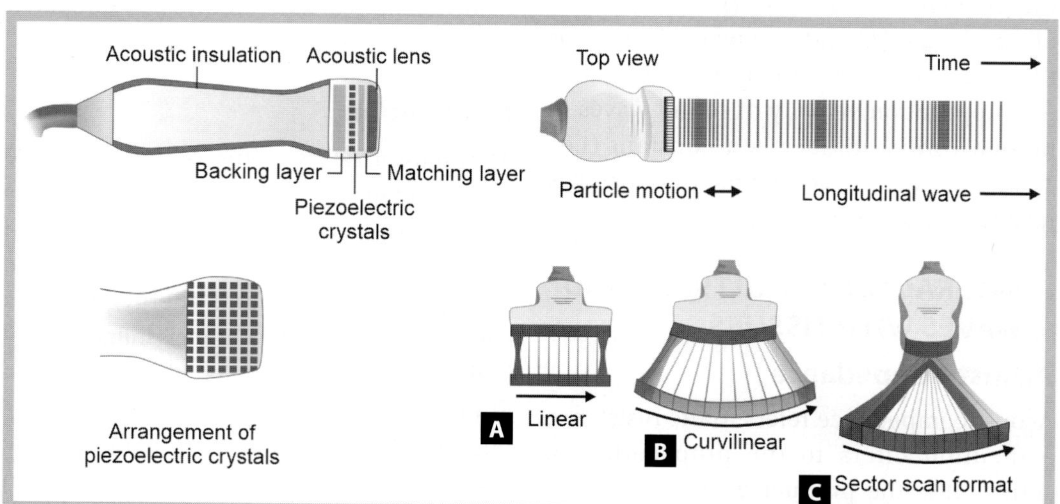


**Figs. 3A to C:** The linear array transducer activates a subgroup of transducer elements to produce an ultrasound beam directed perpendicular to the array. (A) A rectangular field of view is produced; (B) The convex arrangement in the curvilinear probe produces a trapezoidal field of view; and (C) A phased array transducer produces a beam from the near-simultaneous excitation of all array elements. The beam is electronically steered, and a sector scan format is produced.

with or affect the transducer. The *backing layer* suppresses the vibrations of the crystals. By doing so, it allows sound waves to be sent in shorter pulses. This improves the resolution of the image. The *matching layer* reduces the difference in acoustic impedance between the tissue under interest and the crystals. This minimizes the unwanted reflection of the sound waves and ensures sound waves penetrate the tissues.

The simplest ultrasound transducer contains a single piezoelectric crystal and is used for M-mode recordings. To generate a 2D image, mechanical or electronic systems are required to move the ultrasound beam across the desired plane. Typically, transducers consist of multiple crystals (or elements) arranged in a linear array. The sound waves emitted by each crystal combine to form a unified wavefront, which can be more effectively focused and directed compared to using a single crystal.

By adjusting the timing of electrical activation for each crystal in the array, known as a phased array, the beam can be steered without physically moving the transducer. Electronic systems offer advantages over mechanical ones, including the absence of moving parts and the ability to easily manipulate the ultrasound beam for steering, focusing, and narrowing.

Phased-array transducers, which consist of multiple ultrasound crystals arranged for electronic steering without moving parts, are the most commonly used type in clinical echocardiography. The precise timing of the activation of individual transducer elements allows the ultrasound beam to sweep in an arc across the area of interest. This phased-array system enables easy narrowing, steering, and focusing of the beam by varying the sequence of element activation. Electronic beam steering over an arced sector allows for a smaller transducer interface, as seen in transthoracic and transesophageal echocardiography **(Figs. 3A to C)**.

In contrast to echocardiographic imaging, continuous-wave Doppler examinations use two dedicated crystals: (1) Continuously transmits sound waves, while the (2) other continuously receives the returning signals. In pulsed-wave Doppler, a single crystal alternates between transmitting and receiving; it transmits a sound wave and then pauses to receive the returning signal before transmitting again.

Higher-frequency (and lower-wavelength) transducers provide better spatial resolution for imaging. However, due to attenuation, the depth of tissue penetration is directly related to wavelength and inversely related to transducer frequency. As a result, higher-frequency transducers have reduced tissue penetration. The balance between resolution and penetration is crucial in selecting the appropriate transducer frequency for clinical imaging.

## Resolution

The ability of an imaging system to discern two points in space is referred to as resolution. Frequency and wavelength are mathematically related to the velocity of the ultrasound beam within the tissue (approximately 1,540,000 mm/s for human tissue) as follows:

- Velocity of blood = Wavelength (mm) × frequency (Hz)
- Wavelength (mm) = 1,540,000 mm/s/frequency (Hz)
- Wavelength (mm) = 1.54/frequency (MHz)

The resolution of a recording, i.e., the ability to distinguish two objects that are spatially close together, varies directly with the frequency and inversely with the wavelength.

High-frequency, short-wavelength ultrasound can differentiate between objects <1 mm apart. Echocardiographic image resolution typically corresponds to one or two wavelengths. For instance, imaging with a 2.5 MHz transducer achieves a resolution of approximately 1 mm.

In echocardiography, resolution can be classified as axial (along the length of the ultrasound beam), lateral (side-to-side), or elevational (along the thickness of the beam) **(Fig. 4)**.

### *Axial Resolution*

- Axial resolution refers to the ability to distinguish between two structures aligned with the direction of the ultrasound beam.
- It is influenced by the transducer frequency, transducer bandwidth, and the duration/length of the ultrasound pulse.

### *Lateral Resolution*

- Lateral resolution refers to the minimum distance at which two side-by-side structures can be distinguished as separate entities and still produce distinct echoes.
- It indicates the ability to differentiate closely spaced objects that are perpendicular to the ultrasound beam within the imaging plane.
- Lateral resolution is approximately equal to the beam diameter.
- Since the beam diameter changes with depth, lateral resolution also varies with depth. It is most optimal at the focal point, where the beam is at its narrowest.

### *Temporal Resolution*

- Temporal resolution relates to time and refers to the ability to accurately locate moving structures at a specific moment.
- Higher frame rates (more images per unit of time) enhance temporal resolution.
- Temporal resolution, particularly in color Doppler, depends on factors, such as the number of pulses per scan line, line density, imaging depth, and sector size.

## CARDIAC ULTRASOUND IMAGING MODALITIES

Cardiac ultrasound imaging modalities encompass one-dimensional techniques [amplitude Mode (A-mode), brightness mode

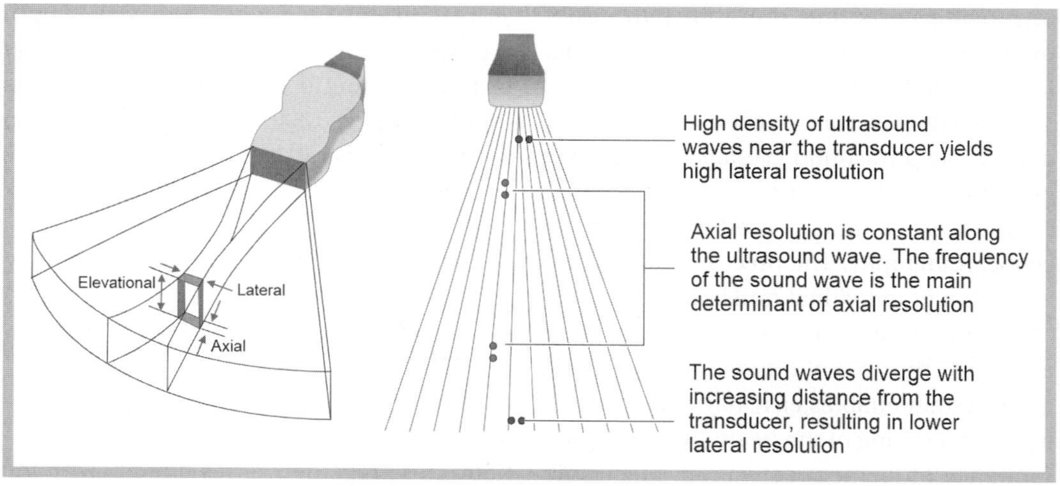


**Fig. 4:** Axial and lateral resolution.

(B-mode), and motion mode (M-mode)], and 2D echocardiography. More recently, three-dimensional echocardiography has also been introduced **(Fig. 5)**.

### Amplitude Mode

In amplitude mode, the returning signal amplitudes are displayed as a series of horizontal spikes along the vertical axis of the display. These spikes represent both the distance to the reflecting tissue and the strength of the returning echoes.

### Brightness Mode

In brightness mode, the amplitudes of returning echoes are displayed as pixels of varying brightness along the vertical axis. The brightness of each pixel correlates with the strength of the returning signal, providing a visual representation of tissue structures.

### Motion Mode

Motion mode (M-mode) enhances B-mode imaging, i.e., it adds temporal information to B-mode; through the sequential display of collected B-mode images. M-mode echocardiography provides a one-dimensional representation of cardiac structures and updates B-mode images at a significantly high frequency **(Figs. 6 and 7)**. This allows for dynamic, real-time imaging. The transducer element captures the reflected energy of the previous pulse before emitting the next one. The frame rate, which is calculated as the reciprocal of the round-trip travel time of the ultrasound pulse, is exceptionally high in M-mode imaging (exceeding 2,000 frames per second). This results in superior visualization of dynamic cardiac motion compared to other imaging modalities. However, M-mode is limited to displaying only axial motion, thus offering a restricted view of cardiac anatomy. Due to its high temporal resolution and ability to accurately depict the timing of cardiac events, M-mode is particularly valuable when used in conjunction with an electrocardiogram.

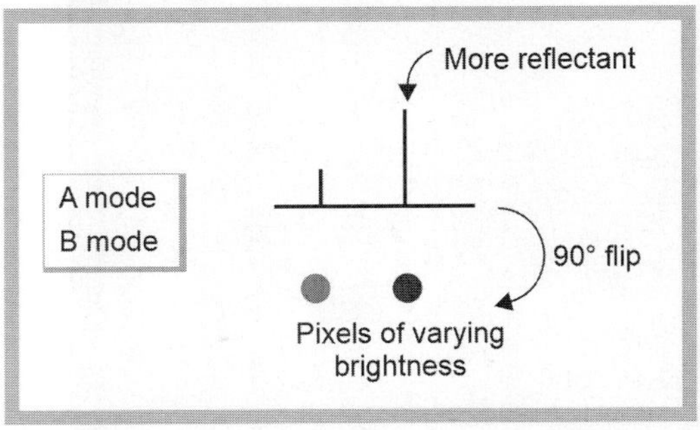


**Fig. 5:** A-mode—amplitude display in which the intensity of the reflected ultrasound wave is displayed as a vertical deflection along the baseline. Reflected ultrasound signals are displayed as spots of varying brightness in B (brightness) mode proportional to the intensity of the reflected signal.

## TWO-DIMENSIONAL ECHOCARDIOGRAPHY

Two-dimensional echocardiography is a modification of B-mode echocardiography and the mainstay of the echocardiographic examination. Instead of repeatedly firing ultrasound pulses in a single direction, the transducer in 2D echocardiography sequentially directs the ultrasound pulses across a sector of the cardiac anatomy. In this way, 2D imaging can display a tomographic section of the cardiac anatomy, and unlike M-mode, it can show shape and lateral motion.

### Principes of Doppler Echocardiography

Two-dimensional imaging, despite its ability to provide detailed anatomic images, does not visualize blood flow. It only displays it as a uniform black area. While both M-mode and 2D echocardiography can create anatomical images of the heart,

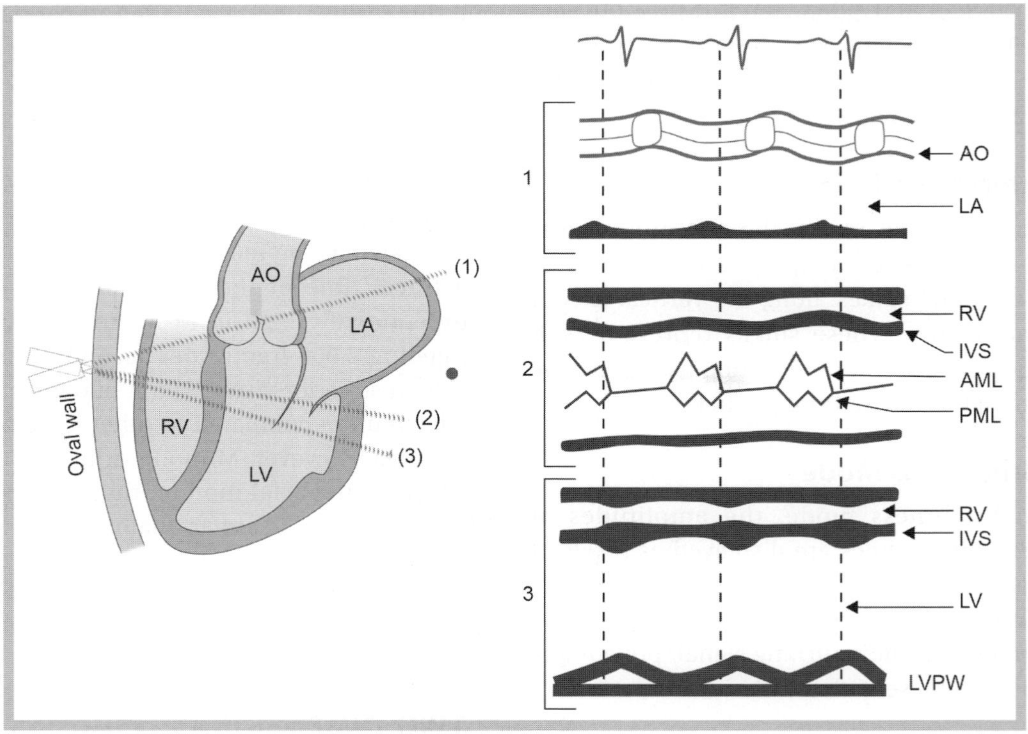


**Fig. 6:** M-mode ultrasonography where a single scan line is emitted, received, and displayed graphically. M-mode provides good temporal resolution and a superior axial resolution to B mode. The image will display all the structures along the ultrasound line. In M-mode ultrasonography, the abscissa represents time and the ordinate shows the distance from the transducer. (B-mode: brightness mode; M-mode: motion mode)

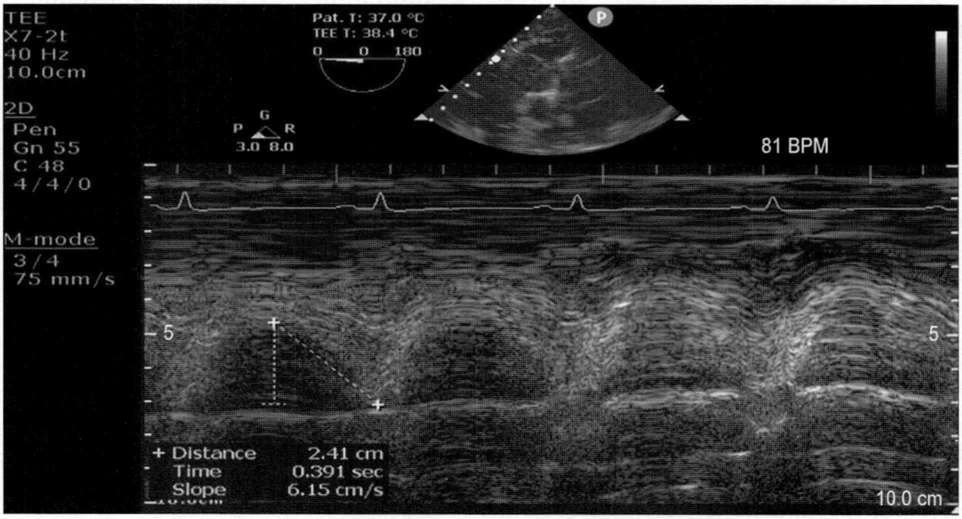


**Fig. 7:** Motion mode (M-mode) at the tricuspid annular plane. The M-mode cursor is placed at the lateral tricuspid annulus.

Doppler echocardiography is utilized to assess blood flow within the cardiovascular system. The color flow display offers various echocardiographic views of blood flow, while spectral Doppler enables quantification of flow magnitude and direction, which is essential for assessing disease severity. Doppler echocardiography relies on detecting frequency shifts in the backscatter signal from moving structures, such as red blood cells.

## BASIC PRINCIPLES

### Doppler Effect

When a moving target backscatters an ultrasound beam to the transducer, the observed frequency changes based on the target's movement. If the target is moving toward the transducer, the observed frequency will be higher than the original transmitted frequency. Conversely, if the target is moving away from the transducer, the observed frequency will be lower. This difference between the transmitted frequency (Fttt) and the received frequency (Frrr) is known as the *Doppler shift*:

$$\text{Doppler shift } [F(d)] = F(r) - F(t)$$

When ultrasound waves are transmitted into the bloodstream, they are scattered by red blood cells, and a portion of this scattered signal is reflected back to the transducer. The strength of these returning echoes is directly proportional to the number of red blood cells reflecting the ultrasound. An increased hematocrit results in more reflecting interfaces and, consequently, a stronger signal. However, if the hematocrit exceeds 30%, the reflected signal strength may decrease due to destructive interference. Modern echocardiographic systems are now designed to detect Doppler signals across a wide range of hematocrit levels. If the red blood cells are stationary, the reflected signal frequency will match the transmitted frequency, resulting in no Doppler shift and a display similar to that of 2D echocardiography.

### Doppler Equation (Table 1)

Blood flow velocity (V) is related to the Doppler shift by the speed of sound in the blood (C) and the intercept angle (ø) between the ultrasound beam and the direction of blood flow. A factor of 2 is applied to account for the "round-trip" transit time of the sound wave to and from the transducer.

$$F(d) = 2 \times F(t) \times [(V \times \cos\theta)]/C$$

By substituting [F(r) – F(t)] for F(d):

$$V = \{[F(r) - F(t)] \times C\}/[2 \times F(t) \times \cos\theta]$$

The angle between the ultrasound beam and the direction of blood flow is crucial for accurate calculation:

- For an angle (ø) of 0° or 180° (parallel to blood flow), cos θ = 1, which maximizes the Doppler shift.
- For an angle of 90° (perpendicular to blood flow), cos θ = 0, resulting in no Doppler shift.
- For an angle up to 20°, cos θ causes only a minimal change (<10%) in the Doppler shift.
- For an angle of 60°, cos θ = 0.50, which means the Doppler shift is reduced by half compared to the maximum value.

The angle (ø) is especially crucial for the accurate assessment of high-velocity jets,

**TABLE 1:** Doppler equation.

| | *0°* | *30°* | *45°* | *60°* | *90°* |
|---|---|---|---|---|---|
| Cos θ | 1 | √3/2 | 1/√2 | 1/2 | 0 |

such as those seen in aortic stenosis and tricuspid regurgitation.

## SPECTRAL DISPLAY

The representation of Doppler data through a time–velocity plot is referred to as a spectral display. Upon receiving the backscattered signal by the transducer, the disparity between the transmitted and backscattered signals is ascertained by comparing their respective waveforms. The Doppler signal, once isolated, and its frequency content is analyzed via the *fast Fourier transform (FFT)* method. This changes the demodulated Doppler signal into its constituent frequency components. This frequency analysis generates a display known as spectral analysis **(Fig. 8)**. Conventionally, in spectral Doppler, time is plotted on the x-axis (horizontal) and frequency shift on the y-axis (vertical). Frequency shifts toward the transducer are represented as "positive" deflections, while frequency shifts away from the transducer are shown as "negative" deflections. The brightness of each frequency shift component illustrates the magnitude (or amplitude) of the received frequencies. Spectral display facilitates measurements such as peak velocity, acceleration, and the velocity-time integral.

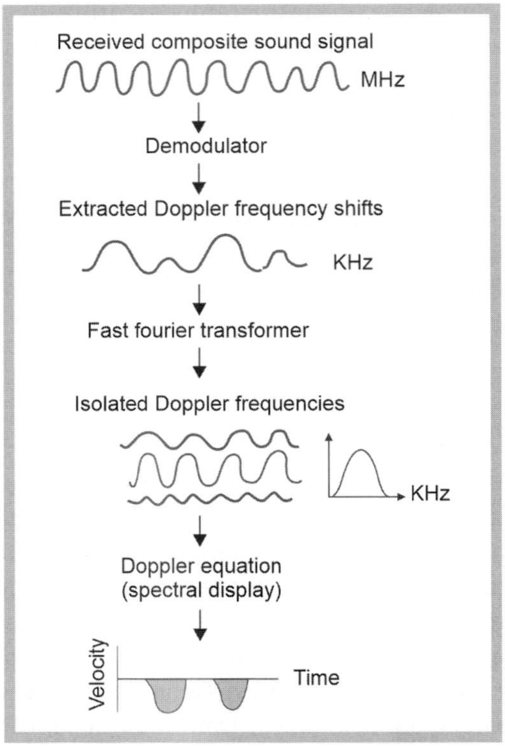


**Fig. 8:** Spectral Doppler display. Fourier analysis is done using an algorithm (FFT) that uses a mathematical tool to extract frequency information from signals. The display thereby generated is called spectral analysis.

## DOPPLER MODALITIES

In clinical practice, pulsed-wave and continuous-wave Doppler are often used alongside 2D imaging. 2D imaging helps identify the area of interest, which is then used to localize the sampling volume in a pulsed-wave Doppler study or to direct the beam in a continuous-wave Doppler study **(Fig. 9)**.

### Pulsed Wave Doppler

Pulsed-wave Doppler allows for the sampling of blood flow velocities at a specific region or sample volume, providing localized measurements. In contrast, continuous-wave Doppler records signal along the entire length of the ultrasound beam. Pulsed-wave Doppler is particularly useful for assessing relatively low-velocity flows, such as those associated with mitral or tricuspid inflow, pulmonary venous flow, and left or right ventricular outflow **(Fig. 10)**.

Similar to 2D imaging, the pulsed-wave Doppler system emits a brief burst of ultrasound toward the target and then switches to "receive mode" to interpret the returning echoes. Given the constant speed of sound (c) in tissue, the time delay for the signal to reach its target and return to the

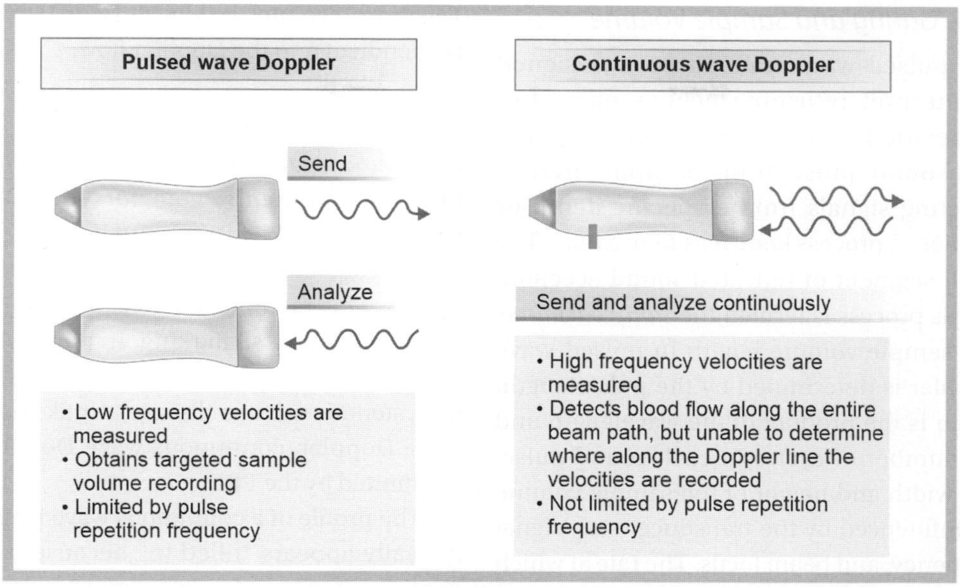


**Fig. 9:** Differences between pulsed wave Doppler and continuous wave Doppler.

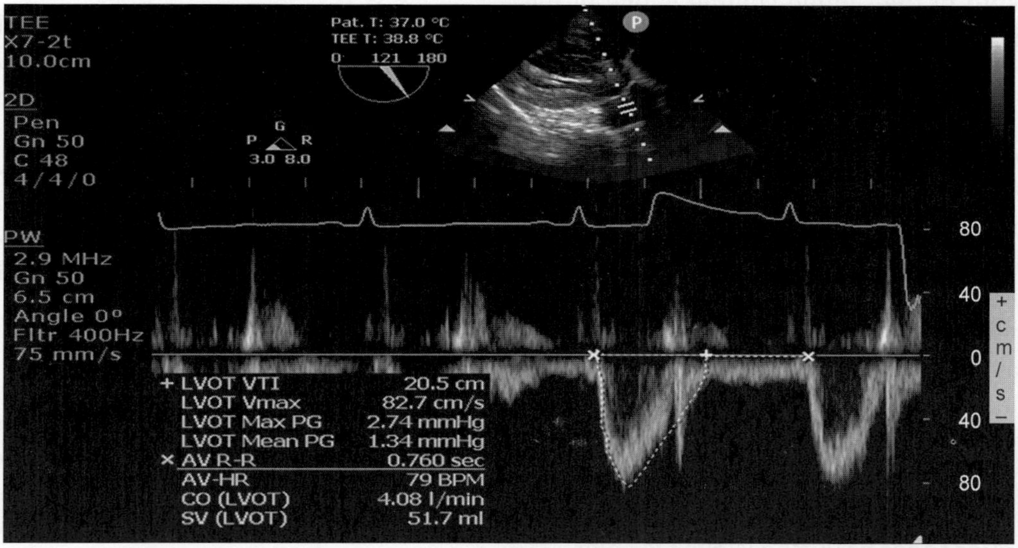


**Fig. 10:** Pulsed wave Doppler showing left ventricular outflow tract velocity time integral (LVOT VTi). The sampling volume is placed at the left ventricular outflow tract. Pulsed wave Doppler obtains targeted sample volume recordings.

transducer depends solely on the distance (d) to the target, calculated as *time delay* = *2d/c*. The use of the same piezoelectric crystal for both transmission and reception of the signal limits the maximum velocity that can be accurately measured with pulsed-wave Doppler to approximately 1.5–1.7 m/s.

### Time Gating and Sample Volume

The pulsed-wave transducer is designed to interpret returning echoes only after a specified time interval following the ultrasound pulse transmission, thereby selecting signals from a specific depth or location, a process known as *time gating*. The small segment of reflected sound accepted by this process is termed the *sample volume*. The sample volume length in pulsed-wave Doppler is determined by the pulse length, which is the product of the wavelength and the number of cycles in each sound pulse. The width and height of the sample volume are influenced by the transducer size, signal frequency, and beam focus. The rate at which the device generates sound bursts is termed the pulse repetition frequency (PRF). The depth of the sample volume is one of the main determinants of PRF.

### Aliasing

To prevent the overlapping of successive Doppler signals, the interval between pulses in a pulsed Doppler system must be adequate. Given the brief time for sound to return, a higher PRF is required. The Nyquist limit, the maximum detectable frequency shift, is half the PRF. If the velocity of interest exceeds the Nyquist limit, aliasing occurs, where the signal first appears in the reverse channel and then cycles back to the forward channel.

### Advantages of Pulsed Wave Doppler

The chief advantage is that it can specify the exact location of where the velocities are to be measured. This is because pulsed wave Doppler sends and analyses ultrasound waves sequentially. The ultrasound machine is designed to omit all signals, apart from those reflected at the specified depth. The sample volume is depicted with two lines perpendicular to the Doppler flow.

### Continuous Wave Doppler

*Continuous-wave Doppler uses two separate ultrasound crystals:* One for continuous transmission of ultrasound signals and another for continuous reception of these signals. This method can measure velocities exceeding 7 m/s, making it particularly valuable for assessing high-velocity flows (e.g., stenotic valvular disease). Unlike pulsed wave Doppler, continuous wave Doppler is not limited by the PRF.

The profile of a continuous wave Doppler typically appears "filled in" because it also captures lower-velocity signals proximal and distal to the point of maximum velocity **(Fig. 11)**. All the velocities from zero to maximum are recorded. It should be remembered that Continuous Wave Doppler positioning should always be interpreted with 2D and color flow mapping to ensure optimal alignment with the flow. The maximum frequency shift depends on the angle of insonation (ø). So, any angle of interrogation of 20° or greater may result in the underestimation of true velocity.

### Color Flow Imaging

Principles of pulsed wave Doppler echocardiography form the basis for color flow imaging. The velocities that are recorded in a given sample volume of pulsed wave Doppler can be represented with a color. If several sample volumes are subjected across several Doppler lines, then we can represent the velocities of the entire area with a color.

Ultrasound pulses are transmitted along each scan line. The signal gets reflected and is received from each sample volume along these lines. Accurate velocity data calculation

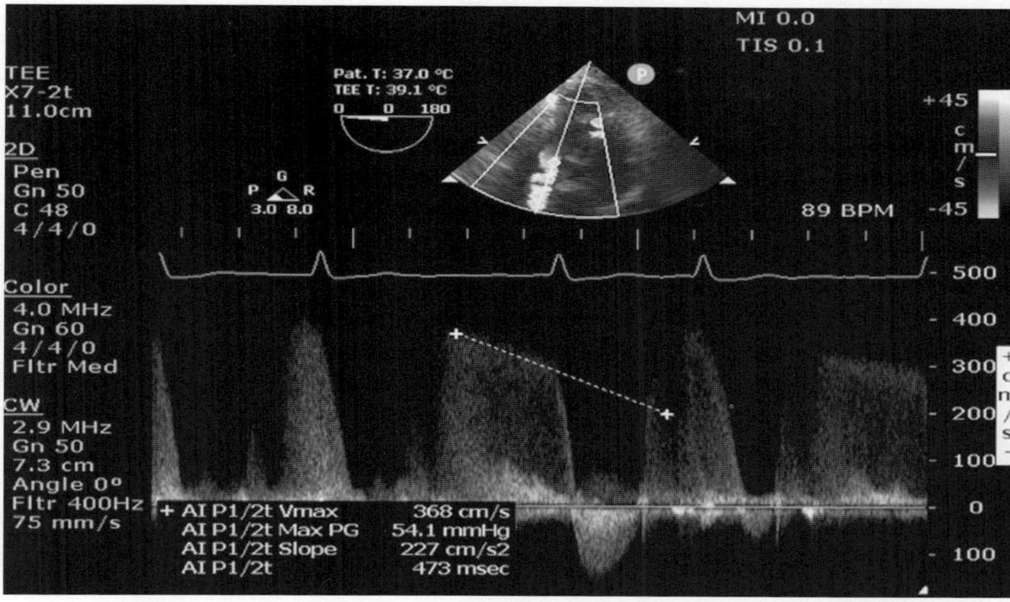


**Fig. 11:** Continuous wave Doppler showing aortic regurgitation. Continuous wave Doppler detects blood flow across the entire beam path.

in Doppler imaging involves multiple bursts along each scan line, known as the burst length. This process is repeated for each scan line across the image plane. Color Doppler provides information about the mean velocity within each sample volume, rather than the maximum velocity. As with pulsed Doppler, color wave Doppler is limited by the Nyquist limit; so, if velocities exceed the Nyquist limit, aliasing occurs.

In color flow imaging, velocities are displayed using a color scale: Flow toward the transducer is shown in red, while flow away from the transducer is displayed in blue.

At the Nyquist limit and its multiples, aliasing is visualized as a reversal in color. Turbulent flow, i.e., velocities are different and directed in different directions, will be depicted as a multicolored mosaic display **(Fig. 12)**.

Color flow imaging is used for screening and evaluating regurgitant flows, assessing intracardiac shunts, and aiding in the alignment of continuous-wave Doppler for velocity measurement. However, it does not provide precise measurements of blood flow velocity or velocity changes throughout the cardiac cycle. Due to these limitations, color flow mapping is primarily used to identify flow abnormalities, which then require further characterization using conventional Doppler methods.

## *Tissue Doppler Imaging*

Tissue Doppler imaging is a variant of pulsed wave Doppler utilized to record myocardial tissue velocity. It applies the same Doppler principles to quantify the higher-amplitude, lower-velocity signals associated with myocardial tissue motion. However, TDI only measures the vector of motion parallel to the ultrasound beam direction. It measures absolute tissue velocity and cannot distinguish between passive motion

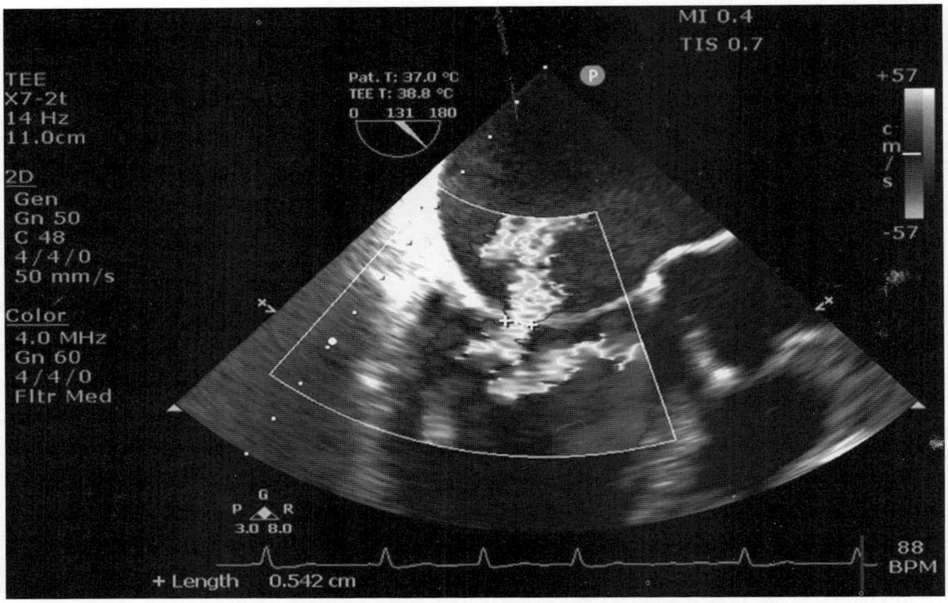


**Fig. 12:** Color flow mapping across the mitral valve showing mitral valvular regurgitation from left ventricle to left atrium. *Flow direction:* In color flow imaging, red indicates flow toward the transducer, while blue represents flow away from the transducer. The color map also adjusts based on flow velocity: High-velocity flow toward the transducer is shown in yellow, high-velocity flow away from the transducer is depicted in cyan and turbulent flow is displayed in green.

(related to translation or tethering) and active motion (fiber shortening or lengthening). TDI can be performed in both pulsed-wave and color modes.

CHAPTER 3

# Basics Including Terminology and Settings

*Gourav Mittal*

## ULTRASOUND KNOBOLOGY

**What is echogenicity?**

- It is the ultrasonologically perceived brightness of a structure.
  - While performing point-of-care ultrasonography (POCUS) structure is usually compared with liver.
    - If a structure is darker than the liver—hypoechoic
    - If it is brighter than the liver—hyperechoic
    - If there is no color—anechoic

## TERMINOLOGY RELATED TO MACHINE SETTINGS (BOX 1)

**BOX 1:** Machine settings-related terminologies.

- *Gain:* White value of the image (increase or decrease)
- *Depth:* Depth of image usually guided by a scale of 1 cm
- *iScan:* Brand proprietary, it automatically optimizes gain and depth
- *Freeze:* For making stand still image
- *Caliper:* To measure distances
- *Still image:* Often labeled save, stores a still photo of your image
- *Clips:* For storing video, usually adjusted either five heartbeats or 3–5 seconds
- *Zoom:* Zooms in on a specific area of the image
- *Cine scroll:* Will replay the last 5 seconds when the machine freeze function on, it is good for reviewing specific structures slowly for measurements

**What are the ultrasound scanning modes used?**

There are mainly three modes available in ultrasound. Amplitude (A) mode, Brightness (B) mode, and Motion (M) mode **(Table 1)**. Doppler mode is another special imaging modality.

1. *A-mode imaging:* (Amplitude modulation)
2. *B-mode imaging:* (Brightness modulation)
3. *M-mode imaging:* (Motion modulation)

### Limitations of Two-dimensional Imaging

- Attenuation
- Tissue properties (fibrosis and calcification)
- Artifacts
- Limited penetration (obesity and narrow imaging window)

### A-mode Imaging: (Amplitude Modulation)

Simplest and oldest mode. It displays a multitude of amplitude spikes of different heights. Only used in Optic nerve examination in current practice. The probe is pulsed with electrical energy of a very short duration lasting a few nanoseconds.

In the human body, ultrasound waves travel at different speeds in different tissues.

**TABLE 1:** Scanning modes.

| *B Mode or two-dimensional (2D)* | *M-mode* | *Doppler modes* |
|---|---|---|
| • At specific frame rate scan lines sequentially sent through a field creates this<br>• Higher frame rates needed for cardiac imaging for resolution | • Precise measurements of change over time<br>• No frame rate as single crystal sends and receives therefore creating a continuous measurement | • Measure the velocity and direction of an object relative to the probe<br>• Doppler change (shift) is calculated in the frequency between the sending and reflected signal<br>– *Direction of the Doppler shift*<br>- Moving toward transducer–increases<br>- Moving away from transducer–decreases<br>– *Amount of the shift:*<br>- Velocity of movement |

It takes a certain time to reach an interface. Depending upon the distance of the tissue from the transducer, reflected sound waves return at different intervals where the probe acts as a receiver. The reflected waves generate a small amplitude (vertical trace) proportional to the strength of the reflected wave. The image consists of an x-axis and a y-axis. The depth of the tissue from the surface is represented in the x-axis, whereas its amplitude is represented in the y-axis. The position of the spikes from the baseline denotes the depths of the corresponding tissue along the beam.

Time-gain compensation is done by the receiver to preferentially amplify ultrasound waves returning from deeper structures so that all the identical interfaces located at different depths produce similar signals **(Fig. 1)**.

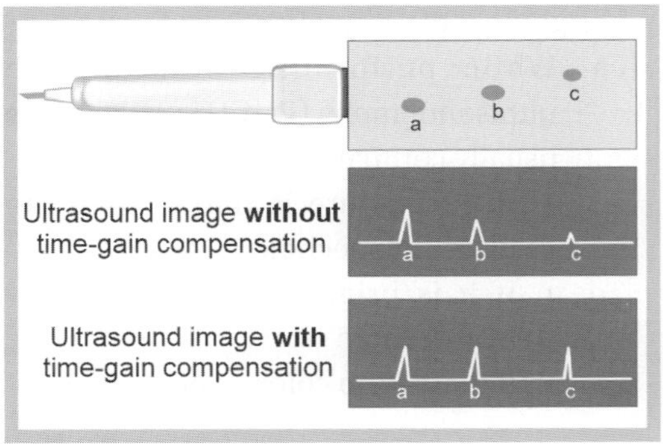


**Fig. 1:** Pictorial depiction of time gain compensation.

## B-mode Imaging: (Brightness Modulation)

This is the most common form of ultrasound imaging used in clinical practice. Unlike in A-mode, images in the B-mode consist of reflected ultrasound waves represented by varying shades of brightness in a grayscale comprising millions of tiny dots ranging from black to white. Brightness depends upon the amplitude or intensity of the reflected US waves. The higher the intensity of reflected waves, the brighter the image, and so on. Depending upon the tissue echogenicity and depth from the transducer, a 2-dimensional image is formed on the screen.

Real-time imaging is possible because of rapid and constant energy pulses. Image is automatically formed in succession due to the high frame rate. The higher the frame rate, the better the quality of real-time imaging of tissues in motion. There are two types of rapid scanners, mechanical or electronic scanning. Most modern scanners currently use electronic scanning to achieve rapid real-time scanning. In electronic scanners, the transducer is made up of numerous separate narrow piezoelectric strips. The distance between each strip is usually about one wavelength in width. These are energized in overlapping groups so that a well-defined ultrasound beam is formed with a focus point. Focal depth can be changed by changing the timing of the applied pulses. Modern scanners also provide the option of multiple zones focusing.

The direction of the ultrasound beam can also be steered electronically. When all the elements are energized simultaneously, the beam travels forward. When they are energized one after the other in a sequence, they reinforce in one direction, and the beam swings to that direction **(Fig. 2)**. Thus, by slightly changing the time delays between subsequent pulses, the entire beam can be made to sweep across a section of the patient.

*Factors determining the effectiveness and quality of real-time imaging:*

- *Scan-line density:* Number of scan lines that pass from the transducer to the patient. They depend on the number of piezoelectric elements in the transducer. To obtain images of high resolution, each frame consists of around 100 lines/frame.

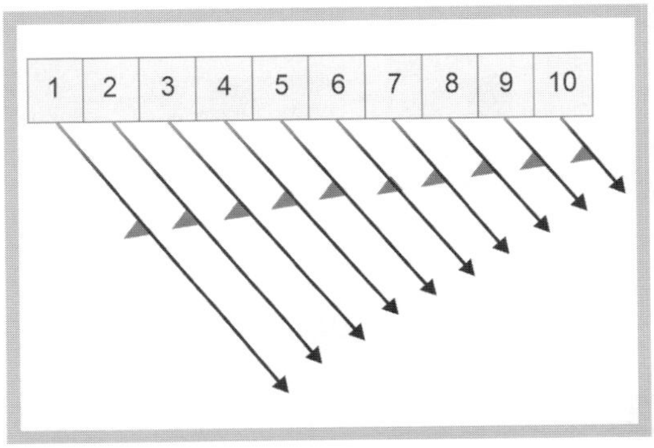


**Fig. 2:** Elements energized one after the other in a sequence.

- *Frame rate:* For real-time imaging, a high frame rate is required. Frame rate × lines/frame = pulse repetition frequency (PRF). For example, at 25 frames/second and scan line density of 100 lines/frame, the PRF is 2.5 kHz.
- *Depth of view:* Each pulse should have sufficient time to allow the return of the reflected beam from the deepest structure before the next pulse is generated. Decreasing the PRF increases the depth of view. Thus, it is not possible to have high scan line density, and high PRF and produce images with a large depth of view. As depth of view × (scan lines/frame) × (frame rate) is a constant, there is a trade-off between PRF and depth of view.

## M-mode Imaging: (Motion Modulation)

Motion modulation is used for imaging of rapidly moving structures, such as cardiac walls, cardiac valves, and fetal heartbeats, and sometimes for non-moving structures such as lungs for detecting pneumothorax. In this mode, scanning starts with B-mode. When a structure of interest is identified, the pointer is moved over it. The line overlying this area of interest is known as line-of-interest. M-mode is activated at this position. From the time of activation, a series of frozen images along the line of interest are stacked one next to each other. Echoes from structures that are not mobile, will be seen as a straight line of uniform color depending upon tissue echogenicity. Echoes from the moving structures are displayed as horizontal moving lines on the screen with the brightness of the line proportional to the intensity of the reflected sound wave and interspacing between the lines depending upon the relative depth between these structures along the line of interest. Even quantitative analyses such as heart rate and flow across cardiac valves are also possible in this mode.

### *M Mode Advantage*

- High temporal resolution
- Good for certain measurements
- Allows measurement of time intervals
- Timing of events

## STEPS FOR IMAGE OPTIMIZATION

- Patient should be placed comfortably.
- The area of scanning should be optimally exposed and positioned.
- Select the appropriate type of transducer. Low-frequency probes for deeper structures, high-frequency probes for relatively superficial structures, phased array probes for cardiac structures, etc.
- Coupling jelly should be used to ensure proper transmission of ultrasound waves to and from the tissue.
- Certain factory presets may come in handy for beginner sonologists. Else, they can be manually adjusted by tweaking variable gain buttons or depth as necessary, so that the reproduced images are neither too dark nor too bright.
- Transducer handling such as optimal pressure, alignment, tilting, and rotation, helps in images with better resolution.
- Further optimization can be done using time-gain correction.
- Special modes of scanning such as Tissue harmonic imaging or Spatial compounding can be used to increase resolution and decrease artifacts.

### Gain

Degree of amplification of returning sound. Increasing gain increases the strength of returning echoes. The gain dial or button lets the sonologist to change how bright (hyperechoic) or dark (hypoechoic) the corresponding image appears on the screen.

### Transducer Handling (Figs. 3A and B)

- Pressure
- Alignment
- Tilting
- Rotation

## DOPPLER

Doppler is used to measure the velocity and directionality of objects

- *Doppler effect:* "Changes in frequency of sound or light wave produced by a moving

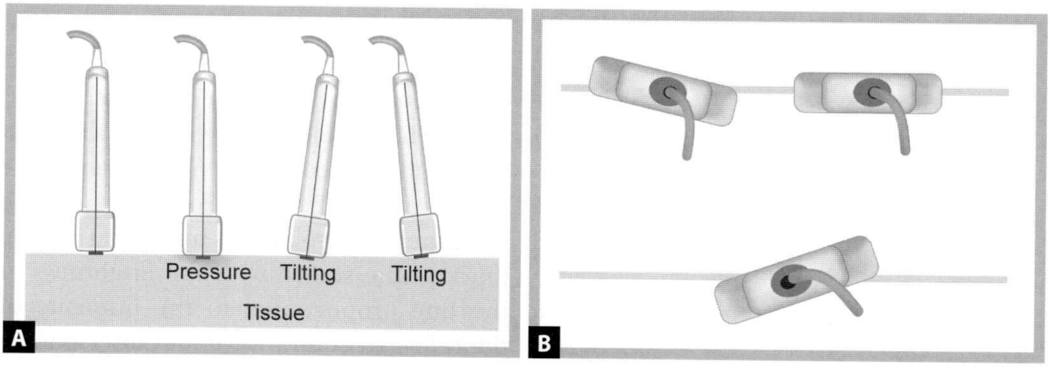


**Figs. 3A and B:** Sideway image showing the movement of the transducer and movement of the transducer from above.

source with respect to an observer" is known as the Doppler effect.

- *Doppler shift:* When a sound wave of a certain frequency (f) hits a stationary object, it gets reflected. This reflected wave has the same frequency as that of the emitted wave. However, when the object is in motion, either toward or away from the source, the frequency of the returning waves (f') may be either higher or lower depending upon the direction of the moving object. This change in frequency (Δf) is called *Doppler shift.* If the frequency of the returning wave is higher than the emitted frequency, it is called a positive Doppler shift. If the frequency of the returning wave is lower than the emitted frequency, it is called a negative Doppler shift. It is directly proportional to the velocity of the moving interface (v) in relation to the transducer and indirectly proportional to the speed of sound (c). It is also affected by the angle at which the interface is traveling (θ). By understanding these principles, the velocity of the moving interface can be calculated by rearranging the formula:

$$\frac{(f - f')}{f} = \frac{(2v) \times (\cos\theta)}{c}$$

$$\Delta f \times c = (f) \times (2v) \times (\cos\theta)$$

$$v = \frac{\Delta f \times c}{2\,(f) \times (\cos\theta)}$$

At extremes of the angle of indentation, i.e., at 0°, cos 0 = 1, and at 90°, cos 90 = 0. By substitution, we can infer that the maximum Doppler shift (Δf) occurs when the angle of indentation is 0° and no Doppler shift at 90°.

## Modes of Doppler Imaging (Table 2)

- Continuous wave Doppler
- Pulsed Doppler
- Power Doppler

### *Continuous Wave Doppler*

The probe uses two angled transducers. Of these, one functions as a continuous

**TABLE 2:** Doppler modes.

| *PWD* | *CWD* | *Color flow Doppler* | *Tissue Doppler imaging* |
|---|---|---|---|
| • Single crystal sending a pulsed signal<br>• Movement is showed around a baseline:<br>– Toward probe—above<br>– Away from—below<br>• Locate flow origin<br>• Not for high velocities as Nyquist limit reached and aliasing will occur<br>• *Uses:* Stroke volume, portal, and hepatic venous flow | • Two crystals. One continuously sends, while other receives<br>• Movement is displayed around a baseline<br>• Cannot measure flow at a specific point<br>• No issue of aliasing and able to measure high flow<br>• *Uses:* TR jet, quantification of AS | • Type of PWD<br>• Assigned as positive and negative Doppler shift:<br>– Red—movement toward transducer<br>– Blue movement away from transducer<br>– Brightness is velocity of flow<br>• *Uses:* Locate blood flow and identify pathologic flow | • Type of PWD<br>• Setting detects the low-frequency change of tissue movement<br>• Measures tissue movement not blood flow<br>• *Uses:* Assessment of diastolic function |

(AS: aortic stenosis; CWD: continuous wave Doppler; PWD: pulsed wave Doppler; TR: tricuspid regurgitant)

transmitting transducer at a certain frequency (f), and the other functions as a continuous receiving transducer which measures the reflected frequency (f'). Doppler shift is calculated electronically (f – f'). Due to the presence of dual transducers, there is continuous and simultaneous transmission and reception of sound waves. When using ultrasound on pulsatile blood flow having a range of velocities, the reflected waves have a spectrum of frequencies in a wide variety because of the Doppler shift. These can be electronically calculated and displayed on the screen on the go. A loudspeaker can be used to hear the Doppler signal. The higher the pitch, the greater is the velocity, the harsher the sound, the more turbulence there is. However, in continuous wave Dopplers, the depth or position of the moving reflector cannot be determined, nor can the flow in two overlapping vessels at different depths along the path of the beam be distinguished.

Continuous wave Doppler is now limited to small handheld portable Doppler equipment for detecting the existence and velocity of flow in the absence of any other data.

### *Pulsed Doppler*

As the name suggests, it uses a pulsed technique, i.e., the transducer is pulsed in small intervals, stimulating piezoelectric crystals to produce ultrasound waves. This is followed by a pause, where reflected waves are received. This continues in a cyclical manner. For further clarity on the direction of the flow, colors are used on grayscale [color Doppler flow imaging (CDFI)] **(Figs. 4A and B)**.

Usually flow toward the transducer is represented by red color, and flow away from the transducer is denoted by blue. However, they can be inverted. The intensity of the color increases with velocity and focal areas of turbulence or stenosis can be seen as color mosaic. Doppler scanning can be combined with B-mode, also known *duplex scanning* **(Fig. 5)**. Together they provide various information including location, depth, velocity, and direction of flow. The intensity of the color increases with velocity and focal areas of turbulence or stenosis can be seen as color mosaic.

The gap between pulses in a pulsed Doppler must be long enough for successive Doppler signals to avoid overlapping. Because

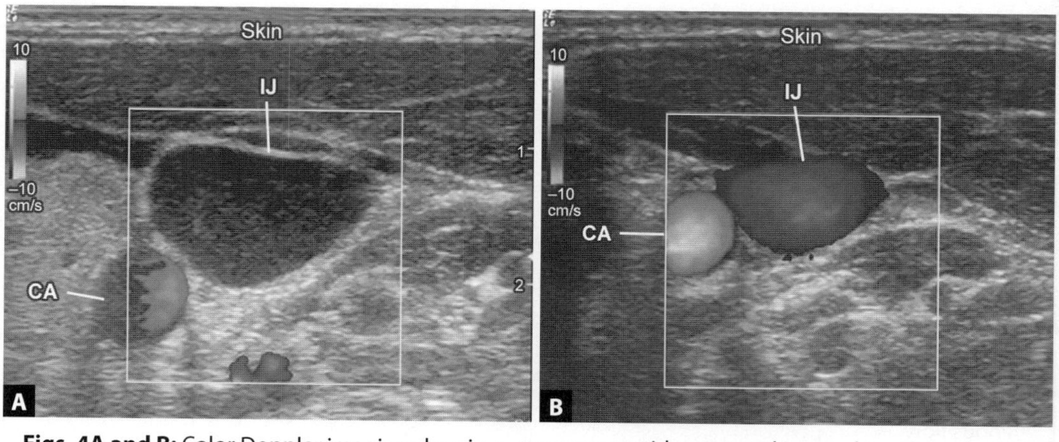


**Figs. 4A and B:** Color Doppler imaging showing common carotid artery and internal jugular vein (IJV). Red depicts flow toward the transducer and blue depicts away from the transducer.

the time it takes for sound to return is short, a higher PRF would have to be set for superficial vessels. Deeper vessels, on the other hand, would require a lower PRF because sound travels farther and takes longer to return from deeper tissues. Low PRF, on the other hand, is linked to a specific phenomenon known as aliasing. Aliasing is the failure to appropriately record sound direction and velocity. Aliasing happens when the PRF is too low and the velocity within the vessel is greater than the PRF **(Figs. 6A and B)**. To prevent it, the PRF should be at least twice the highest Doppler shift frequency produced by the flow, as shown by the Nyquist equation PRF = 2Δf. As a result, the quickest flow that can be correctly measured is velocity which produces a Doppler shift of less than half of the PRF in use. A greater flow velocity causes aliasing, which manifests itself as a wraparound of the maximum velocity on the opposite side of the baseline.

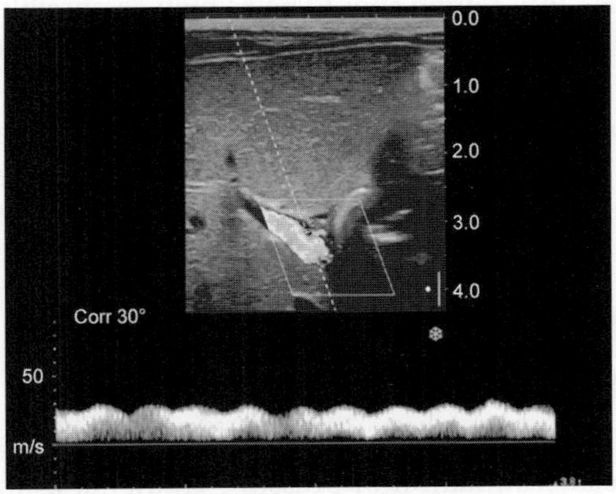


**Fig. 5:** Color Doppler ultrasound image showing the portal venous flow as a colored map over the B-mode image. The obliquely placed box is the color box where any detectable flow is represented in color and the dotted line represents the plane of sample volume. The flow within the sample volume is shown as a graph in the lower part of the image.

Increased PRF reduces aliasing, but it also reduces the depth from which velocity data may be obtained. As a result, measuring fast velocities in deep vessels is frequently impossible. The risk of aliasing can also be reduced by reducing the Doppler shift by using a probe of lower frequency (curvilinear probe over linear probe) or by increasing the angle of insonation (θ). But both these

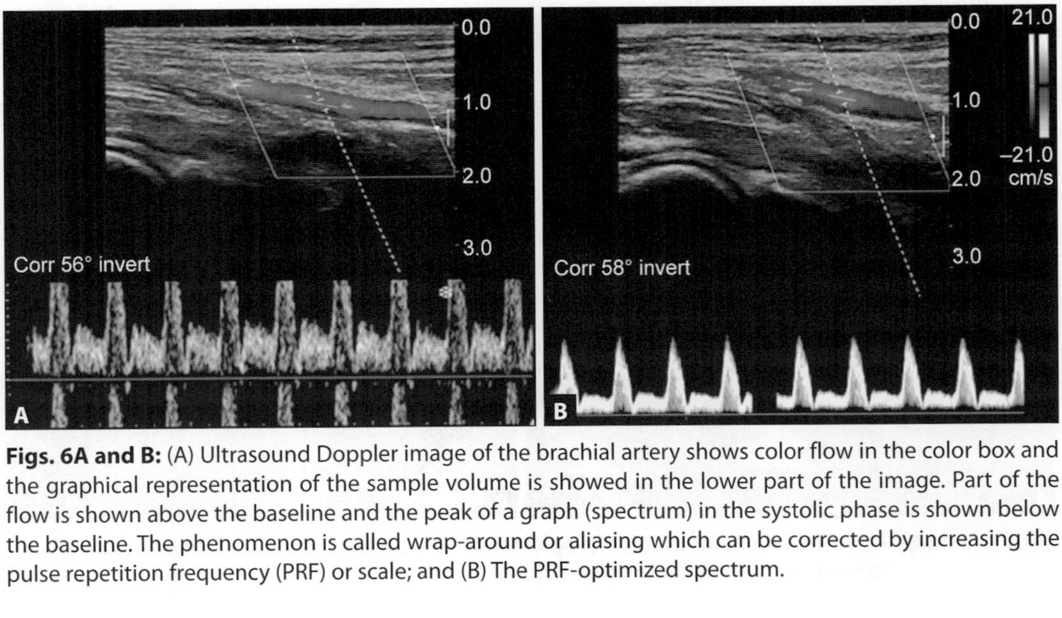


**Figs. 6A and B:** (A) Ultrasound Doppler image of the brachial artery shows color flow in the color box and the graphical representation of the sample volume is showed in the lower part of the image. Part of the flow is shown above the baseline and the peak of a graph (spectrum) in the systolic phase is shown below the baseline. The phenomenon is called wrap-around or aliasing which can be corrected by increasing the pulse repetition frequency (PRF) or scale; and (B) The PRF-optimized spectrum.

modifications increase errors in velocity measurements.

### Power Doppler

Power Doppler imaging is primarily used to identify areas of flow versus no flow. They are highly efficient in detecting even small quantities of flows that are not detected even by color Doppler. It shows the amplitude of the Doppler signal without any direction or velocity of the flow. The amplitude of the power Doppler signal increases as the volume of moving red blood cells in a given sample volume increases, resulting in a brighter hue **(Figs. 7A and B)**.

### Setting Up and Optimizing Doppler Images

- Prior to using CDFI, grayscale or B-mode imaging should be optimized.
- Vessel-of-interest should be visible on the image.
- The vessel of interest should be located optimally, i.e., not too deep.
- Look for areas of constriction, plaque formation, or intimal thickening by scanning the entire vessel in B-mode in longitudinal and transverse sections.
- Activate CDFI. Place sample volume size correctly over the center of the vessel covering two-thirds of the vessel lumen.
- Angle of insonation should be <60°.
- Increase the color gain until the vessel lumen is completely filled without overflowing over surrounding tissues.
- PRF setting should be as high as possible for a giver Doppler study to prevent aliasing.
- To avoid thermal damage, do not utilize Doppler imaging continuously or keep the probe stationary for an extended period of time near soft tissue/bony interfaces.

## FLOW DYNAMICS

### Bernoulli Equation

The simplified Bernoulli equation permits easy estimation of pressure gradients from velocities.

$$\Delta P = 4 \times V^2$$

### Applications of Bernoulli (Table 3)

**What is 3-dimensional echocardiography?**

*Uses:* 3D echocardiography displays images of the heart that contain important new tissue and morphologic information. This new technique is simple, and rapid, and allows

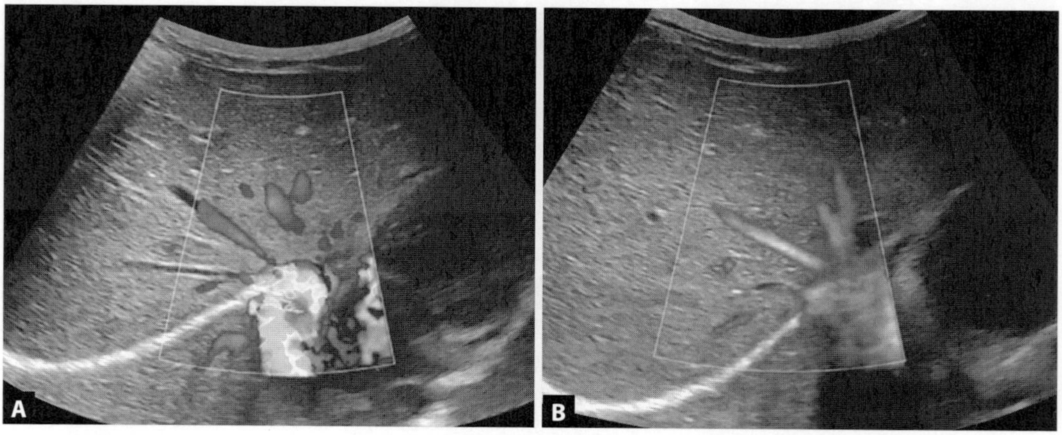


**Figs. 7A and B:** (A) The hepatic veins in color Doppler mode; and (B) Them in power Doppler mode. Power Doppler mode is more sensitive to flow compared to color Doppler mode.

**TABLE 3:** Applications of Bernoulli.

| *Direct (gradients)* | *Indirect (pressure decay)* |
|---|---|
| • Valvular stenosis<br>• Defects (i.e., VSD and coarctation and PDA)<br>• Tricuspid regurgitation signal (sPAP)<br>• Prosthetic valves sites | • Aortic regurgitation quantification<br>• Diastolic function (deceleration time)<br>• dP/dt (contractility)<br>• Mitral stenosis (pressure half-time method) |

(PDA: patent ductus arteriosus; sPAP: systolic pulmonary artery pressure; VSD: ventricular septal defect)

additional clinical information to be obtained in different fields, including evaluation of valve diseases and intracardiac masses, assessment of the volumes and function of the two ventricles, and monitoring of cardiac surgery and new interventional procedures.

## DIFFERENT CLINICAL APPLICATIONS

- Quantification of left ventricular (LV) volumes and function (and shape)
- Quantification of LV mass
- Assessment of regional wall motion of the left ventricle (rest and stress)
- Assessment of LV dyssynchrony
- Quantification of right ventricular (RV) volumes and function
- Evaluation of valve diseases
- Evaluation of congenital heart diseases
- Evaluation of cardiac masses
- Guidance of intracardiac interventions
- Monitoring of cardiac surgery.

CHAPTER 4

# Artifacts in Echocardiography: Implications for Operating Rooms and Critical Care Units

*Amit Kumar Malviya, Vinay Kumar*

## INTRODUCTION

Echocardiography is an invaluable tool in the operating rooms (ORs) and critical care units (CCUs) for the real-time assessment of cardiac function, hemodynamic, and anatomical structures. Despite its widespread use and advanced technology, echocardiography is not without limitations. Artifacts—misrepresentations of anatomical structures—can complicate the interpretation of images and lead to diagnostic inaccuracies. Understanding the common artifacts, their causes, and how to mitigate their effects is crucial for intensivists and anesthesiologists to ensure accurate assessments and patient safety.

Artifacts are frequently encountered during echocardiographic examinations. Understanding the physics and underlying assumptions of ultrasound processing involved in image generation is crucial for the accurate interpretation of two-dimensional (2D) grayscale, spectral Doppler, color flow Doppler, and three-dimensional (3D) artifacts and their clinical implications. Consider the following points:

- *2D grayscale imaging:* Artifacts in 2D grayscale imaging can arise from various sources, such as acoustic shadowing, reverberation, and mirror images. These artifacts can obscure or mimic pathology, so recognizing and differentiating them from true anatomical structures is essential.
- *Spectral Doppler:* Artifacts in spectral Doppler include aliasing, which occurs when the velocity of blood flow exceeds the Nyquist limit, and spectral broadening, which can be due to turbulence or incorrect sample volume placement. Correct interpretation requires understanding these artifacts to avoid misdiagnosis of abnormal flow patterns.
- *Color flow Doppler:* Color Doppler artifacts such as aliasing, color bleed, and shadowing can affect the accuracy of blood flow visualization. Recognizing these artifacts helps in correctly assessing the direction, velocity, and turbulence of blood flow.
- *3D imaging:* In 3D echocardiography, artifacts like stitching artifacts (due to patient or probe movement during acquisition) and volume-rendering artifacts (due to improper gain settings or incorrect spatial resolution) can impact the quality of the 3D reconstruction. Understanding these artifacts ensures a more accurate interpretation of 3D images.

Understanding these artifacts and their sources allows clinicians to adjust their techniques and settings to minimize their impact, leading to more accurate echocardiographic assessments and better clinical decision-making.

Two-Dimensional Grayscale Ultrasound Artifacts Two-Dimensional Grayscale Ultra.

## TYPES OF ARTIFACTS IN ECHOCARDIOGRAPHY (TABLE 1)

### Common Artifacts in Echocardiography

Artifacts in echocardiography can be categorized into those due to technical limitations of the ultrasound system and those arising from patient anatomy or physiology. The most prevalent artifacts include reverberation, mirror image, side lobe, acoustic shadowing, acoustic enhancement, and Doppler-related artifacts.

#### *Reverberation Artifacts*

Reverberation artifacts occur when ultrasound waves repeatedly reflect between two strong reflectors, such as the pericardium, and metallic structures, such as prosthetic valves. This results in multiple, equally spaced echoes on the image, which can mimic structures such as cysts or fluid collections. In the OR and critical care settings, reverberation artifacts are often seen with central venous catheters or surgical instruments, potentially leading to misinterpretation of the pericardial or pleural spaces.

*Management:* Adjusting the transducer position, changing the imaging window, or using harmonic imaging can help reduce reverberation artifacts. Recognizing the characteristic pattern of equally spaced lines can aid in differentiating artifacts from true anatomical structures.

#### *Mirror Image Artifacts*

Mirror image artifacts occur when ultrasound waves reflect off a strong reflector and produce a duplicate image of a structure on the opposite side of the reflector. This is commonly seen near highly reflective surfaces such as the diaphragm and pleura, creating a mirror image of cardiac structures.

*Management:* Awareness of the common locations and appearances of mirror artifacts helps avoid misinterpretation. Altering the angle of insonation or using alternative imaging windows can reduce these artifacts.

#### *Side Lobe Artifacts*

Side lobe artifacts arise from secondary lobes of ultrasound energy that emanate from the transducer and reflect off structures outside the main beam. These can produce spurious echoes, particularly in anechoic regions, such as the cardiac chambers and cysts.

**TABLE 1:** Violations of ultrasound assumptions that lead to artifacts.

| *Assumptions* | *Artifacts* |
|---|---|
| Pulses and echoes travel in straight lines | Refraction |
| Waves are infinitely thin or pulses are extremely small | Beamwidth |
| Echoes return to the transducer after a single reflection | Reverberation, mirror image |
| Echoes originate from the main beam | Side-lobe and grating lobe |
| The depth of an object is directly related to the travel time for an ultrasound pulse to return to the transducer; speed of sound = 1,540 m/s | Refraction |
| Pulses and echoes are attenuated uniformly by all tissues | Shadowing, enhancement |

*Management:* Using higher frequency transducers and adjusting gain settings can minimize side lobe artifacts. Recognizing the characteristic appearance of these artifacts can prevent misdiagnosis.

### *Acoustic Shadowing*

Acoustic shadowing occurs when a structure with high acoustic impedance, such as calcification and bone, completely reflects or absorbs the ultrasound waves, resulting in a shadow behind the structure. In the cardiac context, this can obscure structures posterior to heavily calcified valves or prosthetic materials.

*Management:* Changing the angle of insonation or using different acoustic windows can help visualize structures hidden by acoustic shadowing. Awareness of common causes and appearances of shadowing is essential for accurate interpretation.

### *Acoustic Enhancement*

Acoustic enhancement, or posterior enhancement, occurs when ultrasound waves pass through a fluid-filled structure, leading to increased echo amplitude behind it. This phenomenon is often seen with cysts or fluid collections such as pericardial and pleural effusions and can be mistaken for pathological conditions if not recognized.

*Management:* Recognizing the pattern of increased brightness posterior to fluid-filled structures helps in differentiating true anatomical findings from artifacts.

### *Doppler-related Artifacts*

Doppler echocardiography is prone to various artifacts, including aliasing, clutter, and spectral broadening. Aliasing occurs when the Doppler shift exceeds the Nyquist limit, causing velocities to be displayed inaccurately. Clutter, caused by tissue motion, can obscure low-velocity blood flow signals. Spectral broadening results from turbulent flow or high gain settings, causing a widened Doppler signal.

*Management:* Adjusting the pulse repetition frequency, using low wall filters, and optimizing gain settings can mitigate Doppler artifacts. Understanding the hemodynamics and being familiar with the appearance of Doppler artifacts can prevent misinterpretation.

## ARTIFACTS SPECIFIC TO THE OPERATING ROOM AND CRITICAL CARE UNITS

In the dynamic and challenging environments of ORs and CCUs, certain artifacts are more prevalent due to the presence of various medical devices and the patient's critical condition.

### *Electromagnetic Interference*

Electromagnetic interference (EMI) from electrocautery, pacemakers, and other electrical devices can create artifacts in echocardiographic images. These artifacts typically appear as transient spikes or noise on the image, which can interfere with real-time assessment of cardiac function.

*Management:* Timing echocardiographic assessments to periods when electrocautery is not in use, or temporarily disabling certain devices, can help reduce EMI artifacts. Using shielded cables and maintaining a distance from sources of interference can also be beneficial.

### *Mechanical Ventilation Artifacts*

Mechanical ventilation can introduce artifacts due to lung inflation and deflation, movement of the diaphragm, and changes in intrathoracic pressure. These factors can affect image quality and the appearance of cardiac structures, particularly during transthoracic echocardiography.

*Management:* Coordinating echocardiographic imaging with the respiratory cycle, such as acquiring images during end-expiration, can improve image quality. Transesophageal echocardiography (TEE) may be preferred in mechanically ventilated patients to minimize these artifacts.

### *Motion Artifacts*

Motion artifacts are common in critically ill patients who are often restless or agitated. Patient movement can blur images and create diagnostic uncertainty, especially during transthoracic echocardiography.

*Management:* Sedation, if appropriate, can help reduce motion artifacts. Using faster frame rates and optimizing transducer stabilization can also improve image quality.

# ADVANCED TECHNIQUES TO MITIGATE ARTIFACTS

## Harmonic Imaging

Harmonic imaging enhances image quality by using the harmonic frequencies generated by the tissue itself, rather than the fundamental frequency emitted by the transducer. This technique can reduce artifacts such as reverberation and side lobes, providing clearer images.

### *Management*

Activating harmonic imaging mode on the echocardiography machine can significantly improve image resolution and artifact reduction, especially in difficult-to-image patients.

## Contrast Echocardiography

Contrast agents, composed of microbubbles, can enhance endocardial border delineation, and improve visualization of cardiac structures. This technique is particularly useful in patients with suboptimal acoustic windows or in detecting intracardiac shunts.

### *Management*

Administering contrast agents during echocardiography can help distinguish true anatomical structures from artifacts, improving diagnostic accuracy in the OR and critical care settings.

## Three-dimensional Echocardiography

Three-dimensional echocardiography echo provides volumetric imaging, offering a more comprehensive view of cardiac structures. This advanced technique can help identify and differentiate artifacts that may appear ambiguous in 2D imaging.

### *Management*

Incorporating 3D echocardiography in clinical practice can enhance diagnostic capabilities and reduce reliance on potentially artifact-laden 2D images.

# CASE STUDIES

## Case Study 1: Reverberation Artifact

A 65-year-old male undergoing cardiac surgery was monitored with intraoperative TEE. The images revealed multiple linear echoes in the left atrium, initially concerning for thrombus. Recognizing the pattern of reverberation artifact from the mechanical valve, the anesthesiologist repositioned the transducer, confirming the absence of a thrombus.

### *Management*

Awareness and repositioning of the transducer were crucial in avoiding misdiagnosis.

## Case Study 2: Mirror Image Artifact

A critically ill patient in the ICU showed a duplicated left ventricle on TTE. The duplication was due to a mirror image artifact caused by a highly reflective diaphragm. Adjusting the insonation angle eliminated the artifact, clarifying the diagnosis.

### *Management*

Altering the insonation angle resolved the artifact, ensuring accurate interpretation.

Here is a comprehensive table summarizing various artifacts encountered in echocardiography, particularly focusing on their use in ORs and CCUs.

**Table 2** aims to provide intensivists and anesthesiologists with a clear understanding of common echocardiographic artifacts, their sources, clinical implications, and

**TABLE 2:** Mirror image artifact

| *Type of artifact* | *Source/mechanism of artifact* | *Implications in clinical practice* | *Management of artifact* |
|---|---|---|---|
| Reverberation artifact | Multiple reflections between strong reflectors (e.g., prosthetic valves and pericardial fluid) | Can mimic structures such as vegetations and thrombi, leading to misdiagnosis of endocarditis or thromboembolic events | Adjust transducer position, use different imaging angles, and apply harmonic imaging to reduce artifact appearance |
| Mirror image artifact | Reflection of the ultrasound beam off a strong reflector, creating a duplicate image | Can be mistaken for cardiac masses or additional chambers, complicating the interpretation of cardiac anatomy | Change the imaging angle or use different windows to distinguish real structures from artifacts |
| Acoustic shadowing | Occurs behind highly attenuating structures (e.g., calcified valves and bones) | This leads to a loss of diagnostic information distal to the shadowing structure, potentially obscuring lesions or other pathologies | Optimize gain settings, use alternative imaging planes, and reposition the transducer |
| Side lobe artifact | Off-axis beams that return to the transducer, creating false echoes | This may lead to misinterpretation of the size and shape of cardiac chambers or the presence of pseudomasses | Adjusting the focus, reducing gain, and changing the insonation angle |
| Beam width artifact | Echoes from outside the main ultrasound beam width are included in the image | Can cause false representation of cardiac structures, such as overestimating the size of chambers or vessels | Narrowing the beam width, using different acoustic windows, and optimizing machine settings |
| Range ambiguity artifact | High pulse repetition frequency causes an overlap of echo signals from different depths | Incorrect representation of the depth of structures, potentially leading to inaccurate measurements and assessments of cardiac function | Use lower pulse repetition frequency, optimize depth settings, and ensure proper machine calibration |

*Contd...*

*Contd...*

| *Type of artifact* | *Source/mechanism of artifact* | *Implications in clinical practice* | *Management of artifact* |
|---|---|---|---|
| Doppler aliasing | Exceeding the Nyquist limit in Doppler imaging, causing incorrect velocity measurements | Misinterpretation of blood flow velocities, leading to potential misdiagnosis of conditions such as valvular stenosis and regurgitation | Increase the pulse repetition frequency, lower the baseline of the Doppler scale, or switch to continuous wave Doppler |
| Electrical interference | External electrical sources interfering with ultrasound signals | This can create extraneous lines or patterns in the echocardiogram, potentially leading to confusion or misinterpretation of the cardiac structures | Identify and eliminate sources of electrical interference, ensure proper grounding of equipment, and use filters if available |
| Near-field clutter | High-intensity echoes near the transducer due to ring-down artifact | Obscures near-field structures such as the pericardium and superficial cardiac layers, possibly missing critical findings, such as pericardial effusion and tumors | Adjust gain and depth settings, apply for time-gain compensation, and use higher frequency transducers for better near-field resolution |
| Speckle artifact | Interference of scattered ultrasound waves, producing a granular appearance on the image | Can reduce image quality and clarity, making it difficult to identify subtle pathological changes in cardiac structures | Use speckle reduction algorithms, adjust gain settings, and utilize higher frequency transducers |
| Multipath artifact | Ultrasound waves reflected multiple times before returning to the transducer | This may result in misplaced echoes and inaccurate representation of cardiac anatomy, potentially complicating diagnosis | Change the transducer position, use different imaging windows, and apply harmonic imaging techniques |
| Attenuation artifact | Gradual loss of signal intensity as ultrasound waves pass through tissue | This leads to reduced visibility of structures at greater depths, potentially missing distal pathologies, such as masses and thrombi | Increase overall gain, apply time-gain compensation, and consider using contrast agents to enhance visualization |
| Comet tail artifact | Reverberations within a small, highly reflective structure, such as calcifications | Appears as a series of closely spaced parallel lines, which can be mistaken for pathological structures, such as septal defects and foreign bodies | Adjust the imaging angle, use higher frequency probes, and apply harmonic imaging to reduce the impact of the artifact |
| Blooming artifact | Over-amplification of strong signals, causing adjacent structures to appear larger | Can obscure small structures and complicate the assessment of fine details, such as valve leaflets and small thrombi | Adjust gain settings and use postprocessing software to reduce over-amplification |

management strategies to enhance diagnostic accuracy in critical care and intraoperative settings.

## OTHER COMMON EXTRACARDIAC ARTIFACTS IN CLINICAL PRACTICE

- *A-lines:* Horizontal parallel and evenly spaced echogenic lines, below the pleura. It is created by normally or hyperinflated lung areas.
- *B-lines:* Vertical lines (comet tail artifact) arising from the pleural line.
- Parallel horizontal reverberation artifacts—due to the existence of air within the pleural cavity, which inhibits complete lung expansion.
- *Image artifacts:* Arising due to mechanical ventilation, chest tubes, or electrical interference with monitors, etc.
- *Pseudoflow artifact:* Due to the motion of fluid other than blood, and did not show arterial or venous waveforms, e.g., pericardial effusions.
- Twinkling artifacts—a mosaic of rapidly oscillating blue and red patches of color proximal to highly reflective surfaces, producing patterns that simulate abnormal flow characteristics.

## CONCLUSION

Artifacts in echocardiography can significantly impact the interpretation of cardiac function, especially in the OR and CCUs where timely and accurate diagnosis is essential. Understanding the types of artifacts, their causes, and management strategies is crucial for intensivists and anesthesiologists. Employing advanced echocardiographic techniques and maintaining a high level of suspicion for artifacts can enhance diagnostic accuracy, ultimately improving patient outcomes.

CHAPTER 5

# Basic Echo Views, Their Strengths, and Shortcomings

*Gourav Mittal, Puneet Khanna*

## PREPARATION AND PATIENT POSITION (FIG. 1)

- *Preset of probe:* Cardiac
- Supine
- *Turn to left side:* Parasternal and apical view
- Abduct the patient's left arm—this will open the intercostal spaces
- Marker to the right side of screen. All other modes, it will be left of screen
- *Position:* Ideally left lateral decubitus
- Frequently this position is not possible in intensive care unit (ICU).

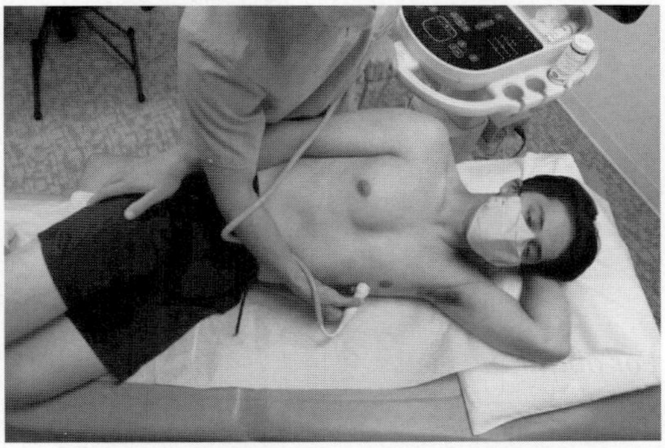

**Fig. 1:** Patient position.

## THREE WINDOWS (FIG. 2)

- *Apical:* Left fourth to fifth intercostal space
- *Parasternal:* Left second to fourth intercostal space
- *Subcostal:* Just below xiphisternum

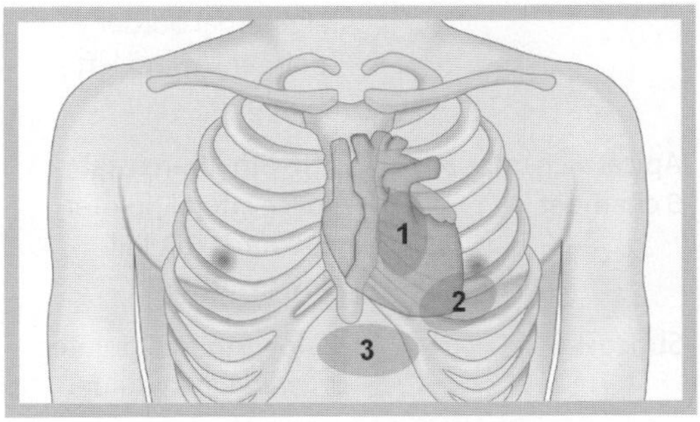


**Fig. 2:** Three windows.

## FIVE VIEWS

- Parasternal long axis
- Parasternal short axis
- Apical four chamber
- Subcostal four chamber
- Subcostal inferior vena cava (IVC)

## ECHO VIEWS

For performing transthoracic echocardiogram (TTE), chest areas are divided into five major zones: Suprasternal, left parasternal, apical, subcostal, and right parasternal **(Fig. 3)**.

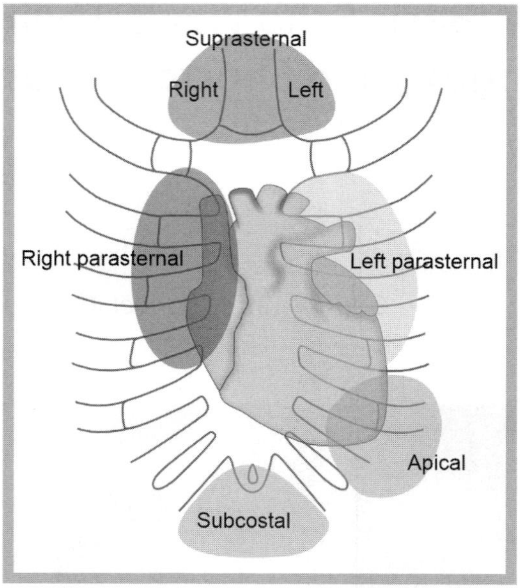


**Fig. 3:** Chest areas.

*For obtaining views:*

| | |
|---|---|
| Parasternal long axis | 2–4th intercostal space left sternal border (pointer toward right shoulder) |
| Parasternal short axis | 2–4th intercostal space left sternal border (pointer toward left shoulder) |
| Apical 4 chamber/ 5 chamber | 4th–5th intercostal space lateral pointer outwards (tilt tail downward) |
| Subcostal | Below xiphoid pointer toward left shoulder |

*Optimization of individual view:*

1. *Parasternal long axis* ***(Fig. 4)****:*
   *View should have:*
   - Visible—LV/RV/LA/aorta, 2 cusps of MV/AV
   - LV should be fully open, apex not visible
   - Septum and posterior LV wall should be horizontal.

   *To optimize:*
   - Stay close to left sternal border
   - To open up LV—small angulation and rotation

   To make LV central and ventricular septum more horizontal—move tail of transducer toward right shoulder.
2. *Parasternal short axis* ***(Figs. 5 to 8)***:
   *View should have:*
   - LV/RV visible, LV totally rounded

   *To optimize*:
   - 20–30° inundation with chest wall
   - Too much MV—tilt tail toward right shoulder
     - To achieve a parasternal short axis (PSAX) view, the probe is rotated clockwise (at the same place where PLAX was achieved) to the left so that the marker on the probe is directed toward the left shoulder of the patient.
     - PSAX can be obtained at three levels basal, mitral level, and mid ventricle level.
     - To achieve the other two views, the probe is titled downward toward the apex of left ventricle.
   - Too much apical view (papillary muscles not visible):
     - Tilt tail away from right shoulder
3. *Apical four chamber* ***(Fig. 9)****:*
   - This is the most common view used to visualize the heart.
   - The probe is placed just lateral to the apex in the left fourth to fifth intercostal space and adjusted to get the view.
   - The probes should be shifted left or right gently to orient the interventricular septum parallel to the screen to get a true four-chamber view.

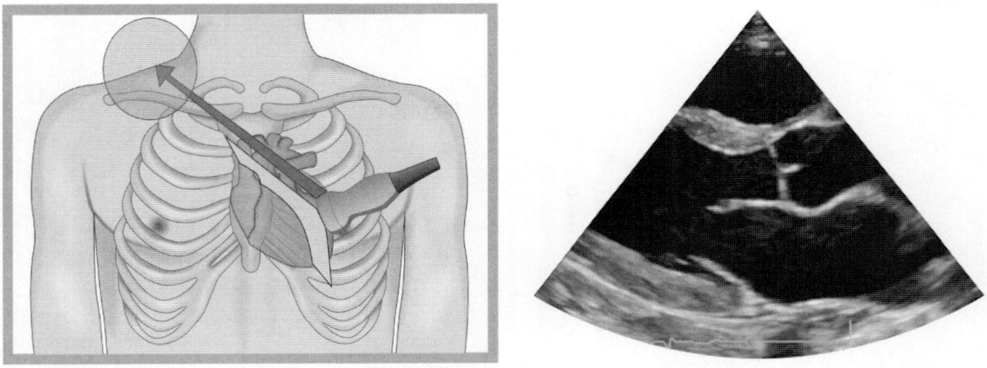

**Fig. 4:** Parasternal long axis.

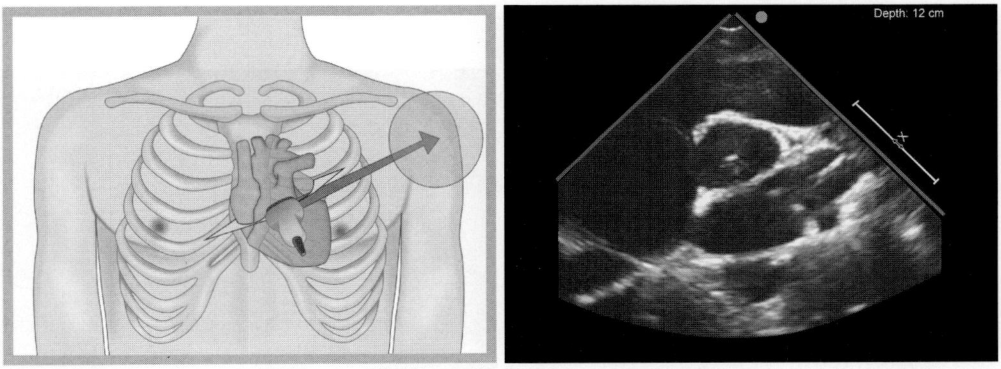


**Fig. 5:** Parasternal short axis—aortic valve level.

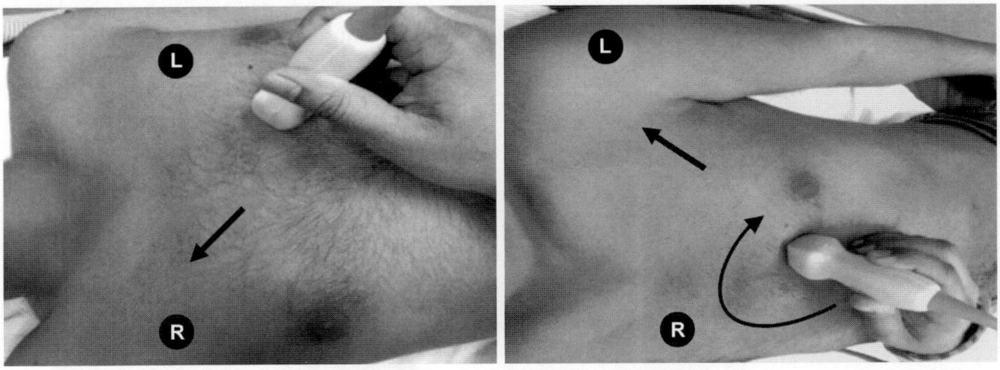


**Fig. 6:** Parasternal short axis (PSAX) view.

*View should have:*

- Apex should be centered
- Intraventricular septum perpendicular
- Lateral wall visible
- Fully open atria without aortic valve and coronary sinus.

*Optimization:*

- If RV in focus—slide laterally
- If diagonal picture—move tail of transducer laterally
- If AV visible—lift up tail
- If coronary sinus visible—lower the tail

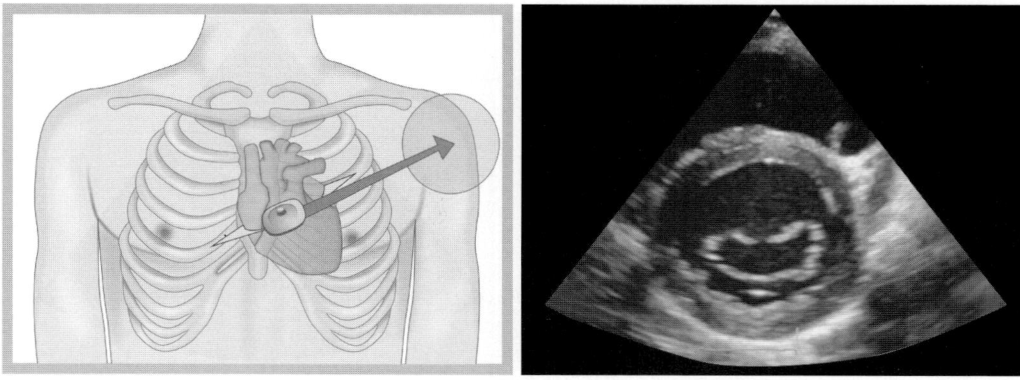

**Fig. 7:** Parasternal short axis—mitral valve level.

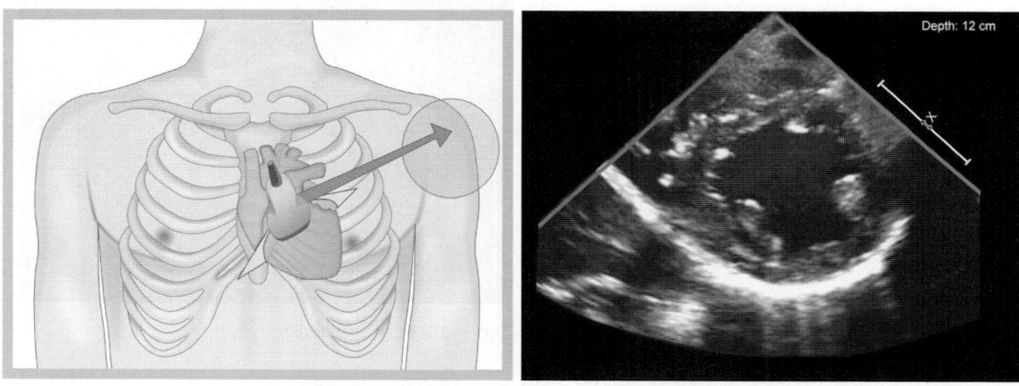


**Fig. 8:** Parasternal short axis—papillary muscle level.

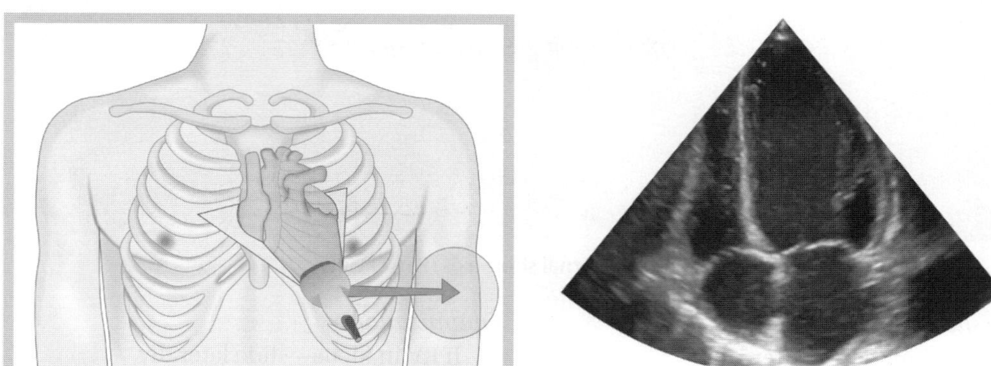

**Fig. 9:** Apical four-chamber view.

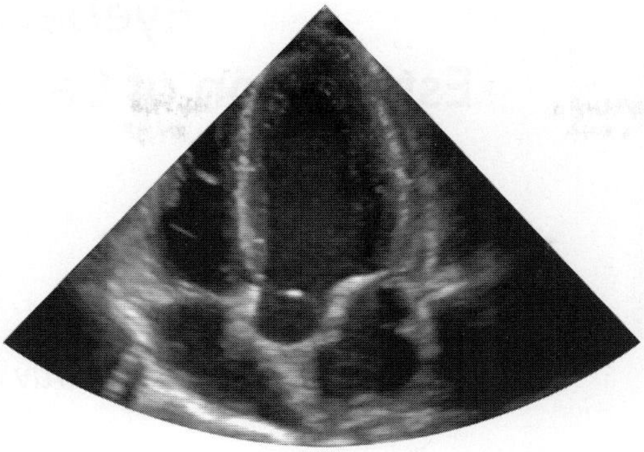

**Fig. 10:** Apical five-chamber view.

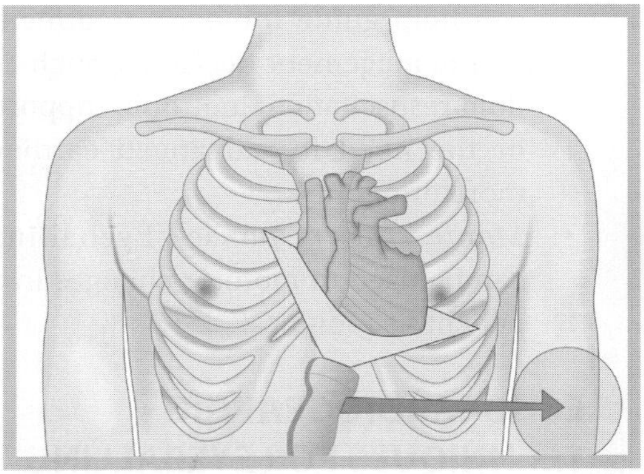

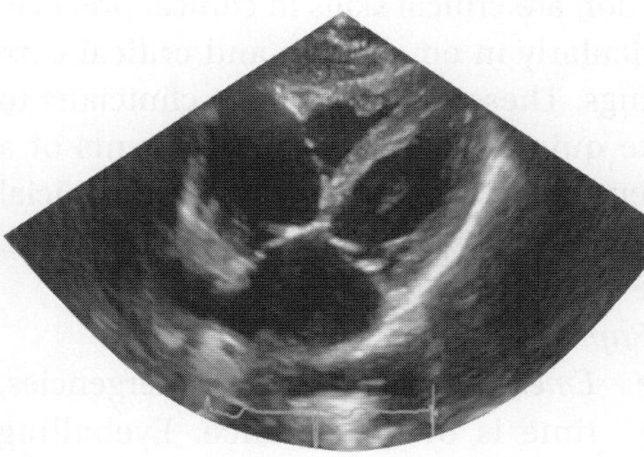

**Fig. 11:** Subcostal view.

*Apical five-chamber **(Fig. 10)**:*

Aortic outflow tract to be clearly visible without cusp of AV

*Subcostal view **(Fig. 11)**:*

*To obtain the view, the probe is placed in the subcostal area with the marker facing left and is tilted upwards to look at the heart.*

All four chambers visible without AV valve.

*Optimization:*

- If chambers are not opening—tilt up/down and 10-degree anticlockwise rotation
- If AV visible—tilt tail upwards
- If lung shadow obstructing—slide probe toward right side

*Please note:* Where ECHO probe is not available, subcostal view can be obtained with curvilinear probe.

CHAPTER 6

# Eyeballing and Gross Estimation of Cardiac Functions

*Gourav Mittal, Puneet Khanna*

## INTRODUCTION

Eyeballing and gross estimation of cardiac function are critical skills in clinical practice, particularly in emergency and critical care settings. These methods allow clinicians to make quick, preliminary assessments of a patient's cardiac status, which can be crucial for timely decision-making and intervention. Here is why these skills are important:

- *Rapid assessment:*
  - *Emergency situations:* In emergencies, time is of the essence. Eyeballing can provide immediate insights into a patient's cardiac function, guiding initial management while more detailed diagnostics are being prepared.
  - *Initial triage:* Helps in quickly determining the severity of a patient's condition and prioritizing care in crowded or resource-limited settings.
- *Bedside utility:*
  - *Point-of-care:* Gross estimation techniques can be performed at the bedside without the need for complex equipment, making them invaluable in settings where advanced imaging is not immediately available.
  - *Noninvasive:* These assessments are noninvasive and can be repeated as needed without causing discomfort or risk to the patient.
- *Clinical decision-making:*
  - *Guiding treatment:* Initial assessments can help guide the early treatment and management decisions, such as fluid resuscitation, inotropic support, or the need for advanced cardiac monitoring.
  - *Monitoring response:* Eyeballing can be used to monitor changes in a patient's condition.

## ECHOCARDIOGRAPHIC TECHNIQUES FOR EYEBALLING AND GROSS ESTIMATION

*Global function:* Visual estimation of ejection fraction (EF), wall motion abnormalities, and overall cardiac contractility.

*Volume status:* Assessing inferior vena cava (IVC) collapsibility and left ventricular (LV) filling pressures.

*However, it has some limitations:*

- *Subjectivity:* Eyeballing can be subjective and may vary between clinicians.
- *Complementary role:* While valuable, it should complement, not replace, more definitive diagnostic tools like formal echocardiography, ECG, and laboratory tests.

*Basics of visual assessment of LV function/ejection fraction* ***(Fig. 1 and Flowchart 1):***

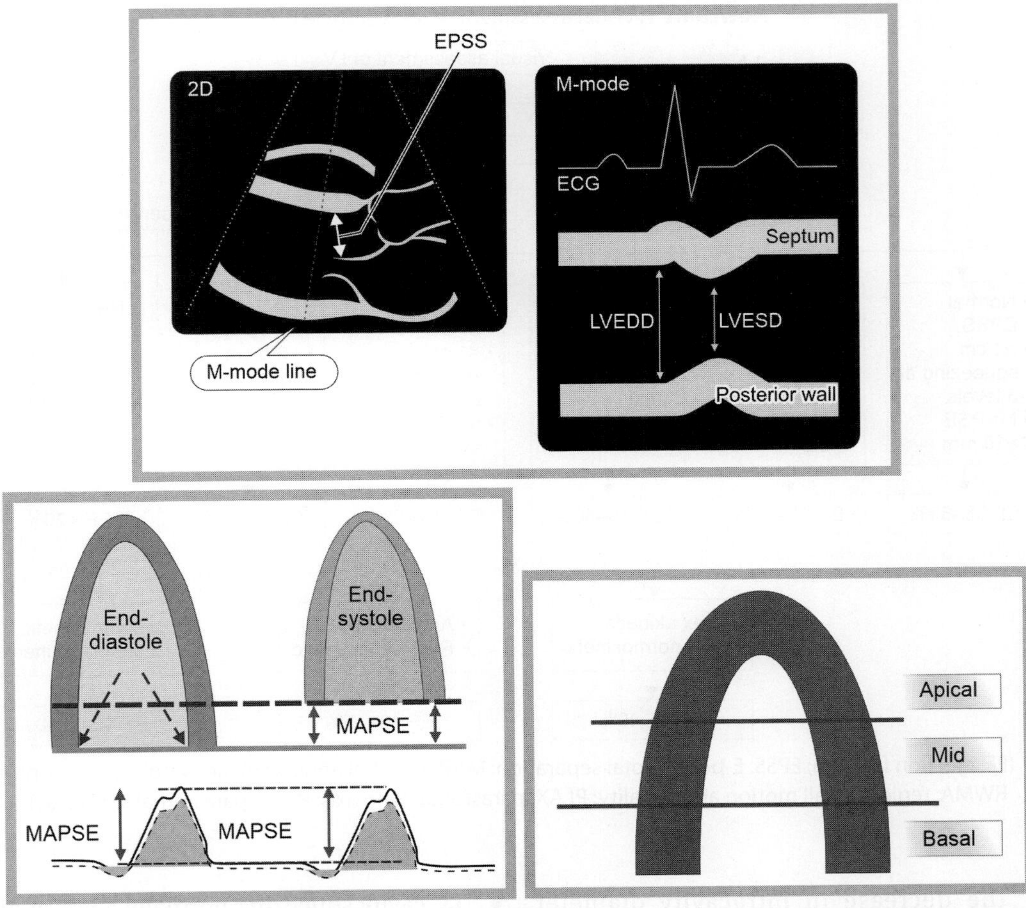


**Fig. 1:** Visual assessment of left ventricle (LV) function/ejection fraction. (EPSS: E-point septal separation; LVEDD: left ventricular end-diastolic diameter; LVESD: left ventricular end-systolic diameter; MAPSE: mitral annular plane systolic excursion)

- *Always check in at least three views:* (1) Preferably parasternal long axis (PLAX), (2) parasternal short axis (PSAX), and (3) apical 4 chamber (A4C). Also include apical 2 chamber (A2C) and apical 3 chamber (A3C) views whenever feasible.
- Try to obtain views that are not off-axis to optimize imaging quality as much as possible.
- Maintain a 3D imagination of cardiac function during the assessment.
- Ensure to check for the presence of regional wall motion abnormality (RWMA).
- *The left ventricle (LV) exhibits three types of movements:* Longitudinal, circular, and rotational. As the severity of impairment increases, each type of movement becomes impaired in sequence: First longitudinal, then circular, and finally rotational.
- Assess longitudinal movement by visualizing mitral annular plane systolic excursion (MAPSE) in the A4C view. Circular movement can be evaluated in the PLAX view by measuring E-point septal separation (EPSS) and observing

**Flowchart 1:** Visual assessment of left ventricle (LV).

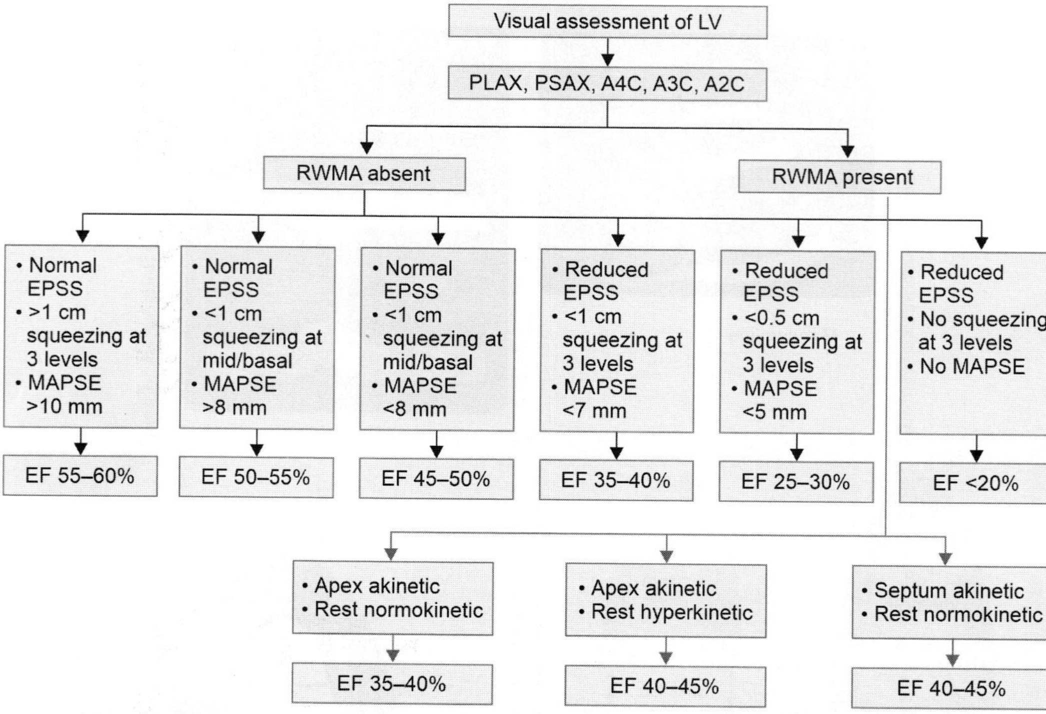


(EF: ejection fraction; EPSS: E-point septal separation; MAPSE: mitral annular plane systolic excursion; RWMA: regional wall motion abnormality; PLAX: parasternal long axis; PSAX: parasternal short axis)

the decrease in intracavity diameter during systole at the level of the papillary muscles, in the A4C view, including the contribution of the apex, mid, and basal segments in contraction.

- *If RWMA is present, identify the affected segment:* Apical, septal, or other regions.

*Gross quantification parameters to be kept in mind before assessing visual function:*

- Good LV function EPSS touches septum (although insensitive to detect decrease in function)
- LV cavity decreasing diameter >1 cm normal (observe at all three level) (use ruler on screen for estimation)
- LV cavity squeezing normally >50% at all three levels apical, mid, basal (apical contribute more in output followed by (f/b) mid f/b basal)
  - If basal and mid gone—reduce EF by 5% each
  - If apical gone—10% reduction in EF

  Look other segment if hyperkinetic—reduction will be less
- MAPSE ≥10 mm indicates a preserved ejection fraction—<7; 10% reduction in EF
- Normal kinesis (LV wall contracting >30%)
- All 3 present, i.e., longitudinal, circular, rotational (usually EF >40%), complete loss of longitudinal (EF ≤30%), complete

loss of longitudinal and circular (EF ≤20%).

- *In presence of RWMA:*
  - APEX akinetic with other hyperkinetic—EF drops by 10–15%
  - APEX akinetic with other normokinetic—EF drops by 15–20%
  - Asynchrony—EF drops by 10%
  - Other segments apart from apex septum 15% reduction in EF
  - Other segment apart from apex/septum 3–5% per segment drop in EF

## CONCLUSION

Eyeballing and gross estimation of cardiac functions are indispensable skills that provide rapid, valuable information in clinical settings. They are essential for initial patient assessment, guiding immediate management, and serving as an educational tool for developing clinical expertise. However, these assessments should be used in conjunction with more detailed and objective diagnostic methods to ensure comprehensive patient care.

CHAPTER 7

# Left Ventricle Systolic Function and Cardiac Output Estimation: Approach and Clinical Application

*Gourav Mittal, Puneet Khanna*

## BASICS

- *Arrangement of myocardial fibers in left ventricle (LV):*
  - *Subendocardial fibers:* Obliquely
  - *Mid myocardial fibers:* Circumferential
  - *Subepicardial fibers:* Obliquely

*Contraction of oblique fibers:* Shortening and twisting

*Contraction of circumferential fibers:* Radial myocardial thickening and reduction in ventricular diameter

*The contractile function can be classified for each wall as:*

- Normal
- Hypokinetic
- Akinetic
- Dyskinetic

## LEFT VENTRICLE FUNCTION ASSESSMENT

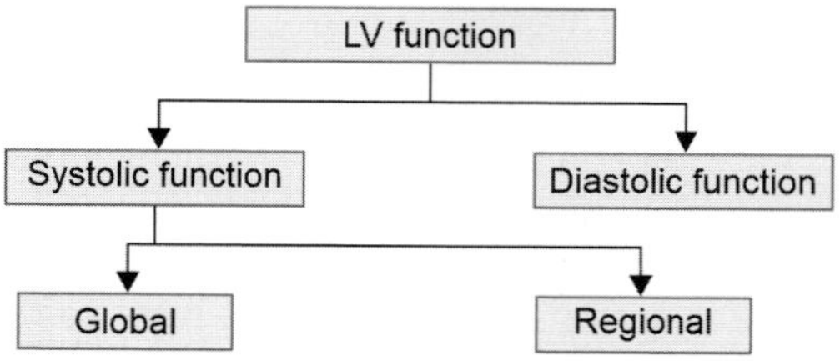


*Left ventricle systolic function (various methods of assessments):*

- Eyeballing
- Standard measurement of dimensions
- *M-mode measurements:* E-point septal separation (EPSS)
- Longitudinal shortening
- Fractional shortening
- Fractional area change

*Left ventricle systolic function in various modes:*

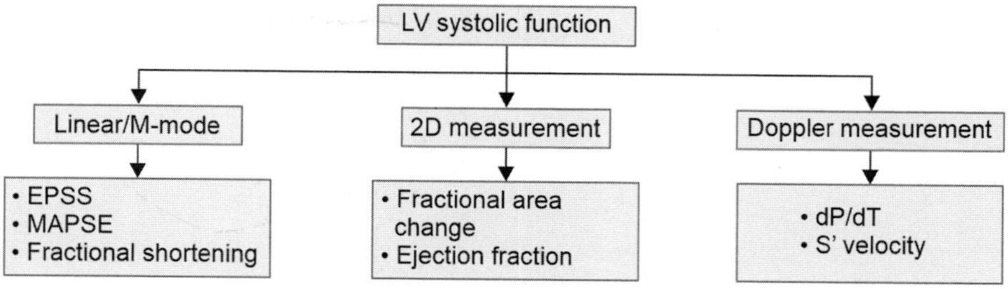


(EPSS: E-point septal separation; MAPSE: mitral annular plane systolic excursion)

- Ejection fraction
- Tissue Doppler
- *Strain measurement:* Longitudinal speckle tracking

*Left ventricle systolic indices:*

- *Dimensions*
- *Linear measurements*
  - Fractional shortening
- *Area measurements*
  - Fractional area change
- *Volume calculations, ejection fraction*
  - Method of disks
  - Teicholz
  - Quinones
  - Area—length
  - 3D volume
  - Mitral motion
  - Mitral annular plane systolic excursion (MAPSE)
- *Spectral Doppler:*
  - Rate of pressure rise (dP/dT)
  - Myocardial performance index (MPI)
  - Velocity circumferential shortening (Vcf)
  - Stroke volume (SV)/cardiac output (CO)
- *Tissue Doppler:*
  - Systolic mitral annular velocity (S')
  - Strain (global longitudinal peak systolic strain)
  - Strain rate

**Left Ventricle Systolic Function: Eyeballing**

*What are we looking for?*

- Inward movement of the endocardium
- Thickening of the myocardium
- Longitudinal motion of the mitral annulus
- Reduced motion of the anterior mitral valve leaflet in parasternal long axis (PLAX)
- The anterior mitral valve leaflet should come within 8 mm of the septal wall in the PLAX view in systole
- Normal motion <8 mm, moderately reduced motion 8–18 mm, severely reduced motion >18 mm
- Geometry of the left ventricle (size and aneurysms)

*Normal left ventricle dimensions and volumes:*

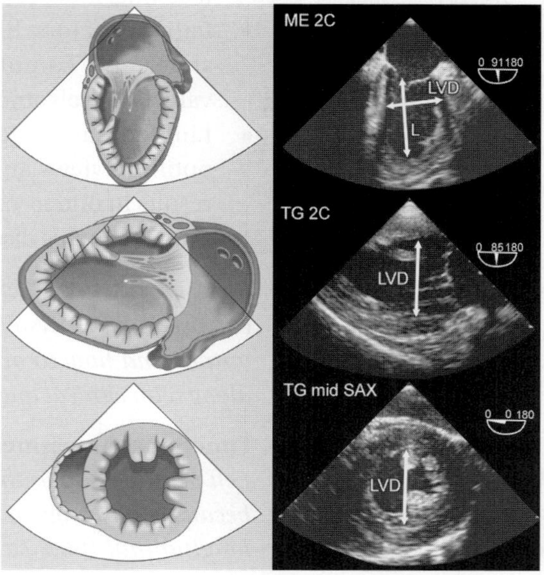

| Normal left ventricle (LV) size | Male | | Female | |
|---|---|---|---|---|
| | Mean ± SD | 2-SD range | Mean ± SD | 2-SD range |
| *LV diameter (LVD):* | | | | |
| Diastole, mm | 50.2 ± 4.1 | 42.0–58.4 | 45.0 ± 3.6 | 37.8–52.2 |
| Systole, mm | 32.4 ± 3.7 | 25.0–39.8 | 28.2 ± 3.3 | 21.6–34.8 |
| *LV volume:* | | | | |
| Diastolic volume, mL | 106 ± 22 | 62–150 | 76 ± 15 | 46–106 |
| Diastolic volume/BSA, mL/m$^2$ | 54 ± 10 | 34–74 | 45 ± 8 | 29–16 |
| Systolic volume, mL | 41 ± 10 | 21–61 | 28 ± 7 | 14–42 |
| Systolic volume/BSA, mL/m$^2$ | 21 ± 5 | 11–31 | 16 ± 4 | 8–24 |

*Left ventricle systolic function although erroneously taken as equivalent to cardiac output has paramount importance for an intensivist/emergency physician in acute care as well as routine care of patient. Admission value and trend over admission has its prognostic as well as therapeutic value.*

*How estimation of above said function could be helpful in acute care settings?*

- Baseline function helpful in predicting outcome of current admission.
- Narrow down differential diagnosis of particular condition by determining whether heart is involved or not, whether involvement is clinically significant or not.
- If it is involved, i.e., function is reduced how to optimize? Fluid, vasopressors, inotropes, inodilators, and mechanical circulatory support have to use over due course of time.
- Identifying need of intervention/interventional cardiology team for certain intervention especially time-sensitive illness like myocardial infarction, severe depressed function requiring mechanical support, huge effusion requiring drainage.

*Some logistic and academic issues create hindrance to application of this knowledge:*

- Nonavailability of echo probe
- Not able to integrate the echo knowledge with clinical application (probably because of work load, reduced bedside teaching, more reliance on digital media)
- Patient factors like obesity, nonstable state, and complex heart lesions like valvular involvement
- Limited knowledge often leads to non-optimize views and wrong interpretation results in under- or overestimation sometimes becomes disastrous.

*First, we discuss different views in which we can ascertain LV systolic function and cardiac output and how to optimize them. Later on, along with clinical query their application.*

**Functional Assessment**

*Left ventricle shows three types of movements because of arrangement of muscle layers, i.e., longitudinal (60% cardiac output), circular (fractional shortening), and rotatory.*

*Principle of LV function:*

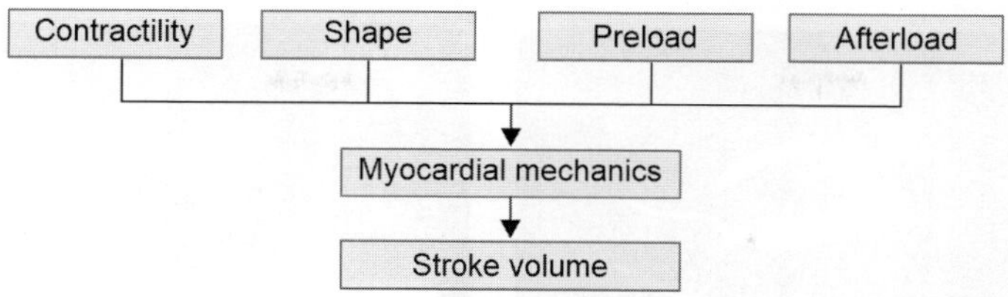


**Pathophysiology of LV Failure: Cascade and Compensatory Mechanisms**

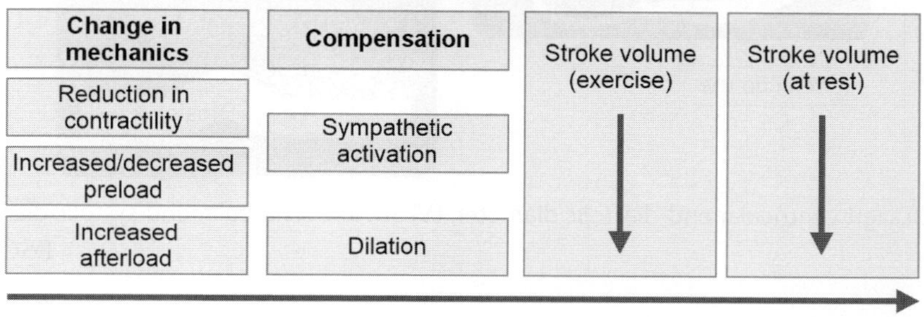


*Quantitative assessment:*

- *Anatomical and load-dependent indices:*
  - Fractional shortening (PLAX)
  - Ejection method (Simpson method) (A4C)
  - MAPSE (A4C)
  - Eyeballing
- *Doppler and load dependent:*
  - Cardiac output (PLAX + A5C)
  - Tei index (Myocardial performance index) (A4C)
- *Doppler and relatively load independent:*
  - Contractility (dP/dT) (A4C)
- *Load dependent:* Where measurements tend to change with loading conditions of heart, i.e., change in preload and afterload.
- *Load independent:* Where measurements tend to remain unaffected with loading conditions of heart, i.e., change in preload and afterload.

*(A) Anatomical and load dependent indices:*

1. *Fractional shortening:* Less technicality and alignment requirement make this way an easier method to obtain LV function. But it is a gross method with its limitations, so while driving ejection fraction from this method, one should be conscious enough to take clinical decision. Load-dependent parameter it is, so if patient is not adequately resuscitated it gives false reading.

   *PLAX view obtained; M mode is applied below opening of mitral valve. We will get 2 dimension of LV, one while contracting other one while relaxing*

*FS = End diastolic LV diameter – End systolic/ End diastolic LV diameter*

| | ***Male*** | ***Female*** |
|---|---|---|
| Normal | 25–43% | 27–45% |
| Mild | 20–24% | 22–26% |
| Moderate | 15–19% | 17–21% |
| Severe | 14% | ≤16% |

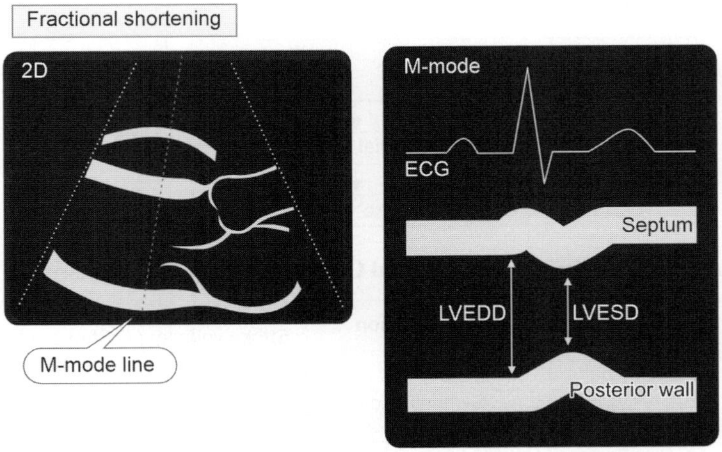


(LVEDD: left ventricular end-diastolic diameter; LVESD: left ventricular end-systolic diameter

ESC/ASE, 2005

*Contraindication:*

- Left bundle branch block (LBBB)/dyssynchrony/pacemaker
- Abnormal septal motion
- Regional wall motion abnormalities
- Inadequate (oblique) M mode orientation
- Poor image quality
- "Pseudoshortening" of the LV (very small ventricle)

  *Ejection fraction can be derived from FS by Teichholz formula = Ejection fraction = 2 *FS*

  Do not use this as this is very crude and using a lot of assumptions.

2. *Ejection fraction (Simpson method):* Apical 4-chamber view, freeze in diastole (MV fully opened) 2D mode, select calculation, under this LV, A4C view end diastolic volume, trace endocardial border of LV cavity including papillary muscle and MV opening. This will give us end diastole volume of LV. Now freeze in systole when both AV and MV closed, select end systolic volume.

*Ejection fraction = Edvol – Esvol/Edvol * 100*

| | ***Values*** |
|---|---|
| Normal | >55% |
| Mild | 45–54% |
| Moderate | 30–44% |
| Severe | <30% |

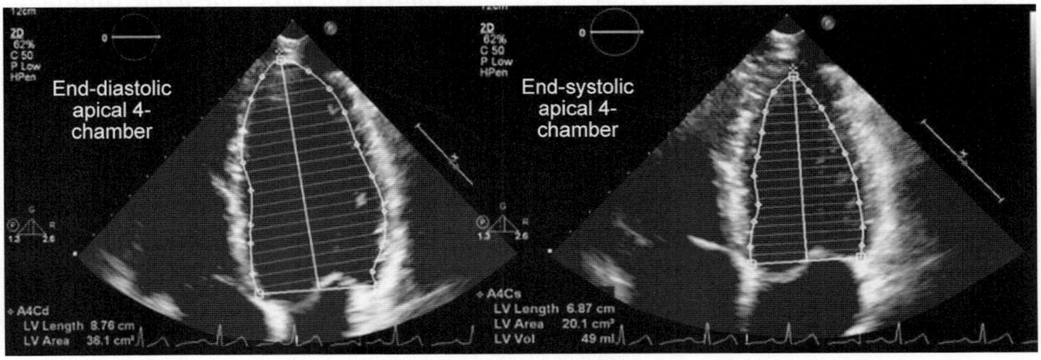

- *Ejection fractions tend to be higher in small ventricles.*
- *Athletes often have ejection fractions in the low normal range.*
- *Ejection fraction does not predict exercise capacity or functional reserve.*
- *Ejection fraction is supernormal in patients with reduced afterload (e.g., mitral regurgitation)*
- *Mitral annulus peak systolic excursion (MAPSE)*

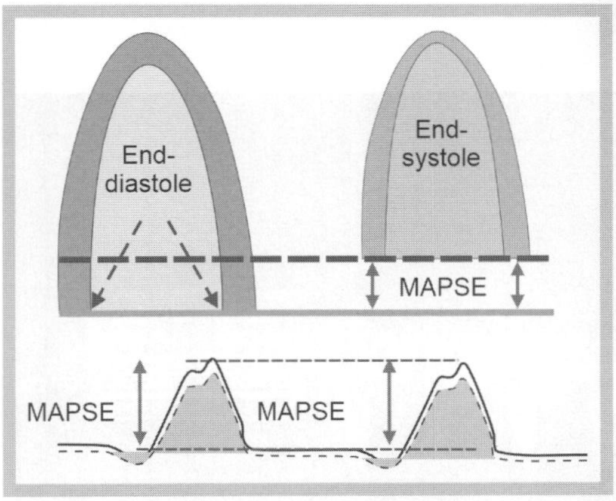


It gives fair estimation of longitudinal contractility of LV.

Which itself contributes to 60% of its output.

A4C view, apply M mode across lateral mitral annulus.

- *M-mode has to be aligned perpendicular to the annulus.*
- *From the lowest point in early diastole to the highest point during systole*
- *The postsystolic motion should not be included in the measurement*
  I. *Average normal values = 12–15 mm*
  II. *≥10 mm indicates a preserved ejection fraction.*
  III. *<8 mm indicates impaired, and <7 mm indicates severely impaired.*

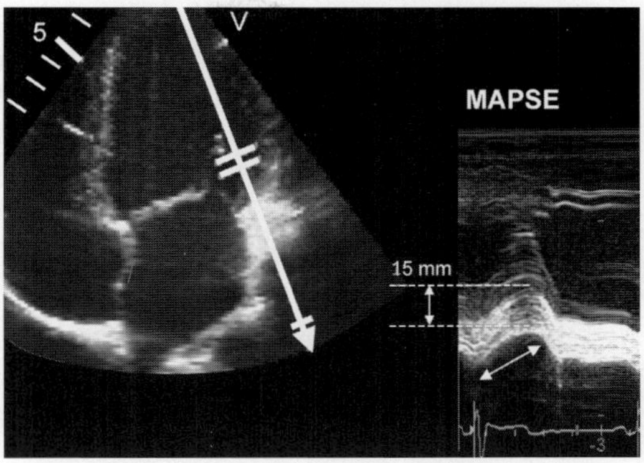


Mitral annular plane systolic excursion can be used for the assessment of prognosis in the following clinical settings:

- Hypertensive heart disease
- *Aortic stenosis:* In particular isolated low-grade aortic stenosis
- Hypertrophic cardiomyopathy
- Myocardial infarction
- Heart failure
- Tetralogy of Fallot
- Atrial fibrillation

*Limitation:* Echocardiographic assessment suffers from angle and load dependence. Consider only one aspect of LV contractility, i.e., longitudinal, during ICU stay loading conditions frequently changes and also vasopressor usage, it underestimates LV function.

3. *Eyeballing:* Left ventricle shows three movements longitudinal, circular, and rotational. As severity of impairment increases each one impaired in sequence longitudinal followed by (f/b) circular f/b rotational.

*Circular and rotational movements can be scanned in PSAX and longitudinal in A4C:*

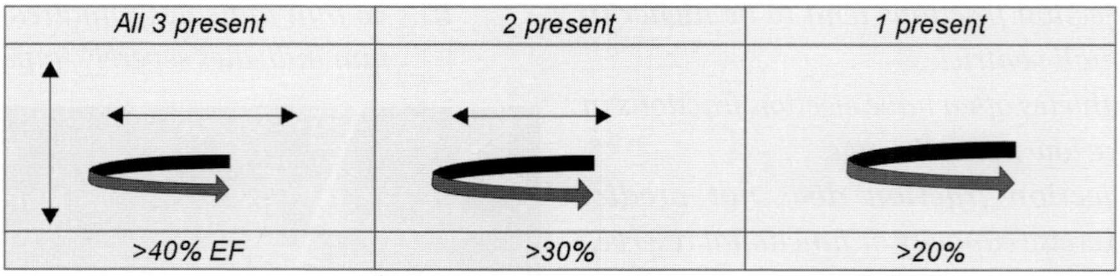


*(B) Doppler and load-dependent parameters:*

1. *Cardiac output:*
   = Stroke volume * Heart rate
   =LVOT VTI * LVOT area * Heart rate
   = LVOT VTI * $\pi D^2/4$ * HR

*For LVOT VTI = A5C view, apply pulse wave Doppler just below aortic valve.*
*For D = LVOT diameter in PLAX view just below aortic valve when fully opened*

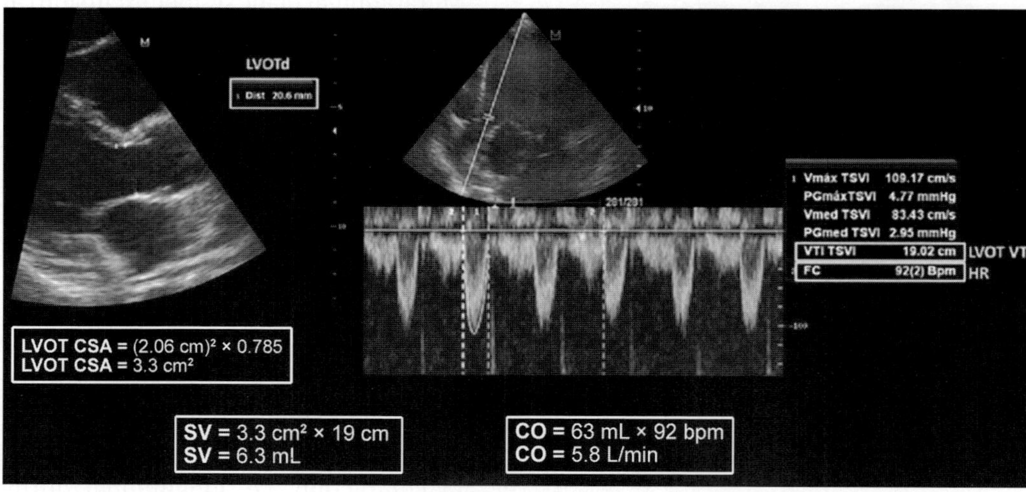


*Limitation:* Operator-dependent measurements, PW Doppler alignment should be <30° from in plane flow. Load-dependent values. Limitation to obtain optimize A5C view.

*Usefulness:* As cardiac output is also dependent on heart rate, despite low stroke volume, CO can be normal if heart rate is >100 bpm. We often measure LV function when patient if hemodynamically unstable, but even during maintained BP LV can be dysfunctional. With this method, we can have fair idea of compensation going on.

2. *Tei index aka myocardial performance index:* The ratio of the time spent in isovolumetric activity divided by the time spent in ventricular ejection. In other words, it is the sum of isovolumic contraction and relaxation times divided by the ejection time.

$$MPI = (ICT + IRT)/ET$$

*ICT:* isovolumic contraction time; IRT: isovolumic relaxation time; ET: ejection time

*A4C PW Doppler across MV will give A*
*A5C PW Doppler across LVOT give B*

$$MPI = A - B/B$$

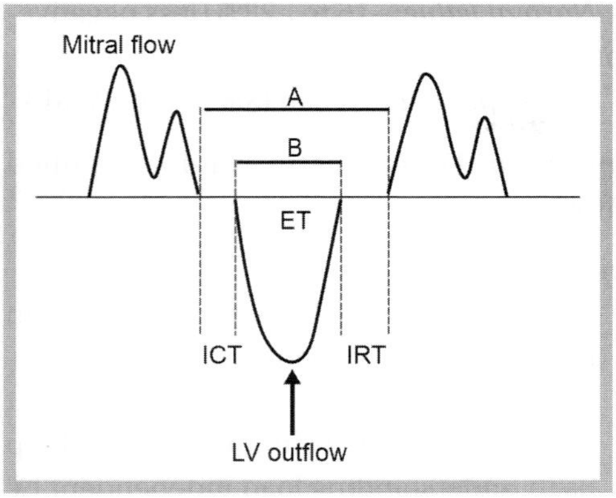


*Interpretation:*

- As systolic function deteriorates, ICT increases and ET decreases ultimately Tei increases.
- Value >0.5 always abnormal.
  Myocardial performance index of >1.14 has been shown to be a powerful and independent predictor of poor clinical outcome in patients with severe left ventricular dysfunction and symptomatic heart failure.

*Advantages of myocardial performance index:*

- Simple to estimate
- Reproducible
- Not affected by geometry
- Assesses global function

*Down sides of MPI:*

- Nonsimultaneous acquisition
- Load dependence
- Variation with heart rate, age and body surface area, and rhythm
- Nonspecific—unable to differentiate between systolic and diastolic dysfunction. There could also be pseudonormalization due to this.

*(C) Doppler and relatively load independent:*

1. *Contractility (dP/dT):* Apical four-chamber view/CW Doppler on mitral regurgitation jet. The dP/dt is calculated by measuring the slope of the initial mitral regurgitation signal between 1 m/s and 3 m/s.
   - *Normal >1,200 mm Hg/s*
   - *Borderline 800–1,200 mm Hg/s*
   - *Reduced <800 mm Hg/s*
   - *Severely reduced <500 mm Hg/s*

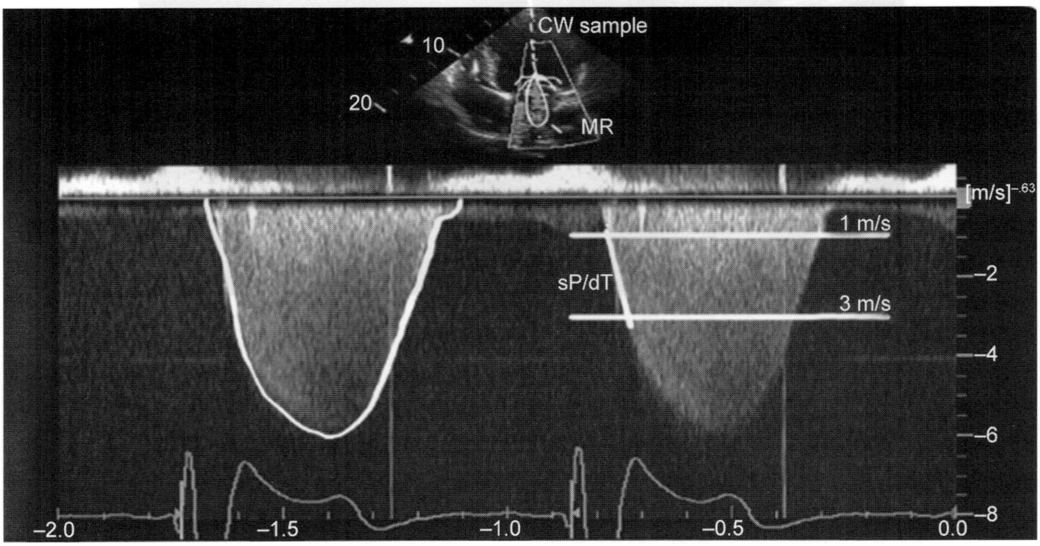

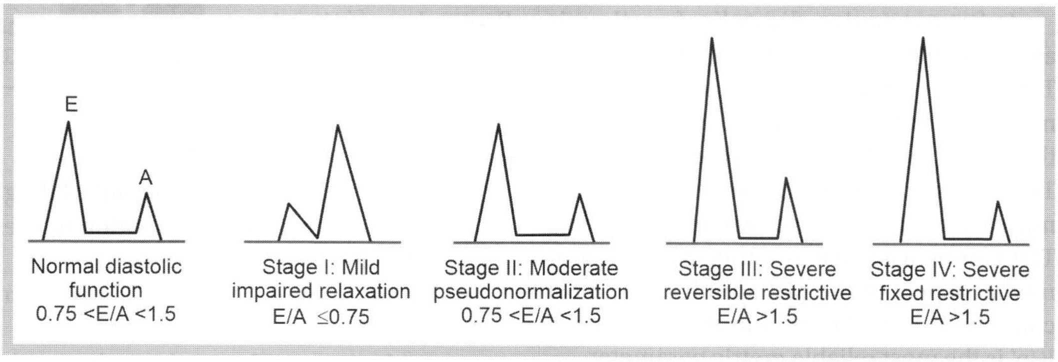


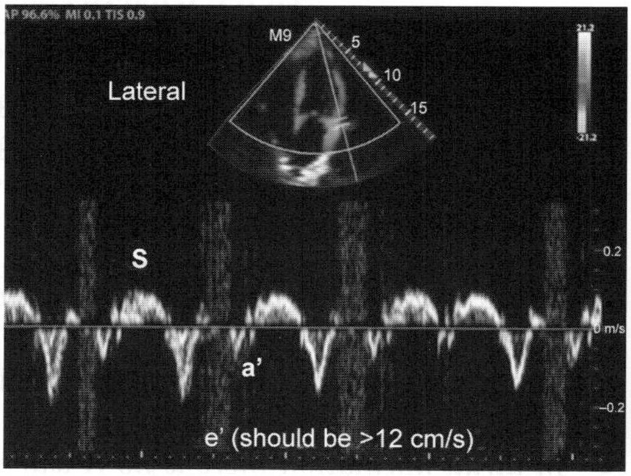


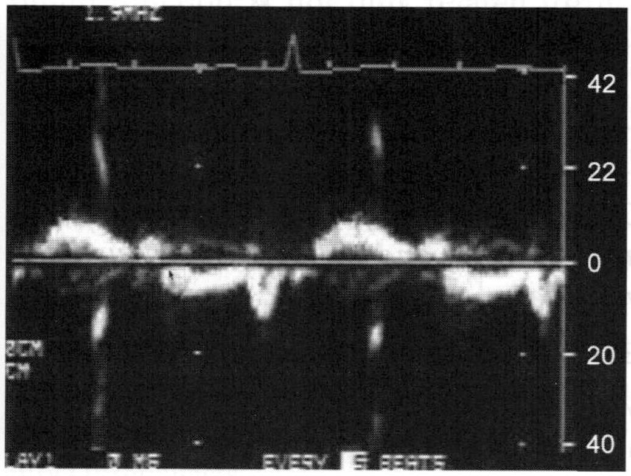


- Place the cursor through the lateral annulus of the mitral valve.
- Set the marker in the thickest part of the annulus.
- Obtain the TDI waveform, save the image
- Identify the e′ wave and the a′ wave.
- *E/e′ Ratio:* Reflects left ventricular end-diastolic pressure (LVEDP)
- *Normally <8:* Elevated >15
- TDI a lateral e′ <10 cm/s and septal <7 cm/s is suggestive of diastolic dysfunction.
- The ratio of E/e′ <8 is normal and a ratio >15 is associated with LV diastolic dysfunction in nonventilated patients.
- A ratio of >12 is sufficient to identify diastolic dysfunction in patients on mechanical ventilation

*ECG correlation*:

*The a′ wave occurs right before the QRS.*

*Measure the e′ peak, save the measurement.*

- Echo assessment of diastolic function is based on the interpretation of a constellation of echo and Doppler measurements.
- No single echo parameter provides a definitive or summary measure of the ventricular PV relationship during diastole.
- If any parameters are abnormal—only reflect isolated changes in relaxation or compliance.
- They are affected by the complex interaction between changes in LV relaxation, LV compliance, LAP, and LA contractility, further complicated by rhythm and loading conditions.

| Optimization of measurements | |
|---|---|
| 1 | Obtain a true apical four-chamber view of the heart that excludes the aortic valve |
| 2 | Reduce the angle between the ultrasound beam and blood flow (visualized with color Doppler mapping) as much as possible (<20°):<br>• *Mitral inflow:* Translate the transducer from the true apical four-chamber view to a slightly more lateral position |
| 3 | *Use a small pulsed-wave Doppler sample volume:*<br>• *Mitral inflow:* 1–2 mm |
| 4 | *Place the sample volume adequately:*<br>• *Mitral inflow:* Between the tips of the mitral leaflets |
| 5 | • Use a sweep speed of 50 mm/s (appreciation of the influence of the respiratory cycle on Doppler velocities) or 100 mm/s (measurement of flow duration or deceleration time)<br>• Use ECG and respiratory tracings, especially in ventilated patients<br>• Set velocity filter as low as possible (200–600 Hz) |
| 6 | Perform all measurements at end expiration (or during apnea) to limit the effects of heart–lung interactions on Doppler velocities |

*Suspected left ventricular diastolic dysfunction (LVDD):*

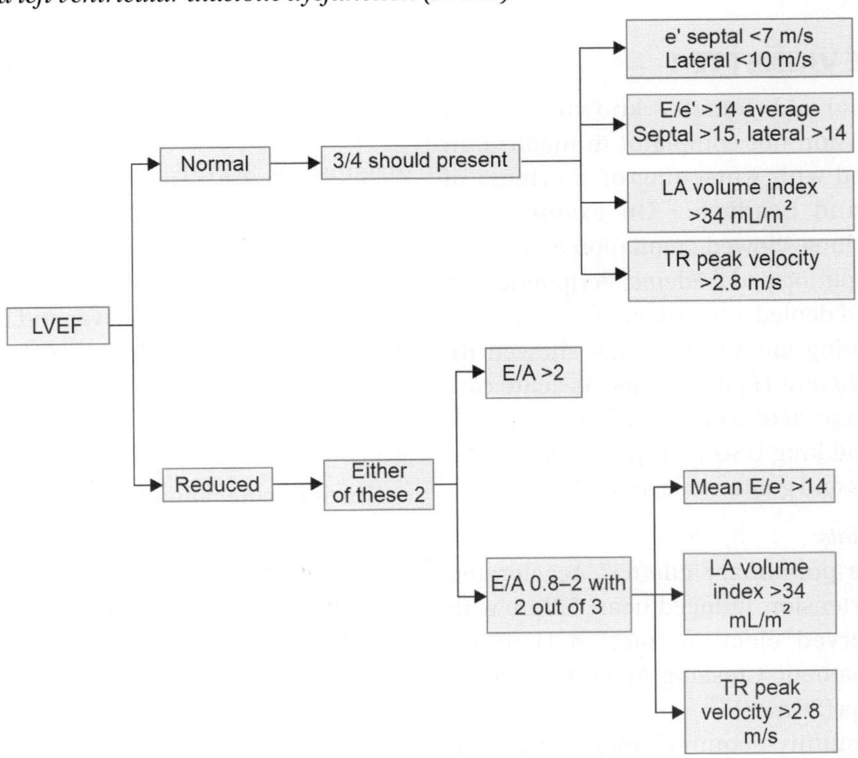


(LVEF: left ventricular ejection fraction)

*Difficult to assess LV volume and TR jet simplified approach as described below:*

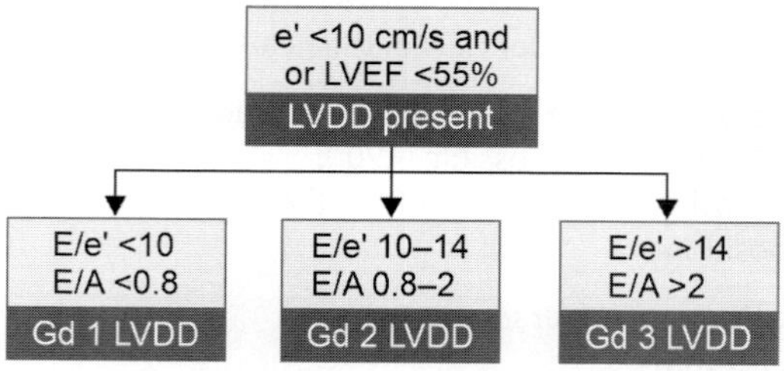


(LVDD: left ventricular diastolic dysfunction; LVEF: left ventricular ejection fraction)

1. Sometimes see E < A in under filled, hyper dynamic hearts

- *If this is the case, the LV appears under filled, high EF, and e >> 10 cm/s*

*For physiological aspect understand as physiology level:*

| | ***Normal*** | ***Grade 1*** | ***Grade 2*** | ***Grade 3*** |
|---|---|---|---|---|
| LV relaxation | Normal | Impaired | Impaired | Impaired |
| Left atrial pressure | Normal | Low or normal | Elevated | Elevated |
| Compliance | Normal | Normal | Reduced | Severely reduced |

## CASE VIGNETTE 1

A 56-year-old female, known case of hypertension not complaint to medication presented with worsening of shortness of breath and headache. On examination, bilateral lung showed crepitation along with bilateral pitting pedal edema. Peripheries are warm and denied any history of fever, cough, and burning micturition. Vital showed BP of 220/120 mm Hg both arms. As acute care physician started basic resuscitation. How 2D ECHO and lung USG help you to determine diagnosis and guide management?

*Differentials:*

- Acute pulmonary edema? Accelerated hypertension-induced heart failure with preserved ejection fraction (HfPEF), Sympathetic Crashing Acute Pulmonary Edema (SCAPE)
- Community-acquired pneumonia with heart failure
- Fluid overload secondary to underlying undiagnosed renal dysfunction.

Acute management if underlying diagnosis is SCAPE or accelerated hypertension, acute care can stabilize patient early and can prevent intubation and subsequent mechanical ventilation.

Relying on history no fever and localizing sign puts infective etiology on backseat, no renal dysfunction and fluid administration also puts fluid overload secondary to renal last D/D.

Having acute pulmonary edema in vision, we can perform echo and lung USG to confirm our diagnosis and guide our management.

Sympathetic Crashing Acute Pulmonary Edema (SCAPE) occurs due to a *vicious spiral* involving increasing sympathetic outflow, excessive afterload, and progressively worsening heart failure. Since SCAPE is a vicious spiral, this may develop very rapidly (hence the terminology "flash pulmonary edema"). With aggressive therapy, it may *resolve* very rapidly as well.

The central, defining pathophysiological feature of SCAPE is pathologically elevated afterload due to systemic vasoconstriction and hypertension.

SCAPE patients may be euvolemic or hypovolemic. The problem is a *shift* of fluid into the lungs, rather than hypervolemia.

Three stages of progression are:

1. *Stage 1:* Distension of small pulmonary capillaries due to increased left atrial pressure
2. *Stage 2:* Interstitial edema
3. *Stage 3:* Flooding of alveolar space causing hypoxia

*ECHO:*

*Views:*

For assessing LV diastolic dysfunction and LA filling pressure:

- A4C LV focused
- Perform systolic function and diastolic function
- Inferior vena cava (IVC) screening for size and variability

*Lung USG:* ≥1 zone with ≥3 B-lines (one positive zone) on each hemithorax

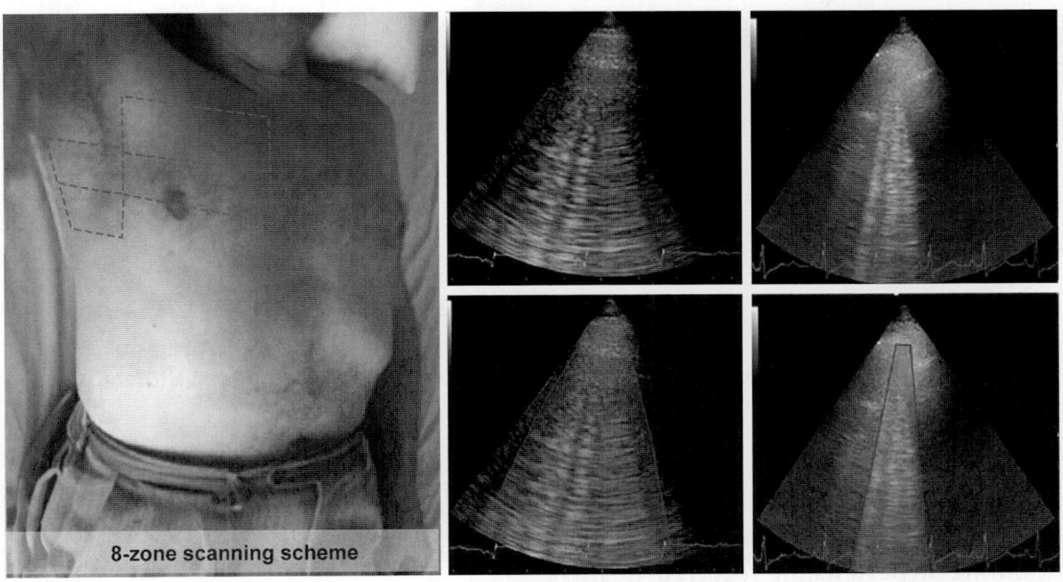

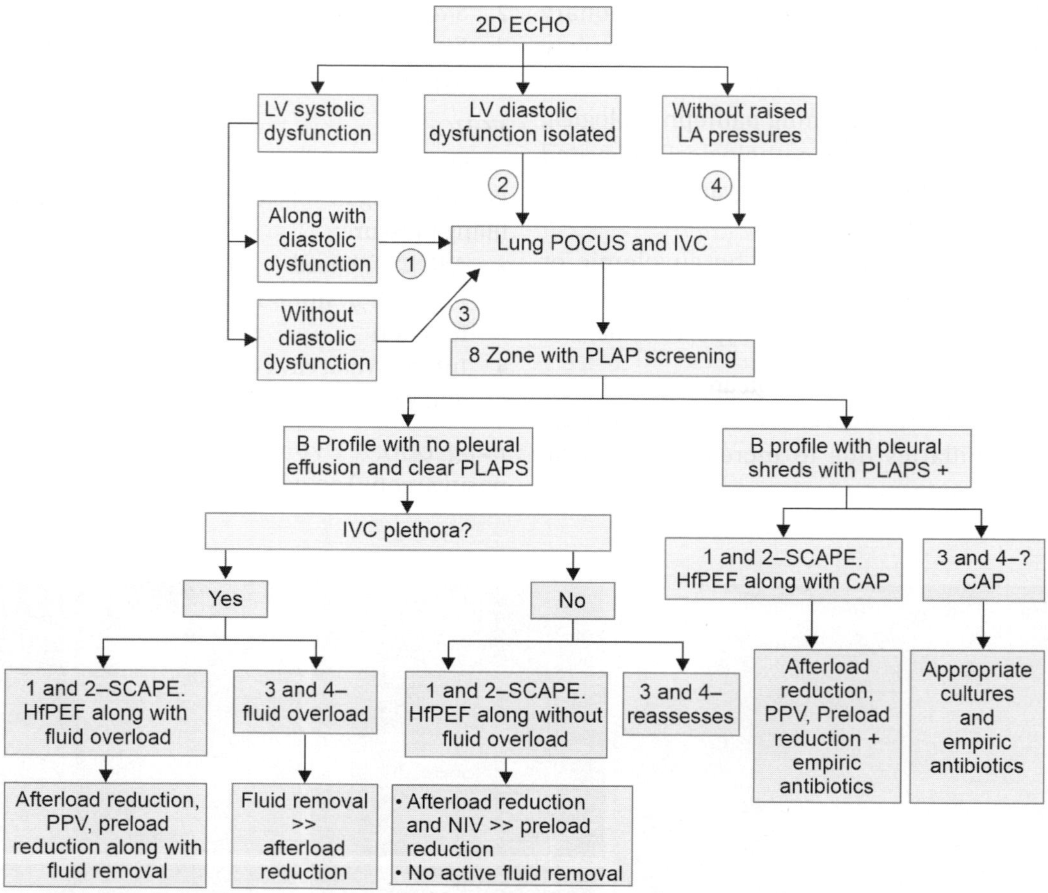


(HfPEF: heart failure with preserved ejection fraction; SCAPE: sympathetic crashing acute pulmonary edema; PLAPS: posterolateral alveolar and/or pleural syndrome; LA: left atrium; LV: left ventricle)

## CASE VIGNETTE 2

A 33-year-old male with known case of long-standing hypertension received positive pressure ventilation for 7 days in view of viral pneumonia and acute respiratory distress syndrome (ARDS). Baseline cardiac functions were normal except presence of LV hypertrophy. After resolution of primary condition you attempted weaning, but he failed 2 SBT trials, work of breathing increased and oxygenation worsens as spontaneous breathing trial attempted. History of long-standing hypertension, grossly positive cumulative positive fluid balance along with gross edematous appearance you suspected weaning induced cardiac dysfunction. How echo will help you to reach diagnosis?

*Answer:*

First we briefly discussed pathophysiology of weaning-induced cardiac failure.

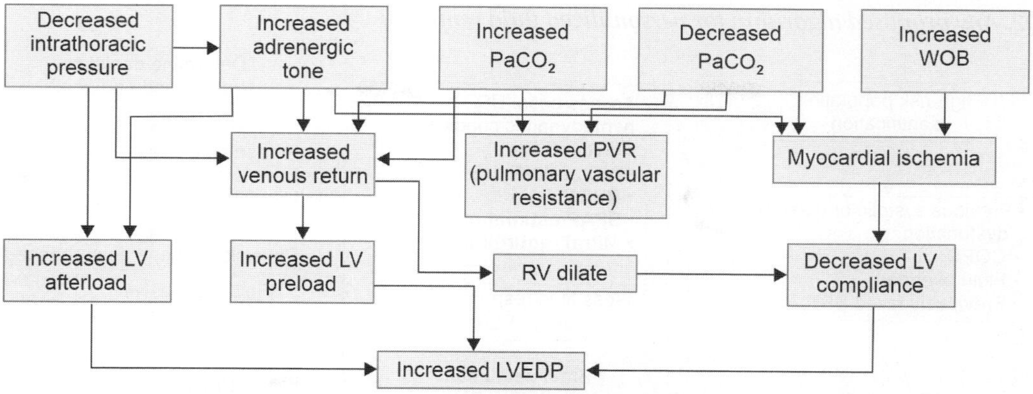


(LVEDP: left ventricular end-diastolic pressure; $PaCO_2$: partial pressure of arterial carbon dioxide; $PaO_2$: arterial oxygen pressure)

*View required:* Similar to previous case

Diagnostic accuracy of 2D ECHO for identifying weaning-induced cardiac dysfunction—E/e′ before SBT >12.5 and >14.5 after SBT have sensitivity of 75% and specificity of 95.8% both increase if clubbed with increased in brain natriuretic peptide (BNP)/pro-BNP >12% after SBT and lung USG (B profile in nondependent area after SBT)

*Q1. How POCUS helps you to manage this case once diagnosis of weaning-induced cardiac dysfunction becomes certain?*

CHEOPS bundle is helpful in managing diastolic dysfunction in ICU.

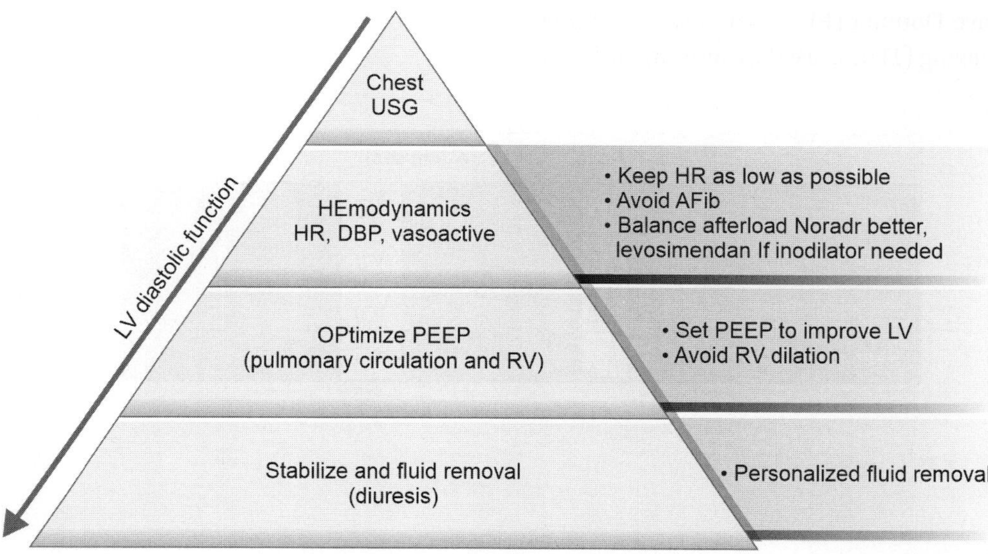


CHEOPS: BUNDLE

(HR: heart rate; DBP: diastolic blood pressure; PEEP: positive end expiratory pressure)

*Q2. Any proposed algorithm for personalized fluid removal?*

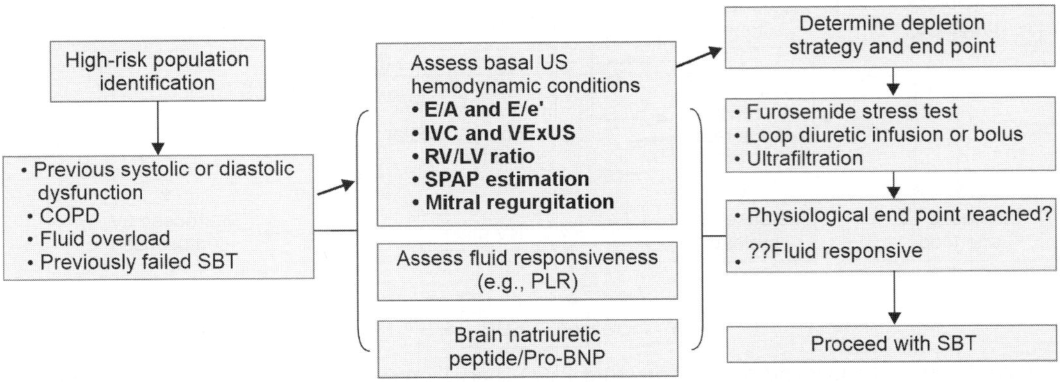


(BNP: brain natriuretic peptide; COPD: chronic obstructive pulmonary disease)

*Points to remember:*

- Diastole is an active energy requiring process. It is not a passive filling of the heart.
- With echocardiography, we can evaluate diastolic function rapidly and non-invasively. A simplified method looking at the mitral valve inflow with pulse wave Doppler (PWD) and tissue Doppler imaging (TDI) is used by most intensivists.
- E/e′ is the most reliable metric parameter.
- Suspect in elderly, diabetic, hypertensive patients.
- One important modifiable factor in weaning failure, always screen for before attempting weaning and look for if weaning failure happened comparing to before weaning E/e′.

| | E–A Ratio | e' (cm/sec) | E/e' |
|---|---|---|---|
| Normal | E>A | >8 | <8 |
| Imparied | A>E (2:1) | | <8 |
| Pseudo-normal | E>A | <8 | 8–15 |
| Restrictive | E>>A (3:1) | <8 | >15 |

CHAPTER 9

# Right Ventricle Function and Pulmonary Arterial Hypertension

*Gourav Mittal, Puneet Khanna*

## RIGHT VENTRICLE DYSFUNCTION

The importance of the right ventricle (RV) and its interactions with pulmonary circulation was first realized by Sir William Harvey in 1616, yet up until the mid-20th century little emphasis had been placed on the RV.

Acute right ventricular failure (RVF) accounts for 2–9% of acute heart failure admissions to hospitals with in-hospital mortality ranging from 5 to 17%.

In the intensive care unit, acute right ventricular dysfunction (RVD) and failure can present in many common critical illnesses, as discussed in **Table 1**.

## ANATOMICAL AND PHYSIOLOGICAL IMPORTANCE IN BRIEF

The RV blood supply is dependent on the dominance of the coronary system. 80%have an RV supplied by the right coronary artery, and 20% by the left coronary artery. Unlike the LV, perfusion of the RV occurs during both systole and diastole **(Table 2)**.

Initially adaptive and accompanied by an increase in contractility and preserved stroke volume (homeometric adaptation)—Anrep. These early compensatory mechanisms are achieved in part by neurohormonal activation with increased adrenergic tone. Neurohormonal activation ultimately becomes maladaptive. Over time, as contractility declines or afterload further increases, the RV must dilate to maintain stroke volume (heterometric adaptation). Right ventricular ischemia may result from a mismatch between increased oxygen demand and reduced coronary arterial perfusion due to increased wall stress with hypertrophy and capillary rarefaction.

## DEFINITIONS RELATED TO RIGHT VENTRICULAR FUNCTION

### Right Heart Failure

A clinical syndrome that reduces the ability to propel blood to pulmonary circulation and may be accompanied by high systemic venous pressures as a result of an alteration of either the structure or function of the right heart circulatory system.

### Acute Right Ventricular Dysfunction

Acute occurrence of RV systolic dysfunction and dilatation as seen on transthoracic echocardiography (TTE). A rise in natriuretic peptides in the absence of LV or renal impairment, or RV strain patterns on electrocardiography (ECG).

**TABLE 1:** Common critical illnesses with RVD and RVF.

| | |
|---|---|
| ARDS | • Pulmonary hypertension and impaired RV perfusion<br>• Uncoupling of the RV from the pulmonary circulation and reduced RV output<br>• RV dysfunction occurs in 22–5,596 of patients with ARDS. RV dysfunction is also independently associated with mortality |
| Myocardial infarction | • Right coronary artery or LCx involvement leads to myocardial damage and an acute decrease in function<br>• Decrease in contractility |
| Pulmonary embolism | Acutely increased RV afterload |
| Pulmonary hypertension | • Remodeling of the pulmonary vasculature and hypoxic vasoconstriction of small pulmonary vessels results in a steady increase in pulmonary vascular resistance<br>• Increased afterload and disruption of neuroendocrine and autocrine signals leading to cardiomyocyte loss, myocardial ischemia, and remodeling |
| With LVAD | The RV has to work harder to match the increased LV output which leads to an effective increase in preload |
| COPD | • Cor pulmonale<br>• Increase in RV afterload due to changes in pulmonary vascular structure and mechanics, and lung hyperinflation |

(ARDS: acute respiratory distress syndrome; COPD: chronic obstructive pulmonary disease; LCx: left circumflex; LV: left ventricle; LVAD: left ventricular assist device; RV: right ventricle; RVD: right ventricular dysfunction; RVF: right ventricular failure)

**TABLE 2:** Comparison in right ventricle to left ventricle.

| | *RV* | *LV* |
|---|---|---|
| Shape | Crescent | Ellipsoidal |
| Structure | 2 layers | 3 layers |
| Free wall thickness | 2–5 mm | 8–10 mm |
| Circulation | Low pressure low resistance | High pressure high resistance |
| Stroke volume | 70–90 mL | 70–90 mL |
| EF | 65% | 70–80% |
| Ventricular pressure diastole | 0–8 mm Hg | 4–12 mm Hg |
| Ventricular pressure systole | 15–30 mm Hg | 90–140 mm Hg |
| Afterload | PVR <250 dynes/s/cm$^{-5}$ | SVR 800–1200 dynes/s/cm$^{-5}$ |
| Adaptation | Tolerant to preload | Tolerant to afterload |

(EF: ejection fraction; LV: left ventricle; PVR: pulmonary vascular resistance; RV: right ventricle; SVR: systemic venous return)

## Acute Right Ventricular Failure

Acute RVD with low cardiac output (CO) and hypoperfusion resulting in multiorgan dysfunction or failure. RVF is a result of the failure of the RV to provide enough blood flow to the pulmonary circulation to accomplish adequate LV filling.

## Volume and Pressure Overload

- *RV free wall thickness:* <5 mm at end-diastole if >5 mm, hypertrophy
- >1 cm—severe hypertrophy.
- *Easy assessment:* Cardiac apex
- *LV usually forms apex*: RV is two-thirds of LV in length

- RV, if it forms the apex, dilated RV
- The end-diastolic area (EDA) of RV is <60% of LV.
- If 60–100%, mild RV dilatation, >100%, severe dilatation
- Shape of RV changes from triangular to circular, when dilated
- Septum—convex toward RV
- RV hypertrophy, a center of mass shifts, and interventricular septum (IVS) is flattened
- RV mass >LV, septum bulges into LV—paradoxical.
- RV systolic pressures can be estimated as right atrial pressure (RAP) + maximal tricuspid regurgitation velocity (TR Vmax).

## ECHOCARDIOGRAPHIC ASSESSMENT: VARIOUS TECHNIQUES (TABLE 3)

- Tricuspid annular plane systolic excursion (TAPSE)
- Fractional area change (FAC)
- S' velocity
- Tei index
- Hepatic venous Doppler
- Two-dimensional (2D) speckle tracking
- Three-dimensional (3D) ejection fraction
    - Normally, RV area or LV area is <0.6 and RV length is <0.6 LV length.
    - The dilatation of RV can be graded as:
        - *Mild:* RV area/LV area = 0.6
        - *Moderate:* RV area /LV area = 1.0
        - *Severe:* RV area/LV area >1.0.

### Causes of Right Ventricular Dilatation and Dysfunction

- Pulmonary artery hypertension
- Coronary artery disease
- Tricuspid or pulmonary regurgitation
- Atrial or ventricular septal defect
- Dilated cardiomyopathy (idiopathic, chemotherapy-induced, pregnancy-induced, etc.)

*The goal of echocardiography:*

- To find whether RVD is present or not
- If present, whether it is acute or chronic
- To assess whether RV is coupled to pulmonary artery circulation or not.

The sections enumerated further will discuss each parameter, how to obtain it, and pitfalls of each one.

**TABLE 3:** RV: Assessment.

| *RV structural parameters* | *RV functional parameters* | *RV afterload assessment* |
|---|---|---|
| Basal RV diameter >42 mm | RV fractional area change ≥35% | Acct <100 milliseconds |
| RV mid diastole diameter >33 mm | MPI >0.43 (PW); >0.54 (TDI) | • Shape of RVOT Doppler envelope<br>• No notch/late/midsystolic |
| RV EDD/LV EDD >0.9 | TAPSE <16 mm | |
| RV/LV EDA >0.6 | S' velocity <10 cm/s | |
| LV eccentricity index >1 | | |
| McConnell's sign | | |
| RV-free wall thickness >5 mm | | |

(EDA: end-diastolic area; EDD: end-diastolic diameter; LV: left ventricle; MPI: myocardial performance index; RV: right ventricle; RVOT: right ventricular outflow tract; TAPSE: tricuspid annular plane systolic excursion; TDI: tissue Doppler imaging)

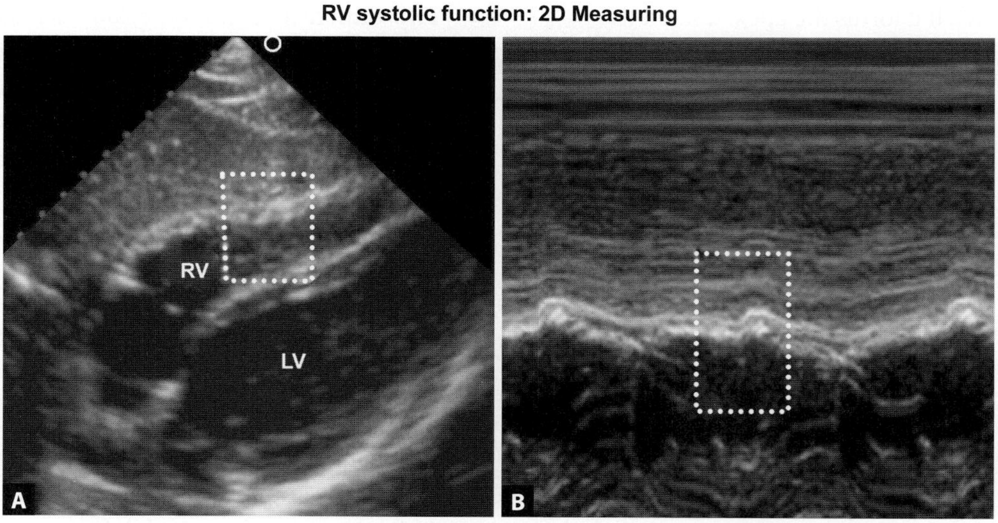


**Figs. 1A and B:** Normal range for RV wall thickness <0.5 cm.

## RIGHT VENTRICULAR FREE WALL THICKNESS (FIGS. 1A AND B)

### Echocardiography Views

Subxiphoid long-axis (SXLA) or parasternal long-axis (PLAX) views.

### Steps

- Acquire a SXLA (preferred) or PLAX view.
- Decrease the imaging depth to have a free wall in the center of the screen.
  - Free wall should be oriented horizontally
- Freeze the B-mode image. Measure in end-diastole [SXLA and PLAX, this corresponds to when the tricuspid valve (TV) and mitral valve have only just closed, respectively]. Exclude trabeculae, papillary muscles, and epicardial fat.
  - SXLA, measure below the tricuspid annulus (i.e., toward the right ventricular apex) at the same distance to where the anterior tricuspid leaflet tip would open in diastole.
  - PLAX, measure at or below the anterior mitral leaflet tip (i.e., toward the left ventricular apex) at a level where the interventricular septum, mitral valve, and posterior left ventricular wall are seen.
- ≤5 mm suggests acute right ventricular dysfunction.
- >5 mm suggests chronic RVD.

## TRICUSPID REGURGITATION PRESSURE GRADIENT

### Echocardiography Views

Parasternal short axis view (PSAX) [at aortic valve (AV) level, A4C, SXLA, and subxiphoid short-axis (SXSA) (at AV level)].

### Steps

- Assess for TR using the color Doppler in the above views.
  - In these views, the transmitter's emitted sound waves are oriented roughly parallel (i.e., 0° angle) to TR flow, which produces the maximal shift in Doppler frequency (cos 0° = 1).
  - For the highest frame rate and image resolution, imaging depth should be

decreased to the minimum required for visualization of the TV and RA. The color Doppler box should only encompass those structures.

- Align the continuous wave Doppler (CWD) beam in the same direction as the TR jet. Place the beam focus within the center of the jet.
  - To avoid underestimation of Doppler frequency, the angle θ between the CWD beam and TR flow should ideally be 0° (i.e., parallel to one another) but is recommended to lie within 20°.
- Press the CWD button again.
  - Use sufficiently high sweep speed (~100 mm/s) to stretch out the waveforms and thereby better discriminate true velocities from sonographic artifacts.
  - Adjust the y-axis scale and baseline so that the waveform takes up as much of the screen as possible without aliasing. This provides for the most precise velocity determinations.
  - To avoid overestimation of TR Vmax, decrease Doppler gain to minimize spectral noise.
- Freeze the frame. Place the cursor at the outer edge of the largest trough to obtain TR Vmax from that particular echocardiographic view.
  - For patients with atrial fibrillation, use the third beat after two consecutive equally-spaced heartbeats, or take the average from at least five heartbeats.

## Pearls and Pitfalls

- Use only when indicated as tricuspid regurgitation peak gradient (TRPG) <46 mm Hg could be seen in normal patients.
- TRPG depends not only on resistance of the pulmonary circulation but also on pulmonary flow and left atrial pressure.
  - High-output (e.g., pregnancy and anemia) or high-volume states (e.g., pulmonary edema), or those with increased pulmonary venous and left atrial pressures (e.g. CHF or mitral valvulopathies), may show elevated TRPG despite low pulmonary vascular resistance (PVR). Moreover, hypoxia from acute respiratory illness leads to pulmonary vasoconstriction and increased PVR, which also increases TRPG.
- In severe RVF, there may not be sufficient systolic force to generate a TR jet. Any measurable TRPG will not reflect the severity of RVD even if PVR is high.
- With severe TR, earlier equalization of right ventricular and atrial pressures in systole results in rapid deceleration of the spectral waveform, which leads to underestimation of TRPG.
- From a technical perspective, an eccentric TR jet (i.e., directed toward the RA's medial or lateral wall) will appear smaller using the color Doppler than a central jet of equal or lower severity (the Coanda effect).
- TR Doppler technique cannot be applied in cases of right ventricular outflow tract (RVOT) obstruction or pulmonary stenosis (which is mostly associated with congenital heart disease). In such cases, the TRPG obtained would reflect blood flow trying to pass through the obstructed RVOT or stenotic pulmonary valve (PV), respectively, and not through the pulmonary atresia (PA) as desired.

## Interpretation

- ≤46 mm Hg (TR Vmax ≤3.4 m/s) suggests acute RVD
- >46 mm Hg (TR Vmax >3.4 m/s) suggests chronic RVD

American Society of Echocardiography (ASE) guidelines prefer using pulmonary artery systolic pressure (PASP) instead of TRPG to evaluate for right ventricular dysfunction. PASP is obtained by adding the estimated RAP to the TRPG (i.e., PASP = 4 × TR Vmax 2 + RAP). In contrast, the 2022 European Society of Cardiology (ESC)/ European Respiratory Society (ERS) and British Society of Echocardiography (BSE) guidelines prefer using TRPG, while omitting RAP due to inaccuracies in its estimation from inferior vena cava (IVC) diameter and respirophasic collapsibility.

## PULMONARY ARTERY ACCELERATION TIME

### Echocardiography View

Parasternal short axis view or SXSA view at AV level for simultaneous visualization of RVOT, PV, and PA.

### Steps

- Acquire a PSAX or SXSA view at the AV level for simultaneous visualization of RVOT, PV, and PA.
    - Depth should be decreased to the minimum required for visualization of these structures.
- Place the pulsed-wave Doppler (PWD) sampling gate in the RVOT 0.5–1.0 cm proximal to the PV's insertion points. Align the beam roughly in the same direction as blood flow.
- Press the PWD button again. The PA systolic ejection waveform appears as a downward deflection on the y-axis.
- Freeze the frame. Use calipers to measure the time interval on the x-axis from the onset of PA systolic ejection to peak velocity [i.e., pulmonary artery acceleration time (PAAT)].

### Pearls and Pitfalls

Precise angulation of the PWD beam is not required for obtaining PAAT. Even if the angle between the beam and the direction of blood flow lies within reasonable deviation from 0°, the shape of the PA systolic ejection waveform will remain the same.

### Interpretation

- ≤60–80 m-sec suggests acute right ventricular dysfunction.
- <105 m-sec suggests chronic right ventricular dysfunction.

The 2022 ESC/ERS and BSE guidelines suggest that PAAT <105 milliseconds increases the probability of pulmonary hypertension (PH) being present.

## 60/60 SIGN

### Steps

- TRPG is obtained from TRVmax
- PAAT is obtained from the PA systolic ejection waveform

### Pearls and Pitfalls

A common misconception is that the 60/60 sign incorporates PASP ≤60 mm Hg, rather than TRPG ≤60 mm Hg as the original studies intended.

### Interpretation

TRPFG <60 mm Hg and PAAT <60 m-sec suggests acute right ventricular dysfunction.

## PULMONARY ARTERY EARLY-SYSTOLIC NOTCHING

Suggests a proximally located, higher-risk PE.

Pulmonary venous congestion alone (without elevated PVR) no mid systolic notching. In PE, the reflection site is located even closer to the RVOT, because of earlier notching on the PA systolic ejection waveform. Therefore, whereas MSN (i.e., in the second half of the waveform) can occur with both proximal PA obstruction (i.e., PE) and peripheral pulmonary obstruction (i.e., PH), "early-systolic notching" (ESN) (i.e., in the first half) is more likely in proximally located, higher-risk PEs.

### Steps

- Generate the PA systolic ejection waveform.
- Evaluate for the presence of ESN.

### Pearls and Pitfalls

Pulmonary valve's opening click on the PA systolic ejection waveform can be a false-positive for ESN.

## McCONNELL'S SIGN

Suggests acute right ventricular dysfunction.

McConnell's sign refers to diffuse hypokinesis of the RV with intact (or "spared") apical systolic contraction. McConnell's sign was 22–29% sensitive and 97–99% specific for PE. Sensitivity rises with proximally located, higher-risk PEs.

### Steps

- Acquire an RV-focused apical four-chamber (A4C) view in which the RA and RV are well visualized.
- Qualitatively assess for McConnell's sign.

### Pearls and Pitfalls

McConnell's sign may also be caused by right ventricular infarction. This supports the proposed mechanism that free wall hypokinesis is caused by reduced right coronary artery (RCA) perfusion.

## RIGHT ATRIAL ENLARGEMENT

### Steps

- Acquire an RV-focused A4C view in which the RA and RV are well visualized.
- Qualitatively assess if the RA appears as large as the LA. Also look for interatrial septal bowing into the LA, particularly at end-systole.
- The right aortic arch (RAA) can also be obtained and compared to the upper limit of normal (i.e., 18 $cm^2$).
  - Trace the RA's blood-tissue interface along the tricuspid annular plane, interatrial septum, superior wall, and lateral wall. Exclude the triangular space between tricuspid leaflet tips and tricuspid annulus, as well as the IVC, superior vena cava, and right atrial appendage.

### Pearls and Pitfalls

The accuracy of linear dimensions is limited by measurements arising from only a single dimension. RAA values are limited by the assumption of a symmetric cavity shape.

*Interpretation:*

- Equal to left atrial size suggests acute right ventricular dysfunction.
- Greater than left atrial size suggests chronic right ventricular dysfunction.

## TAPSE AND TRICUSPID LATERAL SYSTOLIC VELOCITY (S' WAVE) (FIG. 2 AND TABLE 4)

### Echocardiography View: Apical Four-chamber View

Apical four-chamber view (tissue Doppler) in the M mode, the cursor of the echo probe is placed at the lateral annulus of the TV and the excursion of the annulus is measured in the systole. The TAPSE has been correlated with the EF of RV.

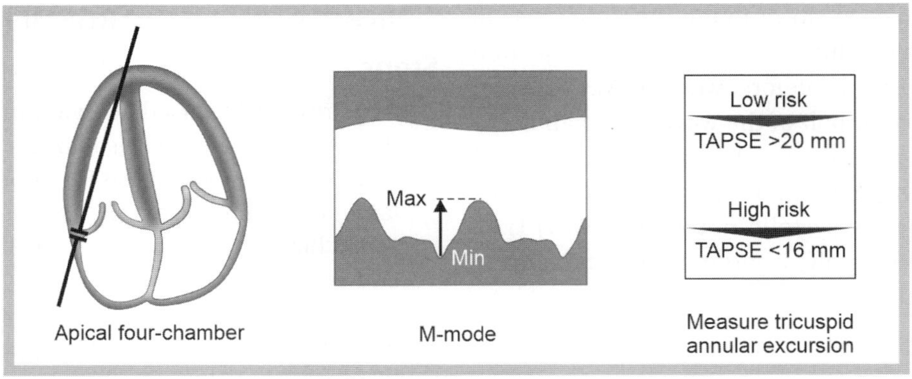


**Fig. 2:** RV systolic function: TAPSE.

**TABLE 4:** Relation between TAPSE and RVEF.

| *TAPSE (mm)* | *RVEF (%)* |
|---|---|
| 20 | 40 |
| 15 | 30 |
| 10 | 20 |
| 5 | 10 |

(RVFF: right ventricular ejection fraction; TAPSE: tricuspid annular plane systolic excursion)

Right ventricular ejection fraction = 2 × TAPSE

Normal right ventricular ejection fraction (RVEF) = 40%.

## Pearls and Pitfalls

- It is angle dependent.
- It evaluates the longitudinal shortening and not the global systolic function of the RV.

## S' Velocity

An S' wave value <9.5 cm/s reflects RV systolic dysfunction.

- Modified 2D TAPSE, deep transgastric (dTG) M-mode TAPSE, and TG M-mode TAPSE.
- Anatomical M-mode gives better alignment
- The septal attachment of the TV is fixed.
- Majority of motion—lateral annulus
- TAPSE measures the systolic excursion.
- After pericardiotomy, the anchor for this movement is lost. Hence, TAPSE becomes less reliable.
- Normal is 20–25 mm. <15—severely depressed

# RIGHT VENTRICULAR MYOCARDIAL PERFORMANCE INDEX

## Echocardiography View

### *Right Ventricular-focused Apical Four-chamber View*

The RV myocardial performance index, also known as the right Tei index, is a measure of both systolic and diastolic RV function. Calculated by dividing the total isovolumic time (isovolumic contraction plus isovolumic relaxation) by the ejection time (ET).

Myocardial performance index

$$= \frac{\text{Isovolumic contraction time (IVCT)} + \text{Isovolumic relaxation time (IVRT)}}{\text{ET}}$$

$$= \frac{\text{TV opening to closure time} - \text{Ejection time}}{\text{Ejection time}}$$

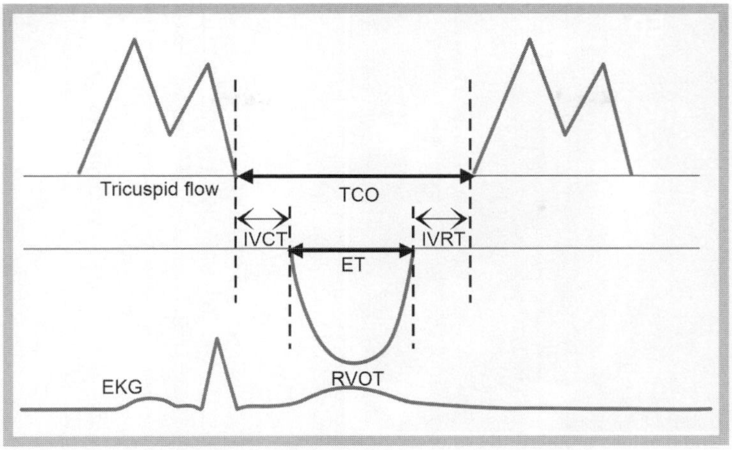


**Fig. 3:** Myocardial performance index (TEI index).

## Normal Myocardial Performance Index for Right Ventricular (Fig. 3)

- Pulse wave Doppler <0.4
- Tissue Doppler <0.55

## Pearls and Pitfalls

- It bypasses the limitations of the complex RV geometry, as it is only derived from time intervals and makes use of no assumption of RV shape.
- It is unreliable in patients with elevated RAP, and irregular rhythms make myocardial performance index (MPI) difficult to calculate.

## Interpretation

Right ventricle MPI are >0.43 using pulsed Doppler and >0.54 using tissue Doppler abnormal.

# RIGHT VENTRICULAR FRACTIONAL AREA CHANGE

## Echocardiography View (Figs. 4A and B)

Right ventricle-focused A4C- laterally displacing and rotating the probe from the standard A4C view until the maximal RV basal and longitudinal diameters are obtained.

Normal >32%
Mild dysfunction 25–31%
Moderate 18–24%
Severe <17%

## Steps

- Manually tracing the endocardial border of the RV in end-diastole and end-systole.
- Calculated as: (End-diastolic area – end-systolic area)/end-diastolic area × 100%.

## Pearls and Pitfalls

- RV FAC reflects both the longitudinal and radial shortening of the RV, but it neglects the contraction of the outflow tract.
- It is load-dependent and potentially difficult to acquire in the case of poor endocardial definition.

## Interpretation

An RV FAC <35% reflects RV dysfunction.

# STRAIN, STRAIN RATE, AND SPECKLE TRACKING (FIGS. 5A TO D)

- Strain is the measurement of myocardial fiber shortening

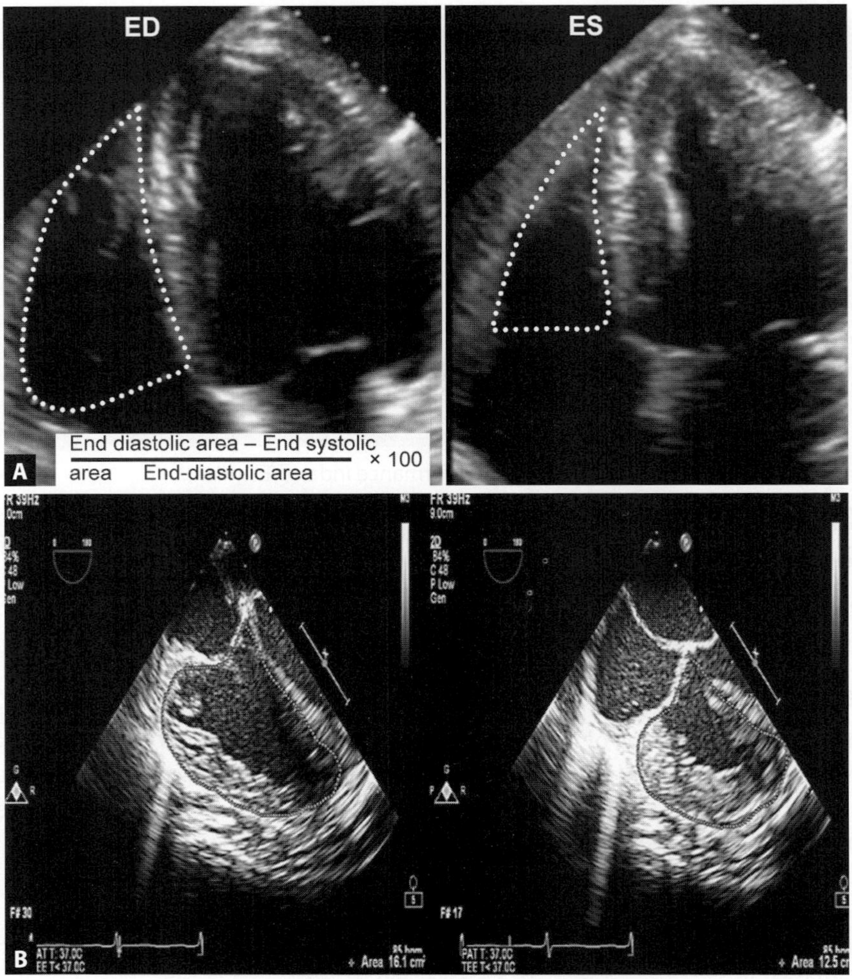


**Figs. 4A and B:** Echocardiography View.
*Note:* RV FAC correlates well with RV ejection fraction.

- Strain rate (SR) is the speed of deformation.
- Strain rate is calculated by measuring myocardial velocities in two regions and dividing the difference by distance (velocity gradient)

$$SR = \frac{Va - Vb}{d}$$

- Speckle tracking—allows myocardial velocity measurement by tracking B-mode speckles.
- B Mode speckles are the naturally occurring acoustic markers within grayscale imaging.
- Longitudinal and circumferential strain—myocardial shortening
  - Negative waveforms in systole
  - Positive waveforms in diastole
- The steeper the strain curve, the larger the strain rate value.
- Impaired function—lowers strain and strain rate.

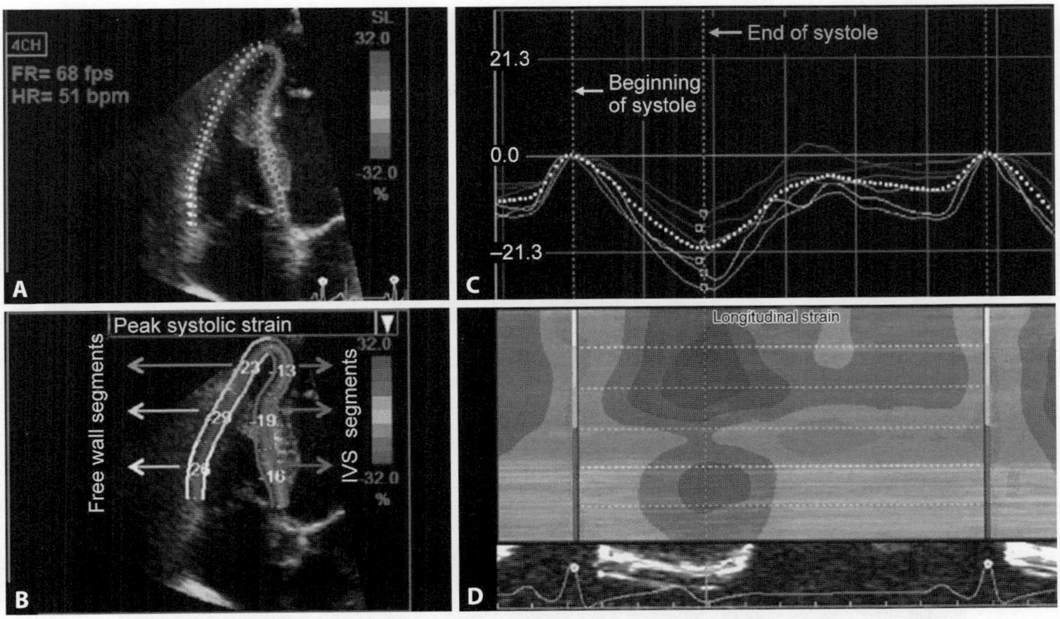


**Figs. 5A to D:** Strain, strain rate, and speckle tracking.

## Hepatic Venous Flow (Figs. 6A to C)

- AR wave—negative wave during RA contraction
- S wave—RA filling from SVC and IVC (TV motion, RA relaxation, and TR)
- V wave—negative at end-systole (RA-RV compliance)
- D wave—RA acts as a passive conduit for RV filling

## Right Ventricular Diastolic Function

- Doppler evaluation of transtricuspid flow velocities.
- Unlike LV, significantly affected by respiration and the larger size of TV
- Spontaneous breath augments RV diastolic filling by 20% during inspiration.
- Similar to LV
- E/A wave <0.8 and >2 are abnormal.

## Right Ventricular Failure

### *Cardiac Conditions*

- Coronary artery disease (RV infarction)
- Valvular heart disease
- Cardiomyopathy (ischemic and dilatative)
- Heart surgery (CABG, AVR, and MVR)
- Heart transplantation
- Post-left ventricular assist device (post-LVAD)

### *Extracardiac Conditions*

- Pulmonary embolism
- Lung disease [chronic obstructive pulmonary disease (COPD) and acute respiratory distress syndrome (ARDS)]
- Primary PH
- Sepsis
- Lung transplantation
- Post-thromboendarterectomy

***Note:* RVF rarely occurs in the setting of normal PVR!**

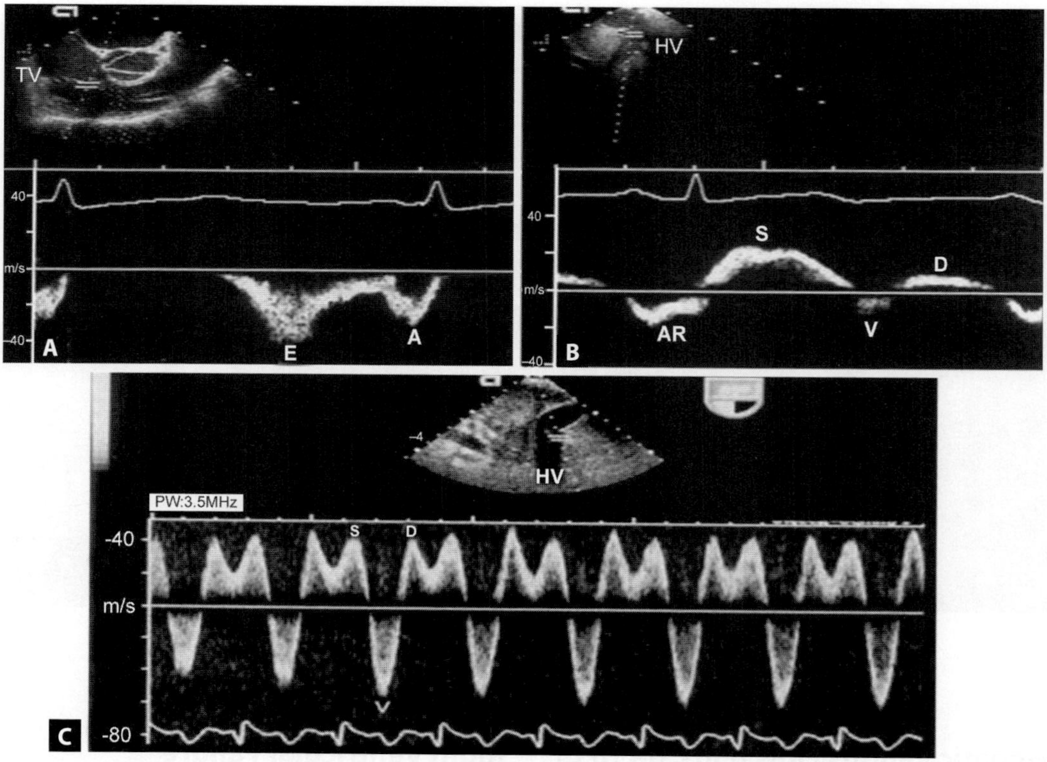


**Figs. 6A to C:** (A) Normal transtricuspid Doppler flow velocity profile; (B) Normal hepatic venous Doppler flow velocity profiles; and (C) Prominent hepatic flow reversal at end-systole (V) in a patient with decreased right ventricular compliance. (A: late diastolic velocity; AR: atrial contraction flow reversal; (D) antegrade flow during right ventricular filling; E: early diastolic velocity; HV: hepatic vein; S: antegrade early systolic flow; TV: tricuspid valve)

## Right Ventricular Dysfunction in Acute Pulmonary Embolism

- Echo RVD is present in 30–56% of normotensive patients with PE.
- All-cause 30-day mortality rate is 5.4–10%, and in-hospital mortality rate directly attributed to PE was 1.1–3.3%
- Cardiogenic shock occurs in ~5% of acute PE cases with a 90-day mortality rate of >50%.
- RV cannot acutely overcome a systolic pulmonary artery pressure (PAP) >50 mm Hg.
- Conversely, acute-on-chronic RVF can tolerate significantly higher PAP.

## Right Ventricular Dysfunction in Acute Respiratory Distress Syndrome

- Mechanisms of ARDS-induced acute RVD include hypoxic/hypercarbic vasoconstriction, an increased alveolar dead space, pulmonary microthrombi, and proinflammatory cytokine activation.
- Both PH and RV contractile impairment are the main factors involved in RVD. Four predictors of acute RVD in ARDS:
  1. Pneumonia-induced ARDS
  2. Partial pressure of oxygen ($PaO_2$)/$FiO_2$ ratio <150 mm Hg
  3. Partial pressure of carbon dioxide ($PaCO_2$) ≥48 mm Hg

4. Driving pressure (plateau pressure – total positive end-expiratory pressure) ≥18 $cmH_2O$.

## Right Ventricular Dysfunction in Right Ventricular Myocardial Infarction

- Right ventricular myocardial infarction (RVMI) can be complicated by acute RVD in 30–50% of patients with inferior wall ST-elevation MI.
- Severe hypotension and low CO are present in 10% on admission
- RV tolerates ischemic injury better than LV.
- The RCA usually is the culprit vessel in RVMI, and proximal RCA occlusions-more extensive RV myocardial necrosis.
- Acute outcome of patients with RVMI is primarily determined by the amount of accompanying LV necrosis.

## Right Ventricular Dysfunction in Pulmonary Arterial Hypertension

Echocardiographic evaluation of right ventricular function in pulmonary arterial hypertension **(Table 5 and Box 1)**.

# CLINICAL CASE SCENARIOS

## Case 1

A 45-year-old male diabetic and hypertensive controlled on medications, presented with shortness of breath and febrile illness. He deteriorated over 3 days and got intubated due to raised oxygen demands and is currently

**TABLE 5:** Echocardiographic evaluation of right ventricular function in pulmonary arterial hypertension.

| 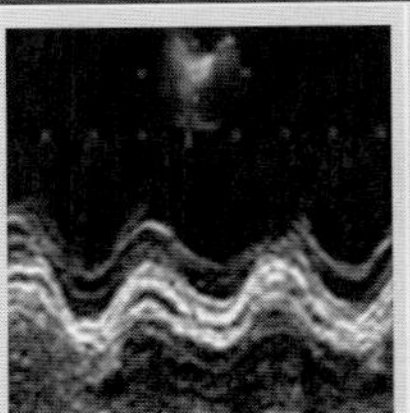 | 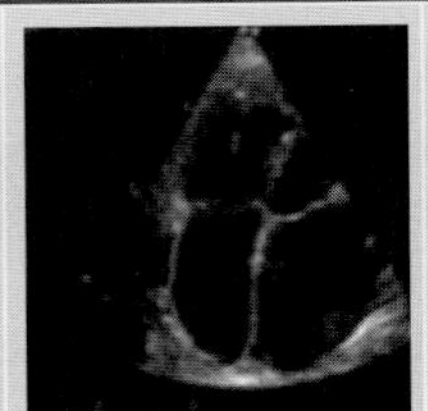 | 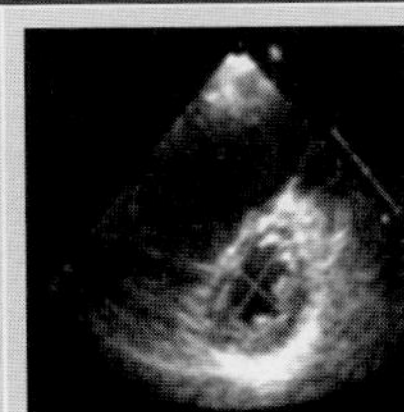 | 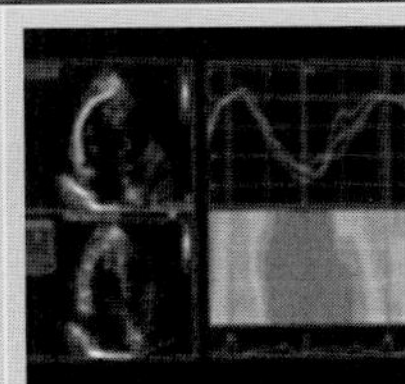 | 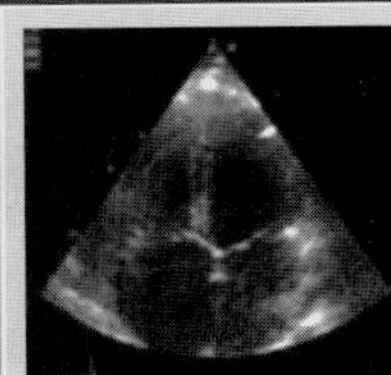 |
|---|---|---|---|---|
| ***TAPSE*** | ***RA area*** | ***Eccentricity index*** | ***RV LSS*** | ***RVFAC*** |
| Measures the right ventricular longitudinal shortening and is a surrogate of systolic function obtained using M-mode of the lateral tricuspid annulus from the 4CV. Systolic dysfunction is likely when TAPSE is <17 mm | Measured at end-systole, just prior to TV opening, in the 4CV. Values >18 $cm^2$ are considered abnormal | Defined as the anteroposterior diameter (green line) to the septolateral diameter (blue line). Normal values are <1.1 | • Images are obtained from the RV-focused apical view<br>• The endocardial border is traced and after manual adjustment of the wall thickness, the software automatically generates the averaged peak systolic strain | Obtained from the 4CV. Defined as *[(end-diastolic area – end-systolic area)/end-diastolic area] of × 100%.* Care must be taken to trace the free wall beneath the trabeculations. The lower reference value for normal RV systolic function is 35× |

(4CV: four chamber view; LSS: longitudinal shortening; LV: left ventricle; RA: right atrium; RV: right ventricle; RV FAC: right ventricular fractional area change; TAPSE: tricuspid annular plane systolic excursion)

**BOX 1:** Echo features of pulmonary arterial hypertension.

- Right atrial enlargement
- Right ventricular enlargement/dilatation—D-shaped LV on the short axis
- Right ventricular hypertrophy
- Significant tricuspid regurgitation—(TR jet estimated RVSP is $4V^2 + RAP$)
- Right ventricular dysfunction
- Pulmonary regurgitation—PR jet estimated mPAP and PAEDP
- Reduced RV outflow tract velocity, short acceleration time
- Dilated IVC not collapsing with respiration (if patient not ventilated)
- Patent foramen ovale (bubble contrast used)
- Pericardial effusion
- Dilated pulmonary arteries

(IVC: inferior vena cava; LV: left ventricle; mPAP: mean pulmonary arterial pressure; PAEDP: pulmonary artery end-diastolic pressure; PR: pulmonary regurgitation; RV: right ventricle; TR: tricuspid regurgitation)

on lung protective ventilation. Started having hemodynamic instability not responding to fluid and vasopressors. Worsening liver enzymes and worsening edema raise doubt about RV dysfunction **(Table 6)**.

**Q1. How will you proceed with TTE to rule out RV dysfunction?**

**Ans.**

*View needed:* RV-focused A4C, PSAX AV valve view, and PSAX MV view.

*Parameters needed:*

- RV dilation—RVEDA/LVEDA
- RV function impairment—TAPSE
- RV PA coupling—TAPSE/PASP ratio
- PA flow characteristics—PAAT, MSN, PAAT/RVET ratio

Acute respiratory distress syndrome has several reasons to have RV failure including—MV, high peep, hypoxemia, hypercarbia, sepsis, and left heart failure preexisting or due to sepsis-induced **(Table 7)**.

**TABLE 6:** Mechanisms and targeted management in specific clinical scenarios of acute RV failure.

| *Clinical scenario* | *Mechanism* | *Treatment* |
|---|---|---|
| Right ventricular infarct | Decreased RV contractility | Early myocardial reperfusion (percutaneous coronary intervention and systemic thrombolysis) |
| Pulmonary embolism | Increase RV afterload (mechanical obstruction and vasoconstriction) | • Systemic anticoagulation, systemic or catheter-directed thrombolysis, embolectomy<br>• Parenteral prostanoids (with or without inhaled pulmonary vasodilators |
| Decompensated PAH | Increase RV afterload | |
| ARDS | Increasing RV afterload/decreasing RV contractility | Limiting Vt and PEEP, avoiding hypoxia, hypercapnia, and acidosis |
| Noncardiac surgery | Acute PH, decreasing RV contractility (RV infarct) | Pulmonary vasodilators, myocardial reperfusion, inotropic drugs |
| Cardiac surgery | Volume overload, myocardial ischemia, preexisting RVD, and arrhythmias | Diuretics, inotropic drugs, cardioversion, antiarrhythmic drugs |

(ARDS: acute respiratory distress syndrome; PAH: pulmonary arterial hypertension; PEEP: positive end-expiratory pressure; RVD: right ventricular dysfunction; Vt: tidal volume)

**TABLE 7:** Echocardiographic evaluation of RV dysfunction.

| | | |
|---|---|---|
| Pericardial fluid >5 mm in diastole<br>Pericardial effusion<br>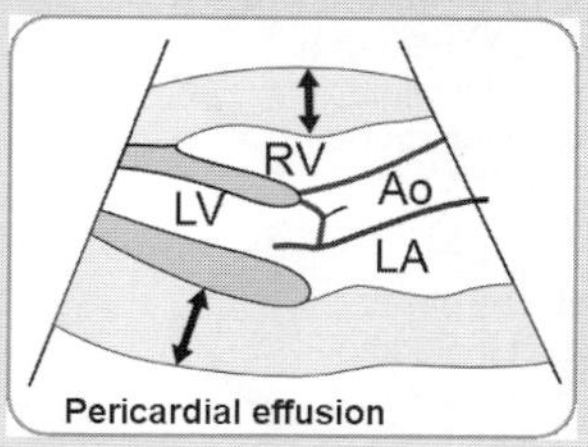<br> | RV wall thickness >5 mm<br>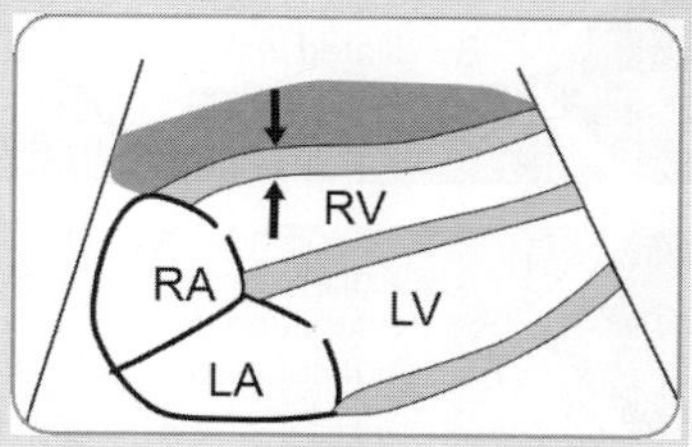<br> | Inferior vena cava diameter >21 mm, inspiration collapse <50% suggests high RA pressure<br>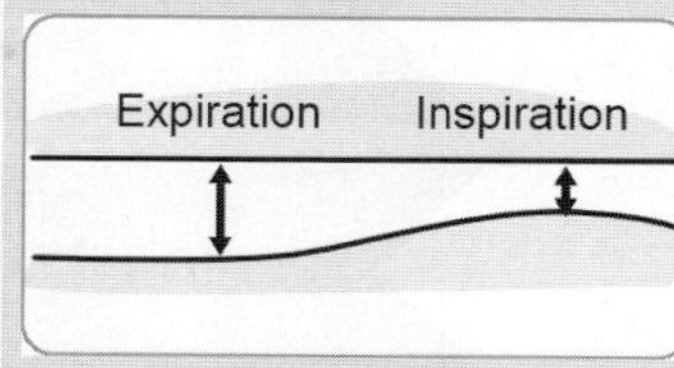<br> |
| Tricuspid regurgitation peak systolic velocity of TR >2.8 m/s<br>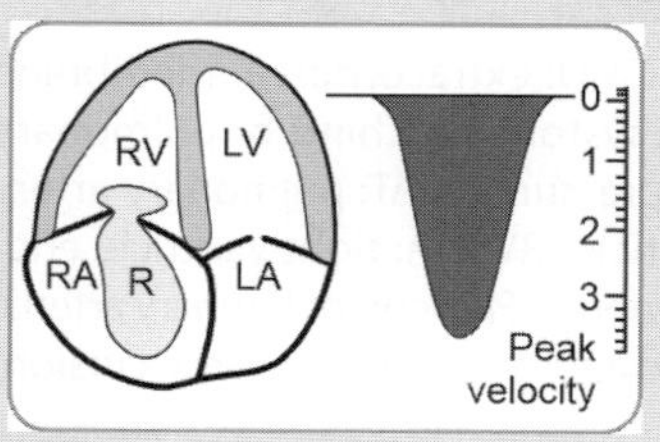<br> | Tricuspid annular plane systolic excursion TAPSE <17 mm<br>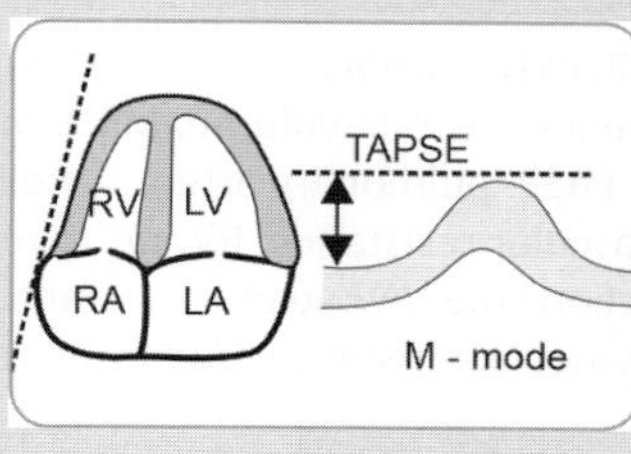<br> | • RV dilation<br>• RV EDD/LV EDD >1.0<br>• RV basal diameter >41 mm<br>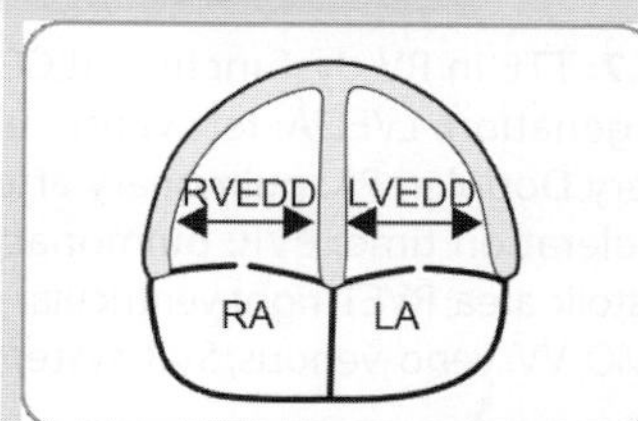<br> |
| RV fractional area change, FAC <35%<br>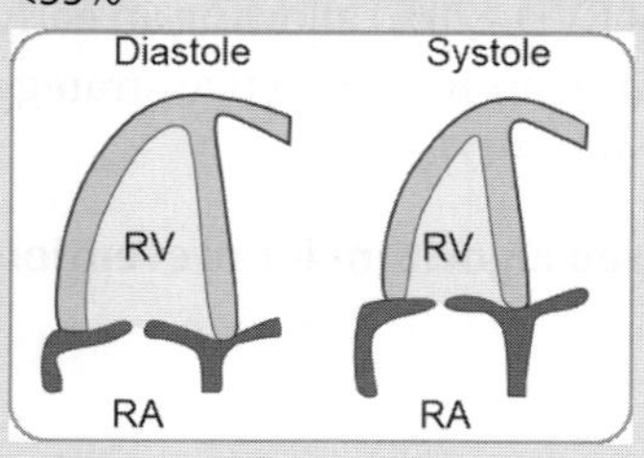<br> | Ventricular interdependence: Septal shift, D-shaped LV<br>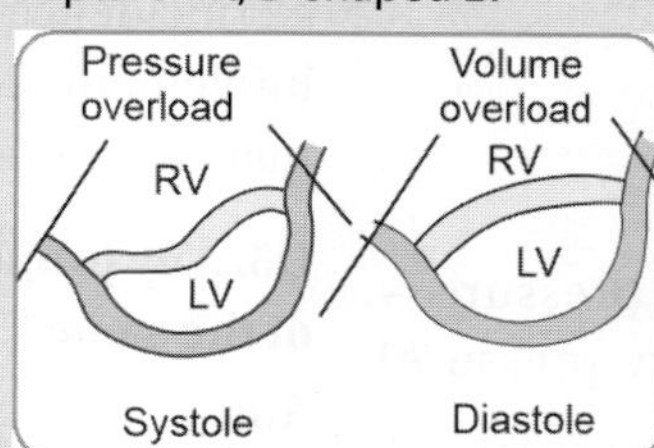<br> | Systolic S′ velocity of tricuspid annulus <9.5 cm/s by DTI<br>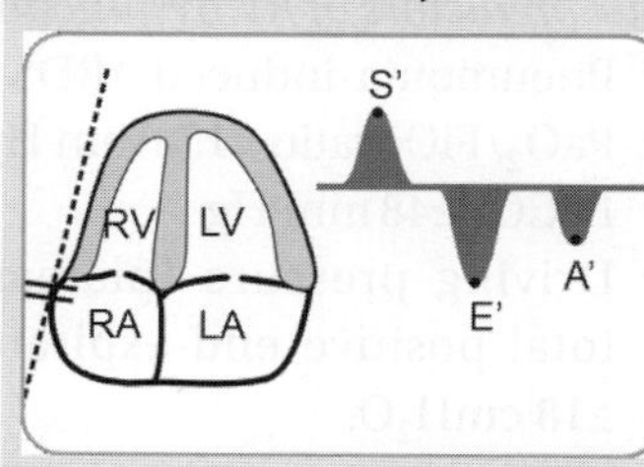<br> |
| Longitudinal strain of RV-free wall <20%<br>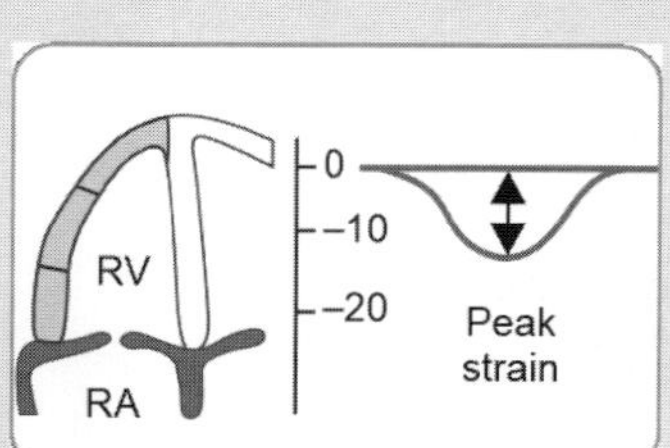<br> | Right ventricular index of myocardial performance, RI MP >0.54 by DTI<br>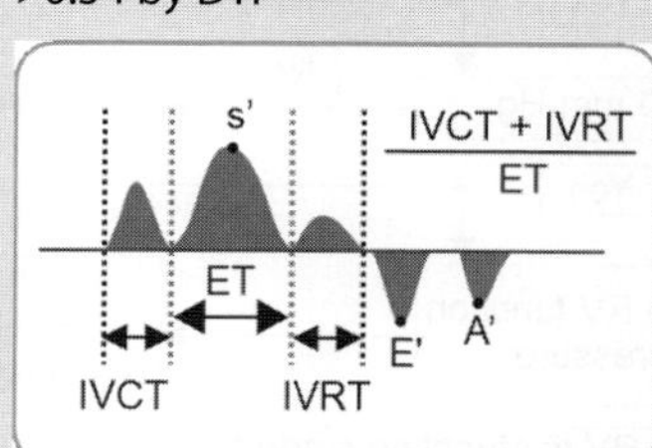<br> | 3D RV ejection fraction <45%<br>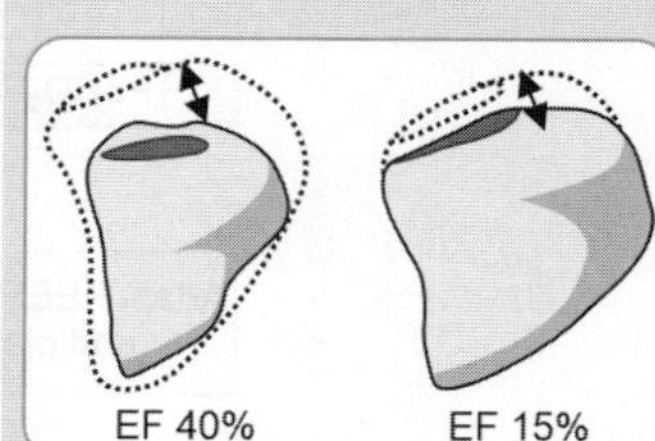<br> |

(DTI: Doppler tissue imaging; FAC: fractional area change; LV: left ventricle; LV EDD: left ventricular end-diastolic diameter; RA: right atrium; RV: right ventricle; RV EDD: right ventricular end-diastolic diameter; TAPSE: tricuspid annular plane systolic excursion; 3D: three dimensional)

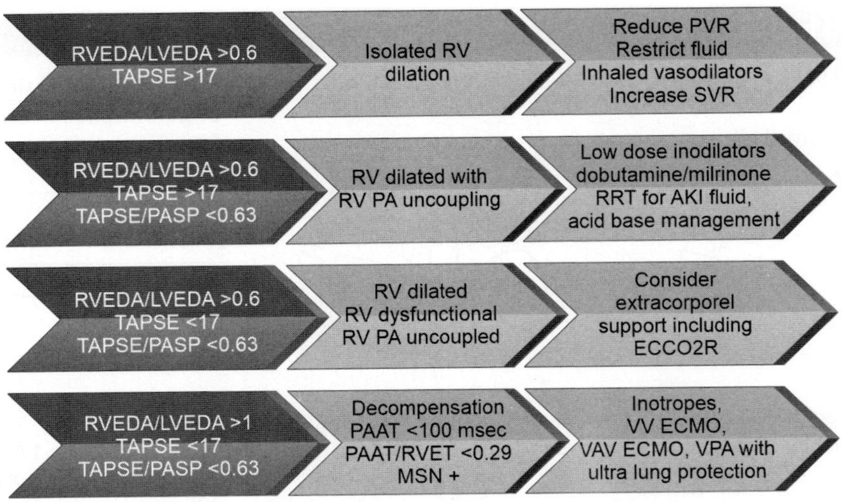


**Fig.7:** TTE in RV dysfunction. (ECCO2R: extracorporeal $CO_2$ removal; ECMO: extracorporeal membrane oxygenation; LVEDA: left ventricular end-diastolic volume; MSN: mid systolic notching of pulmonary artery Doppler; PA: pulmonary artery; PASP: pulmonary artery systolic pressure; PAAT: pulmonary artery acceleration time; PVR: pulmonary vascular resistance; RV: right ventricle; RVEDA: right ventricle end-diastolic area; RVET: right ventricular ejection time; VAV: veno-arterial and venous; VPA: veno pulmonary arterial ECMO; VV: veno-venous; SVR: systemic vascular resistance; TAPSE: tricuspid annular plane systolic excursion)

**Q2. Can we predict RVD or failure in ARDS?**

**Ans.**

*Four predictors of RV dysfunction:*

1. Pneumonia-induced ARDS
2. $PaO_2/FiO_2$ ratio <150 mm Hg
3. $PaCO_2$ ≥48 mm Hg
4. Driving pressure (plateau pressure – total positive end-expiratory pressure) ≥18 $cmH_2O$.

Routine echocardiography is recommended in all ARDS patients with a score ≥2 (incidence of RVD ≥20%) allowing an early implementation of an RV-protective strategy that might prevent RVD)

**Q3. Any proposed algorithm for prevention of the same?**

**Ans.**

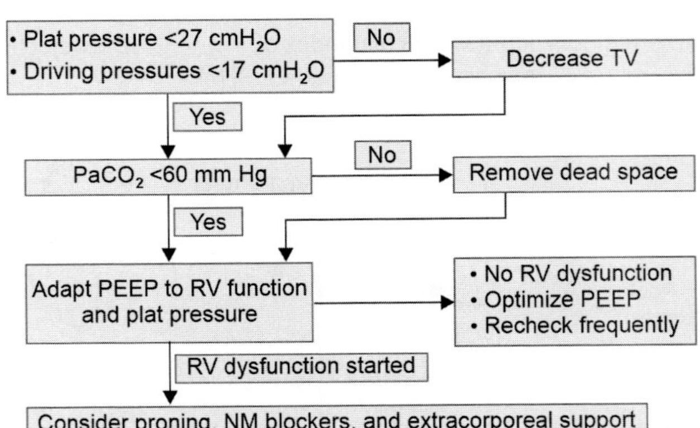


(LV: left ventricle; NM: neuromuscular blockers; PEEP: positive end-expiratory pressure; RV: right ventricle; TV: tricuspid valve)

## Case 2

A 65-year-old male, a chronic smoker with a family history of dyslipidemia, presented to the emergency department with mild chest discomfort, and signs of peripheral hypo perfusion. After stabilization started on vasopressors, ECG showed some ST elevation in V1, high-sensitivity troponin I (hsTrop I) was unremarkable at this point, you suspect RVMI.

**Q1. How TTE 2D echo will help in diagnosing infarction?**

**Ans.**

Right ventricle infarction can present as an isolated event or in the presence of left ventricle involvement.

| *RV involvement* | *Prevalence* | *Infarct related artery* | *Clinical course* | *Prognosis* |
|---|---|---|---|---|
| Inferior MI | • Inferoposterior MI up to 50%<br>• Anterior MI <10% | RCA (LCX) | Return to baseline in weeks to month | Benign |
| Predominant LV shock | • Inferoposterior MI 34%<br>• Posterior MI 17% | • RCA 28%<br>• LCX 14% | 1-year mort RCA 32% LCX 67% | Inferior is better than anterior |
| Predominant RV shock | 5% of all cardiogenic shock | RCA 96% | In hospital mortality 53% | Similar to LV shock |

(LCX: left circumflex; LV: left ventricle; MI: myocardial infarction; RCA: right coronary artery; RV: right ventricle)

Clinical suspicion with clear lung fields, shock without a clear-cut rise in cardiac enzymes, and borderline ECG, echo can give us clues behind the etiology of shock. Although the geometry of RV makes echocardiography less reliable for RV infarction but when clinical conditions clubbed with ECG with echo findings can save time to wait for the rise in cardiac enzymes to rise and get targeted treatment.

Interestingly, the RV appears to behave differently in response to myocardial ischemia compared to the LV with a higher chance of recovery. Several features suggest that RVD due to RVMI is more commonly mediated by ischemic stunning of viable myocardium rather than overt infarction with irreversible myocardial necrosis:

- Reduced myocardial demand of RV due to less stroke work
- Systodiastolic coronary perfusion
- Collaterals from the left coronary system
- Increased coronary flow and decreased myocardial oxygen consumption due to nitric oxide during hypoperfusion

Infarction causes pump failure without change in afterload conditions unless LV is involved and decreased contractility reduces the RV output subsequently leading to LV preload and output without intrinsic decrease in LV function.

*Views needed:* RV-focused A4C and PSAX MV view

*Findings:*

- RV-free wall regional wall motion abnormality
- TAPSE <17 mm
- Reduced FAC, dilation of RV
- Displacement/hypokinesia interventricular septum
- Dilated IVC

*Caution:*

- RV cannot be completely visualized in any single 2D echocardiographic view.
- Echocardiographic abnormalities can be temporary and resolve within a few hours.

- Therefore, information from all available acoustic windows is necessary for the complete assessment of the RV.

**Q2. Management goals and how echo at bedside can guide for volume resuscitation?**

**Ans.**

| | |
|---|---|
| Early recognition | ST elevation in II, III, aVF, right precordial leads and clinical signs of right heart failure (excluding papillary muscle or septal rupture, tamponade), 2D ECHO |
| Early reperfusion | Primary angioplasty, thrombolysis |
| Adequate RV preload | Volume maintenance |
| Reduction of RV afterload | Inotropes, balloon counterpulsation |
| Preservation of RV synchrony | Atrioventricular block/bradycardia |
| Avoid | Vasodilators, nitrates, morphine, beta blockers |

Volume resuscitation can be a double-edged sword while managing RV infarction. Understanding the pathophysiology of ventricular interdependence and echo findings can guide us when to stop further administration of fluid.

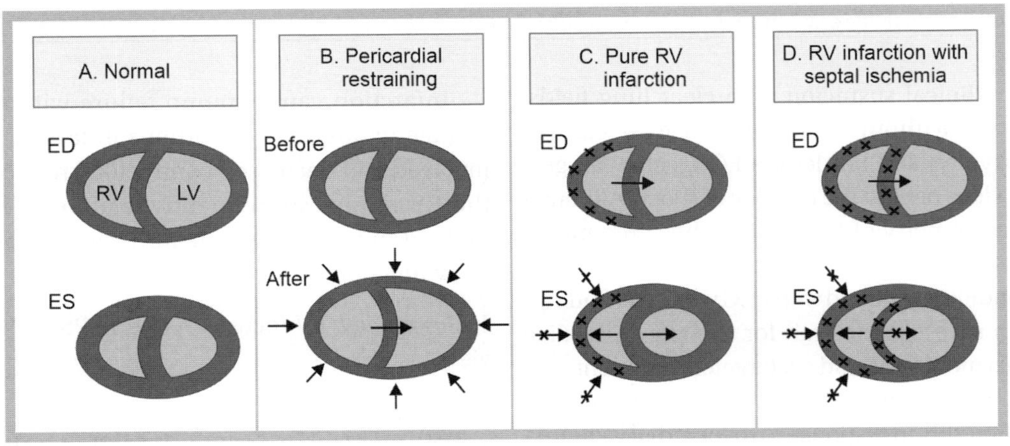


Two physiological concepts explaining the detrimental effects of excessive volume loading. (A) Normal ventricle: At end-systole (ES), the right ventricular (RV) free wall moves toward the septum. (B) Pericardial restraining effects (above, before volume loading; below, after excessive volume loading): RV dilatation, as a result of excessive volume loading, can lead to the elevation of intrapericardial pressure, increase in pericardial constraint (arrow), and change of geometry due to interventricular septum shift. These changes contribute to the low-output state by decreasing left ventricular (LV) distensibility, preload, and ventricular elastance. (C and D) Role of the interventricular septum. (C) At ES, the RV-free wall moves toward the septum. At end-diastole (ED), the RV dilates during diastole and the septum reverse curves toward the volume-reduced LV. At ES, the septum thickens but moves paradoxically into the RV, displacing the RV volume despite RV-free wall dyskinesis. (D) Septal ischemia depresses septal contraction and global LV function, resulting in LV dilatation. The septum stops thickening and there is increased systolic septal displacement into the RV. Pansystolic septal thinning and more extensive paradoxical displacement are associated with further depression of RV performance.

**Q3. Enumerate complications of RV MI.**

**Ans.**

- Atrioventricular blocks
- Arrhythmias (bradyarrhythmia or tachyarrhythmia)
- Vasovagal symptoms
- Hypotension
- Cardiogenic shock
- Ventricular septal defect
- Pericarditis ± pericardial effusion
- RV thrombus
- Tricuspid regurgitation
- PH
- Right heart failure
- Atrial fibrillation

## Case 3

A 55-year-old male without any known comorbidity presented with pain abdomen and obstipation. Subsequently diagnosed with perforation peritonitis went into septic shock managed with adequate antibiotics and mechanical ventilation. Clinically and biochemically improved but requiring vasopressors and evidence of venous congestion without lung congestion was noted. Suspected RV dysfunction, performed DVT scan was negative as an intensivist.

**Q1. How echo can be helpful in diagnosing sepsis-induced RV dysfunction?**

**Ans.**

Sepsis or septic shock can cause RV and or RV compromise either isolated or in combination.

| *Function* | *Pathophysiology* | *EF* | *CO* |
|---|---|---|---|
| LV systolic dysfunction | • Reduced contractility/increase LVESV<br>• EF may appear normal falsely (very low SVR)<br>• LV dilation may occur | ↓/– | ↑ |
| LV hyper dynamic function | • Hyper dynamic contractility<br>• Pseudo hypertrophy of LV<br>• If preload is normal—CO elevated<br>• Reduced LVESV | ↑ | ↑/↓ |
| Dynamic LVOT obstruction | • Anterior movement of the mitral valve against IVS<br>• Severely reduced CO | ↑ | ↓ |
| LV diastolic | • Impaired relaxation<br>• Reduced LVEDV | ↓/– | ↓ |
| RV dysfunction | • Reduced contractility of RV, increased RVESV<br>• RV dilation reduces LV filling<br>• Reduced LVEDV and reduced CO<br>• LV dysfunction may co-occur | ↑/↓ | ↓ |

**Q2. Echocardiographic findings in this case?**

**Ans.**

Clinical suspicion and comparison with baseline echo will give us a fair enough idea for RV involvement in sepsis.

*RV focused A4C:*

- B mode—increased RV/LV size ratio, and fractional area change (FAC) <35%
- M mode and TDI at lateral tricuspid annulus (TAPSE) <1.6 cm, TDI S'<10 cm/s

Right ventricular dysfunction has a prognostic valve and is associated with high mortality.

**Q3. Discuss about therapeutic implications of RV dysfunction.**

**Ans.**

Fluids—administer fluids with caution as a dilated RV with poor systolic function and high afterload will often have difficulty accommodating an increase in volume.

- RVD is a demonstrated predictor of a lower probability of fluid responsiveness
- Prioritization of vasopressors like vasopressin

*Nutshell:* TTE for RV dysfunction

Transthoracic echocardiographic parameters of RVF:

- TAPSE <17 mm
- FAC <35%
- Systolic S' velocity of the tricuspid annulus <9.5 cm/s
- Pericardial fluid >5 mm in diastole
- RV wall thickness >5 mm
- IVC diameter >21 mm and inspiration collapse <50%
- TR peak systolic velocity >2.8 m/s
- RV/LV end-diastolic diameter >1.0
- RV basal diameter >41 mm, ventricular independence (septal shift and D-shaped LV)
- RV index of myocardial performance (RIMP) >0.54

*Management:*

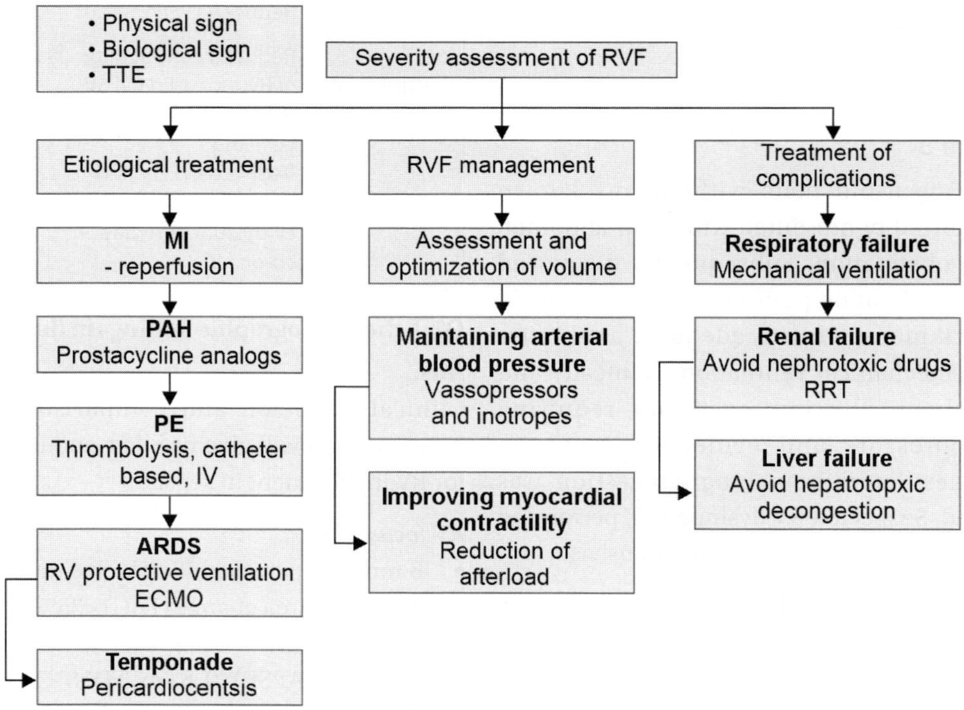


(ARDS: acute respiratory distress syndrome; IV: intravenous; ECMO: extracorporeal membrane oxygenation; MI: myocardial infarction; PE: pulmonary embolism; RRT: renal replacement therapy; TTE: transthoracic echocardiogram)

*In case of refractory RV failure:*

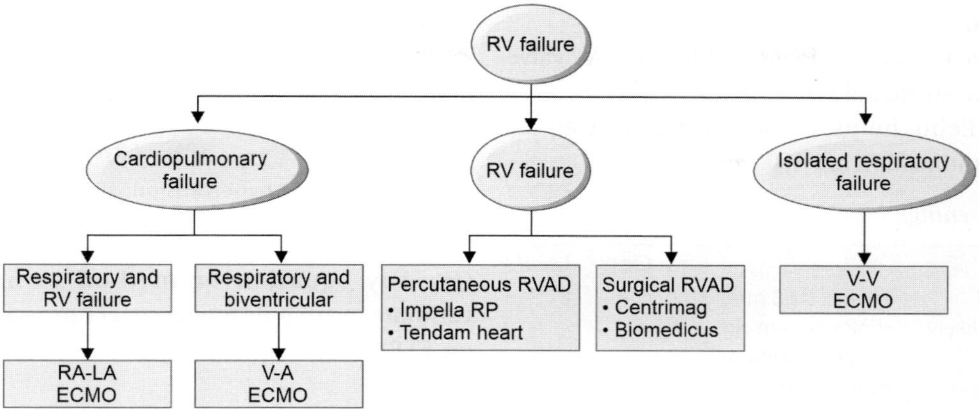


## Case 4

A 45-year-old female known case of connective tissue disorder with mild PAH on home oxygen therapy presented with worsening pedal edema and right upper quadrant pain. No history of fever, or worsening cough; however, history of decreased urine output and drowsiness is there.

**Q1. Do you suspect worsening PAH as the cause of deterioration? How will you proceed and how echocardiography help to formulate a management plan?**

**Ans.**

Background of PAH with worsening congestion and symptoms of reduced cardiac output without history suggestive of infective etiology.

*Differential diagnosis:*

- Worsening PAH
- Community-acquired pneumonia worsening existing PAH
- New onset LV dysfunction-related worsening of PAH

Before we proceed to our case let us briefly about the classification of PAH according to the World Health Organization (WHO):

- *Group 1:* Idiopathic
- *Group 2:* Left heart related
- *Group 3:* Associated with lung pathology/ hypoxia
- *Group 4:* Associated with pulmonary artery obstruction
- *Group 5:* Unclear/multifactorial

**Q2. How echo and POCUS helpful in reaching or ruling out differentials?**

**Ans.**

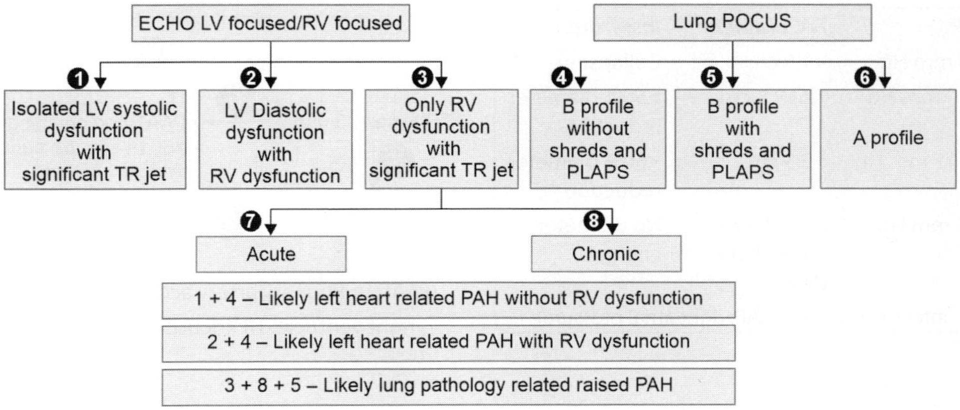

**Q3. How PAH is quantified on echo?**

**Ans.**

*View needed:* RV-focused A4C, SAX AV valve view, subcostal IVC

Echo helps in screening as well as quantification of PAH

*Screening:*

| | | *Class* | *Level* |
|---|---|---|---|
| PH unlikely | TR max ≤2.8 m/s, sPAP ≤36 mm Hg with no additional echo findings* | I | B |
| PH possible | TR max ≤2.8 m/s, sPAP ≤36 mm Hg with additional echo findings* | IIa | C |
| | TR max 2.9–3.4 m/s, sPAP 37–50 mm Hg with/without additional echo findings* | IIIa | C |
| PH likely | TR max >3.4 m/s, sPAP >50 mm Hg, with/without additional echo findings* | I | B |

*Additional echo findings—IVS flattening, short pulmonary vein acceleration time, PA-dilatation.
(sPAP: systolic pulmonary arterial pressure; TR: tricuspid regurgitation)
*Note:* Systolic PAP (sPAP) = $4\ TR\ Vmax_2 + RAP$

**Q4. How RAP can be estimated?**

**Ans.**

| *RAP* | *IVC diameter* | *Inspiration* |
|---|---|---|
| 0–5 mm Hg | <1.5 cm | Collapsing |
| 5–10 mm Hg | 1.5–2.5 cm | >50% diameter reduction |
| 10–15 mm Hg | >2.5 cm | <50% diameter reduction |
| >20 mm Hg | IVC dilated + liver vein dilated | No diameter change |

(IVC: inferior vena cava; RAP: right atrial pressure)

**Q5. How you will quantify PAH on echo?**

**Ans.**

| | |
|---|---|
| Mild PAH | sPAP >40 mm Hg |
| Moderate PAH | sPAP >50 mm Hg |
| Severe PAH | sPAP >60 mm Hg |

(PAH: pulmonary hypertension; sPAP: systolic pulmonary artery pressure)

**Q6. Any equation or method to have estimate mean pulmonary artery pressures on TTE?**

**Ans.**

*View needed:* SAX AV valve view

PWD at pulmonary valve-PAAT – pulmonary acceleration time, PR jet max velocity if present.

mPAP = 4 × maximum pulmonary regurgitation velocity.

mPAP = 79 – 0.45 × (pulmonary acceleration time) (Mahan's regression equation).

**Q7. How TTE help to delineate whether RV involvement is acute or chronic?**

**Ans.**

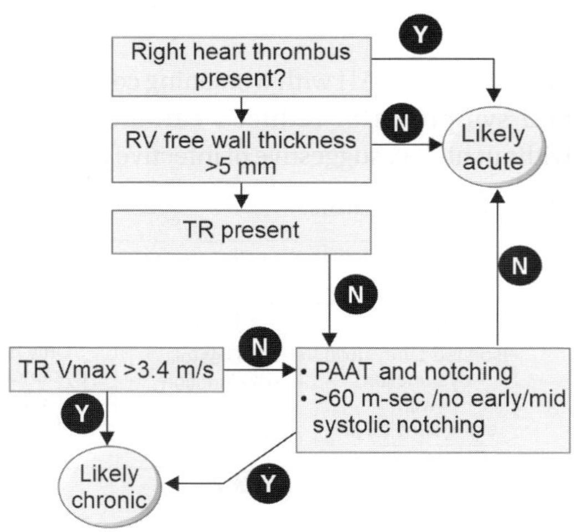


(PAAT: pulmonary artery acceleration time; RV: right ventricle; TR: tricuspid regurgitation)

**Q8. Our case has idiopathic PAH with pericardial effusion with RV failure. Enlist three common mistakes one could commit while managing.**

**Ans.**

| *Avoid* | *Management* |
|---|---|
| Pericardiocentesis for effusion | Target RV afterload with medical management of PAH |
| Volume loading | Target RV afterload with medical management of PAH + diuresis to normalize CVP |
| Mechanical ventilation | Target RV afterload with medical management of PAH |

(CVP: central venous pressure; PAH: pulmonary arterial hypertension; RV: right ventricle)

CHAPTER 10

# Clinically Relevant Stenotic Lesion (Mitral and Aortic) Algorithm Along with Step-By-Step Approach

*Gourav Mittal, Puneet Khanna*

## SEVERAL KEY ASPECTS IN ASSESSING A STENOTIC LESION USING ECHOCARDIOGRAPHY IN CRITICAL CARE

When assessing a stenotic lesion using echocardiography in critical care, several key aspects are typically evaluated:

- *Severity of stenosis:* Echocardiography can help assess the degree of narrowing in the vessel or valve. This is often quantified by measures, such as the pressure gradient across the stenotic lesion and the area of the narrowed passage.
- *Hemodynamic consequences:* Echocardiography can evaluate the impact of the stenotic lesion on cardiac function and hemodynamics. This includes assessing changes in blood flow patterns, chamber pressures, and cardiac output.
- *Structural changes*: Echocardiography allows visualization of structural changes associated with the stenotic lesion. For example, in valvular stenosis, it can show thickening, calcification, or restricted motion of the affected valve leaflets.
- *Complications:* Echocardiography helps detect any complications arising from the stenotic lesion, such as secondary effects on other cardiac structures or the development of conditions, such as heart failure.
- *Monitoring response to treatment:* In critical care settings, echocardiography is often used to monitor the response to treatment interventions, such as medications and mechanical interventions, such as angioplasty and valve replacement.

## MITRAL STENOSIS

### Effects of Mitral Stenosis Intensivists Should Know

- Left atrial (LA)–left ventricular (LV) gradient
- Elevated pressure in LA
- Elevated pressure pulmonary capillaries
- Pulmonary congestion/edema
- Pulmonary hypertension (PHT)
- Right ventricular dilatation
- Tricuspid regurgitation
- Right heart failure
- Atrial fibrillation (AFib)

## MORPHOLOGICAL AND FUNCTIONAL ASSESSMENT OF THE MITRAL VALVE BY TRANSTHORACIC ECHOCARDIOGRAPHY

To assess the mitral valve, transthoracic echocardiography (TTE) requires the following views:

- Parasternal long-axis (PLAX) and parasternal short-axis (PSAX) views
- Apical four-chamber (A4C) and two-chamber (A2C) views

## FACTS AND VALUES REGARDING MITRAL VALVE STENOSIS

- *Normal valve area:* 4–6 $cm^2$.
- *In mitral valve stenosis:* The valvular orifice becomes reduced. The leaflets typically appear thickened due to fibrosis and calcification, and the commissures are often fused. The subvalvular apparatus also gets involved, showing retraction and fusion of the chordae.

## MORPHOLOGICAL ANALYSIS

Morphological analysis includes:

- *Leaflet thickening:* Usually more pronounced at the free edge in cases of rheumatic disease.
- *Chordal changes:* Includes thickening, shortening, and degree of fusion.
- *Altered leaflet movement:* The anterior mitral leaflet (AML) often folds inward, resembling a "hockey stick."
- *Commissural fusion:* Fusion of the commissures can be observed.

## CONTINUOUS WAVE DOPPLER ECHOCARDIOGRAPHY

- *Measurement:* Assesses mitral flow velocity. Using the Bernoulli equation, this measurement is converted into mean and maximum gradient values.
- *Considerations:* The gradient may be overestimated if severe mitral regurgitation is present, or if there is increased cardiac output or restrictive diastolic patterns.

## VALVE AREA CALCULATION METHODS

### Planimetry

- *Method:* Involves measuring the valve area in the diastole using the PSAX view or a focused mitral valve view.
- *Challenges:* Accurate alignment of the scan to the valve is crucial. An oblique view can lead to an overestimation of the valve area.

### Pressure Half-time

- *Definition:* The time required for the early diastolic pressure gradient to decrease from its maximum value to half of that value. This time increases with the severity of mitral stenosis.
- *Measurement:* Use the A4C or A2C view. Place a volume sample through the mitral orifice, parallel to the flow, with sampling facilitated by color Doppler. The PHT is calculated by the echocardiography machine once the maximum and minimum velocities are identified.
- *Calculation:* Valve area = 220/PHT.
- *Considerations:* Various factors, such as reduced left ventricular compliance or severe aortic regurgitation, can influence the PHT and cause overestimation of the valve area. Rapid increases in cardiac output, due to inotropes or volume loading, can also shorten PHT.

### Continuity Equation

- *Principle:* Based on the conservation of mass, this method assumes that the flow volume through the mitral valve equals the cardiac output, in the absence of regurgitation and shunts.
- *Formula:* Area MV × MV velocity time integral (VTI) = Area left ventricular outflow tract (LVOT) × LVOT VTI, thus Area MV = Area LVOT × (LVOT VTI/MV VTI).
- *Application:* The cardiac output is usually calculated at the LVOT or, in cases of aortic regurgitation, at the pulmonary valve. The continuity equation does not rely on transvalvular pressure gradients, left

ventricular compliance, or hemodynamic changes. The absence of regurgitation is essential for the validity of this method.

## CLINICAL SCENARIO

A 23-year-old young female 34 weeks pregnant uncomplicated antenatal care (ANC) course presented with gradual worsening of dyspnea on exertion, cough with frothy secretions, and increased work of breathing. She denied any significant past cardiac history or any long-term illness during childhood. During resuscitation, she developed an irregularly irregular rhythm with hemodynamic instability with a heart rate (HR) >150 beats/min. Some diastolic murmur was heard at the mitral area on auscultation.

**Q1. How to manage Arterial fibrillation and role of TEE?**

**Ans.**

Confirm AFib [irregularly irregular rhythm, absence of P wave on electrocardiogram (ECG)], electrical cardioversion is the choice of therapy however concerns are of thromboembolism especially if underlying valves are involved. If Afib <48 hours in onset risk of thromboembolism is very low, so can go ahead with cardioversion. But if the duration is unknown or >48 hours, the risk is somewhere around 6%, different approaches are advocated to proceed:

- Anticoagulants for 4 weeks then cardioversion followed by continuation of anticoagulation based on risk involved.
- Screen with TEE for thrombus, and anticoagulation acutely followed by cardioversion.

In an acute condition like the above either a second approach if time permits and expertise is available or go ahead with TTE and cardioversion followed by TEE to weigh the risk of thromboembolism.

**Q2. Stenotic lesion of MS how you will quantify in the presence of AFib?**

**Ans.** Various modifications are advised for the quantification of MS in the presence of AFib **(Tables 1 and 2)**

**Q3. How echo findings help to ascertain rheumatic heart disease (RHD) as a cause for this?**

**Ans.**

- *Typical features of mitral stenosis:* Doming of the anterior leaflet, thickening of leaflet tips
- Thickened aortic valve (AV) (AV involvement)
- Reduced left ventricular function (high risk of AFib)
- Enlarged left atrium, AFib
- PHT
- Aortic regurgitation
- Tricuspid stenosis
- Left atrial thrombus

**TABLE 1:** Modification of method required in the presence of AFib.

| *Method* | *Modification* |
|---|---|
| Planimetry | Several different measurements (use average) |
| Mean gradients | Average five cycles with small variations of R-R intervals close to normal heart rate |
| Pulmonary hypertension (PHT) | Avoid mitral flow from short diastoles/average different cardiac cycles |

**TABLE 2:** Values of the above methods for quantification of severity.

| *Mean gradient quantification* | *Planimetry quantification* |
|---|---|
| • Mild (mm Hg) = <5<br>• Moderate (mm Hg) = 5–10<br>• Severe (mm Hg) = >10 | • Normal ($cm^2$) = 4–6<br>• Mild ($cm^2$) = >1.5<br>• Moderate ($cm^2$) = 1–1.5<br>• Severe ($cm^2$) = <1 |

**Q4. Any scoring that will determine whether percutaneous treatment will be helpful?**

*Wilkins Score*

*Grading of aortic valve pathology:*

- *Grade 1:* The valve is highly mobile, with only the leaflet tips restricted. The leaflets are near normal in thickness, measuring 4–5 mm. There is a single area of increased echo brightness, and minimal thickening is observed just below the mitral leaflets.
- *Grade 2:* The mid and base portions of the leaflets have normal mobility. The midleaflets are normal, but there is considerable thickening of the margins, measuring 5–8 mm. Scattered areas of brightness are confined to the leaflet margins. The thickening of the chordal structures extends to one-third of the chordal length.
- *Grade 3:* The valve continues to move forward in diastole, mainly from the base. Thickening extends through the entire leaflet, measuring 5–8 mm. Brightness extends into the mid portions of the leaflets. Thickening is extended to the distal third of the chords.
- *Grade 4:* There is no or minimal forward movement of the leaflets in diastole. There is considerable thickening of all leaflet tissue, >8–10 mm. Extensive brightness is seen throughout much of the leaflet tissue. There is extensive thickening and shortening of all chordal structures, extending down to the papillary muscles.

## AORTIC STENOSIS

### Natural History of Aortic Stenosis

Once a patient with aortic stenosis (AS) has symptoms, it is progressive, and survival will not be significantly improved without valve replacement **(Fig. 1)**.

*Hemodynamic effects of AS intensivists must know* ***(Flowchart 1)****:* Patients with AS have an increased afterload, which results in LV pressure overload. Left ventricular hypertrophy is a compensatory mechanism (reduces wall stress).

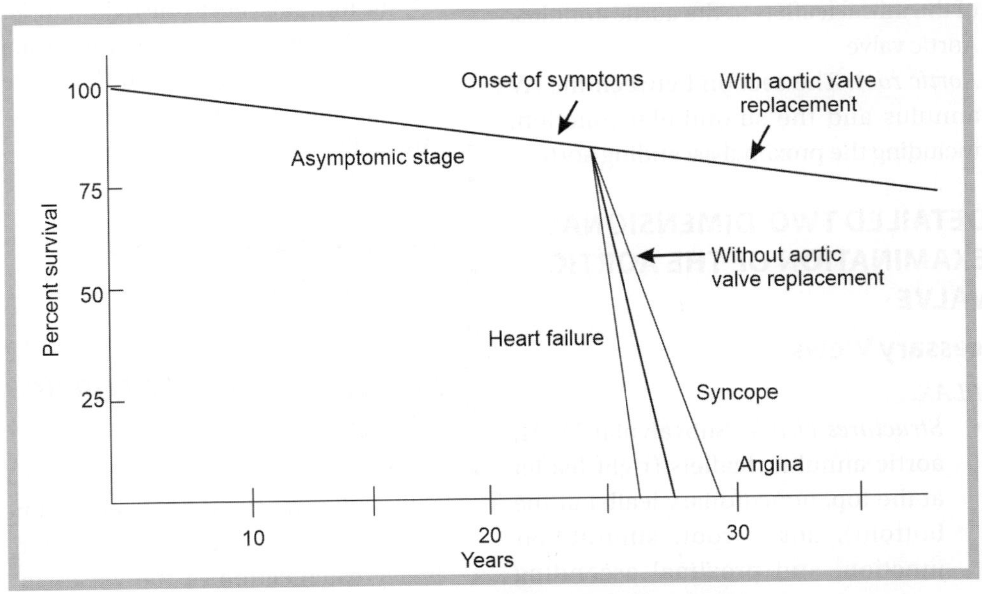


**Fig. 1:** Natural history and progression of aortic stenosis (AS).

**Flowchart 1:** Hemodynamic effects of AS.

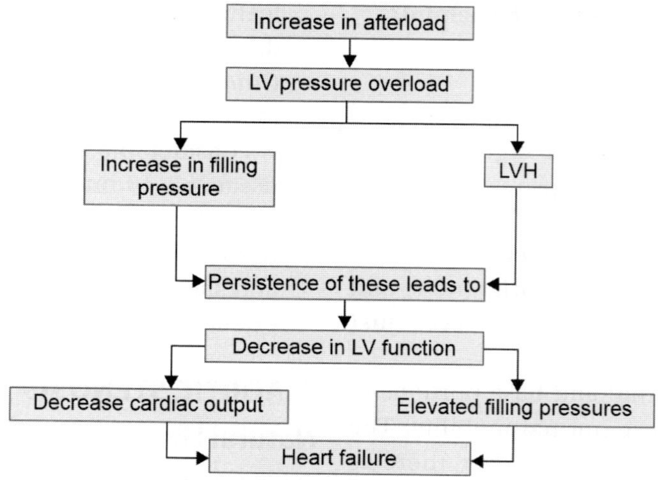


(AS: aortic stenosis; LVH: left ventricular hypertrophy; LV: Left ventricle)

## ECHOCARDIOGRAPHIC ASSESSMENT OF THE AORTIC VALVE

### Components of the Left Ventricular Outflow Tract

- *Subvalvular LVOT:* The part of the left ventricle (LV) extending from the free edges of the mitral leaflets to the aortic annulus.
- Aortic valve
- *Aortic root:* The section between the AV annulus and the sinotubular junction, including the proximal ascending aorta.

## DETAILED TWO-DIMENSIONAL EXAMINATION OF THE AORTIC VALVE

### Necessary Views

- *PLAX:*
    - *Structures visible:* Subvalvular LVOT, aortic annulus, leaflets (right leaflet at the top, noncoronary leaflet at the bottom), aortic root, sinotubular junction, and proximal ascending aorta.
    - *Annular diameter:* Typically, ≤2.5 cm.
    - *Leaflet characteristics:* Normally thin (<2 mm) and mobile.
    - *Normal mesosystolic cusp separation:* ≥2 cm.
- *PSAX:*
    - *Appearance:* The AV appears as a star-shaped orifice, with the right leaflet at the top (adjacent to the right ventricular outflow tract), the noncoronary leaflet at the bottom left, and the left leaflet at the bottom right.
- Apical five-chamber view (A5C)
- Subcostal View

### Doppler Assessment of Aortic Stenosis (Table 3)

*See* **Table 3**.

## QUANTIFICATION OF AORTIC STENOSIS

- *Planimetry (TEE):* Planimetry using TEE is typically employed because Planimetry using TTE is often impractical due to heavy calcification of the valves in AS, making it difficult to trace the AV orifice.

- Pressure gradients
- *Calculated using the simplified Bernoulli equation:* Gradient = 4 × $Vmax^2$
  - *Considerations:*
    - Gradients are influenced by HR and stroke volume.

**TABLE 3:** Doppler assessment while evaluating aortic stenosis.

| | |
|---|---|
| Color wave Doppler | • Color Doppler aliasing caused by high-velocity jet (stenotic turbulences)<br>• Look for the origin of the aortic stenosis jet to exclude LVOT obstruction (SAM/membrane) |
| CWD/ PWD | • Measurement of maximum and mean velocity gradient across the aortic valve<br>• Measurement of LVOT velocity (PW Doppler)<br>• Diastolic dysfunction (filling pressure, indirect sign of severity, correlation with symptoms (PW Doppler)<br>• Elevated pulmonary pressure is a sign of left heart failure (CW Doppler) |

(CW: continuous wave; LVOT: left ventricular outflow tract; PW: pulsed wave; SAM: systolic anterior motion)

    - Jet velocity is elevated (>2 m/s) when aortic valve area (AVA) is <2–2.5 $cm^2$.
- *Continuity equation* ***(Fig. 2)***
- *LVOT width measurement:*
  - Measured in the PLAX, slightly proximal to the AV.
  - Place the pulsed wave (PW) Doppler sample in the LVOT in the A5C.

## PRACTICAL CONSIDERATIONS FOR DETERMINING PRESSURE GRADIENTS

- Align the Doppler beam parallel to the stenotic jet and optimize the angle.
- Assess gradients from various windows, including apical, suprasternal, and right parasternal views.
- Position the continuous wave (CW) Doppler focus on the AV.
- In cases of AFib, average the gradients over multiple beats and include the PW-LVOT velocity.
- For patients with bicuspid AS and severe AS, often characterized by eccentric AS jets, the highest gradient is typically

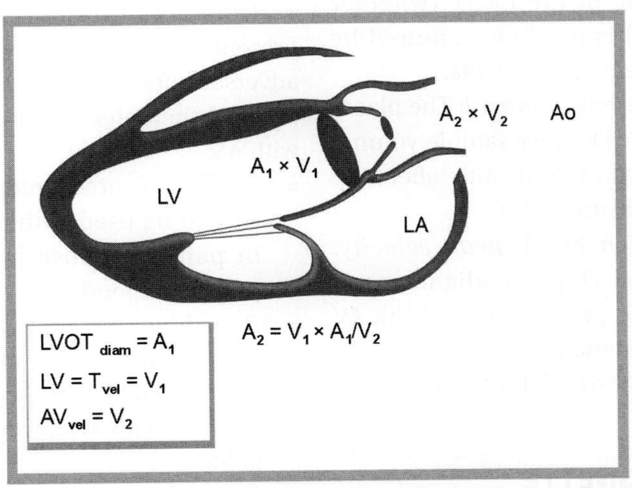


**Fig. 2:** PLAX view and equation of continuity. ($AV_{vel}$: aortic valve velocity; LV: left ventricle; LVOT: left ventricular outflow tract; PLAX: parasternal long axis)

**TABLE 4:** Severity of AS on the basis of mean gradient, area, and jet velocity.

| | *Mild* | *Moderate* | *Severe* |
|---|---|---|---|
| Mean gradient | <25 mm Hg | 25–40 mm Hg | >40 mm Hg |
| AVA | >1.5 cm$^2$ | 1–1.5 cm$^2$ | <1 cm$^2$ |
| Jet velocity | <3 m/s | 3–4 m/s | >4 m/s |

(AS: aortic stenosis; AVA: aortic valve area)

measured from a right parasternal approach.
- High cardiac output states (e.g., in young or anxious patients, hyperthyroidism, fever, or dialysis shunts) may result in flow velocities exceeding 2 m/s, which can mimic AS.

*Measurement of LVOT width is most critical for the calculation of the AV area. Small measurement errors result in large differences.*

## LIMITATIONS OF THE CONTINUITY EQUATION

- *Measurement of LVOT may be difficult:* Accurate measurement of the left ventricular outflow tract (LVOT) can be challenging.
- *Geometry of LVOT not fully appreciated:* The true shape of the LVOT (whether round or oval) is not fully captured by simple distance measurements.
- *PW sample volume positional:* The placement of the PW Doppler sample volume is crucial and can significantly affect the accuracy of measurements.
- *Underestimation of AV peak velocity:* In cases where Doppler alignment is suboptimal, the peak velocity of the AV may be underestimated.

Severity of AS on echocardiography **(Table 4)**.

## CLINICAL VIGNETTE

A 56-year-old male history of TIA twice and intermittent chest pain presented with chest pain, cold peripheries, and hypotension, ECG showing left axis deviation along with LVH and stain pattern. He had a history of cough with expectoration since 2 days and high-grade fever. On auscultation you heard abnormal heart sounds at the aortic area during systole, you suspected valvular involvement.

**Q1. When will you suspect low gradient AS? And how will you proceed?**

**Ans.**

Aortic valve area (AVA) ≤1 cm$^2$ (≤0.6 cm$^2$/m$^2$) along with mean pressure gradient ≤40 mm Hg **(Flowchart 2)**.

**Q2. What is the medical management of the condition?**

**Ans.**

*Management of Hypertension in Aortic Stenosis*

Concomitant hypertension and AS present a "double load" to the LV, which can adversely affect ventricular function. Various medical therapies can pose risks to patients with AS:

- *Diuretics:* Diuretics reduce preload, so they should be used with caution, especially in patients whose hemodynamics are preload dependent.
- *Beta-blockers:* Beta-blockers reduce contractility and may be risky for overloaded LV. They should be avoided in patients with symptomatic AS and heart failure.
- *Vasodilators:* Vasodilators (such as hydralazine, nitroglycerin, and nifedipine) can reduce systemic blood pressure

**Flowchart 2:** Differentiating LFLG AS from others.

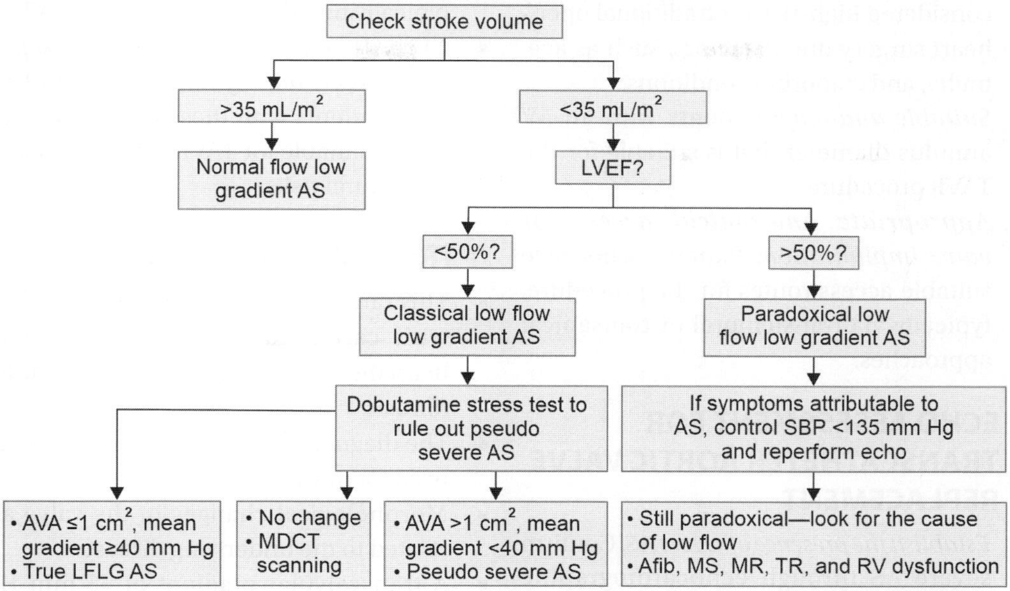


(AVA: aortic valve area; LFLG: low flow low gradient; LVEF: left ventricular ejection fraction; MDCT: multi-detector computed tomography; MS: mitral stenosis; RV: right ventricular; TR: tricuspid regurgitation)

and coronary artery perfusion pressure in the presence of fixed valvular stenosis. These agents should be avoided or used with caution.

- *Angiotensin-converting enzyme (ACE) inhibitors* and *angiotensin receptor blockers (ARBs):* ACE inhibitors and ARBs tend to be well tolerated in patients with moderate and asymptomatic severe AS.

*Management of Heart Failure in Aortic Stenosis*

- *Combination therapy:* A combination of a diuretic and an ACE inhibitor or ARB is recommended. These should be started at low doses with gradual titration.

**Q3. What are the indications for surgery/ interventions in AS?**

**Ans.**

- *Symptomatic patients with severe AS:* Patients presenting with symptoms such as dyspnea, syncope, or angina.
- *Symptomatic patients with severe AS and reduced LV function:* Patients with severe AS and a reduced left ventricular ejection fraction (EF) of <50%.
- *Asymptomatic patients with severe AS and abnormal exercise test:* Asymptomatic patients who demonstrate abnormalities during an exercise test.
- *Concurrent cardiac surgery:* Patients undergoing other cardiac surgeries [e.g., coronary artery bypass grafting (CABG) and ascending aorta surgery].

**Q4. What is transcatheter aortic valve replacement (TAVR), in what subset of patients you will consider it, and how does echo help in TAVR?**

*Transcatheter aortic valve replacement* is a minimally invasive procedure used to replace a stenotic AV without open-heart surgery.

*Consider TAVR in:*

- *Symptomatic/severe AS:* Patients exhibiting symptoms of severe AS.

- *High-risk patients:* Patients who are considered high-risk for traditional open-heart surgery due to factors, such as age, frailty, and comorbid conditions.
- *Suitable anatomy:* Patients with an AV annulus diameter that is suitable for the TAVR procedure.
- *Appropriate anatomical access for valve implantation*: Patients who have suitable access routes for the procedure, typically via transfemoral or transapical approaches.

## ECHO ASSESSMENT FOR TRANSCATHETER AORTIC VALVE REPLACEMENT

- *Establish the presence of severe AS:* Confirm severe AS through echocardiographic evaluation.
- *Assess annular dimension during systole:* Measure the annular dimension in a zoomed Parasternal long-axis view (PLAX) to ensure accurate valve sizing.
- *Undersizing risks:* Device migration or significant paravalvular aortic regurgitation.
- *Oversizing risks:* Underexpansion, reduced durability, and increased vascular access complications.
- *Assess the extent and distribution of calcification:* Evaluate the calcification around the AV to aid in procedural planning and risk assessment.
- *Exclude patients with bicuspid valves:* Bicuspid valves, which have an elliptical orifice, may predispose to incomplete valve deployment, and these patients are typically not ideal candidates for TAVR.
- *Exclude patients with basal septal hypertrophy and dynamic LVOT obstruction:* Patients with these conditions may not be suitable for TAVR due to increased procedural risks.

## TRICUSPID STENOSIS

- This rare condition is typically associated with carcinoid syndrome, rheumatic heart disease, or Löffler's endomyocardial fibrosis.
- The diagnostic approach is similar to that used for mitral stenosis.
- Morphological changes in the valve are related to the underlying disease.
- A transvalvular gradient of >5 mm Hg, measured by CW Doppler, indicates severe impairment.
- Severe tricuspid stenosis results in caval congestion.

## PULMONARY STENOSIS

- Often linked to Noonan's syndrome.
- In addition to congenital forms, pulmonary stenosis can be caused by carcinoid syndrome or rheumatic disease.
- Among congenital forms, the subvalvular type, often associated with Fallot's tetralogy, is the most common and includes a dynamic obstruction component.
- The right ventricle thickens in response to the obstruction.

CHAPTER 11

# Clinically Relevant Regurgitant Lesion (Mitral, Aortic, and Tricuspid)

*Gourav Mittal*

## REGURGITANT LESIONS

Valvular pathology, whether it is primary or secondary, possesses a significant hemodynamic implication especially in critically ill patients. Early picking up the disease modifies intensivist hemodynamics goal, directs toward specific treatment being it a supportive or targeted treatment, and leads to better optimization. We here going to discuss two important valvular lesions, i.e., mitral regurgitation (MR) and aortic regurgitation (AR), how they impact hemodynamics, how one should identify them, identifying whether they are significant or not, grade them, likely etiology and possible management.

## MITRAL REGURGITATION

### Hemodynamics in Mitral Regurgitation

Mitral regurgitation presents with varying hemodynamic profiles depending on the duration and severity of the condition:

- *Acute MR:*
  - *Ejection fraction:* High
  - *Left ventricle size:* Normal or slightly enlarged (unadapted)
  - In acute MR, the sudden volume overload leads to an increase in ejection fraction without significant ventricular dilation initially.
- *Chronic MR:*
  - *Ejection fraction:* "Supranormal" (above normal)
  - *Left ventricle size:* Dilated (adapted)
  - Chronic MR results in prolonged volume overload, causing the left ventricle to adapt by dilating to accommodate the regurgitant volume. The ejection fraction may initially be supranormal due to increased contractility.
- *Decompensated MR:*
  - *Left ventricle size:* Significantly enlarged
  - *Ejection fraction:* Begins to decrease as the ventricle becomes decompensated from chronic overload.

### Mitral Valve Apparatus Anatomy

The mitral valve (MV) apparatus consists of several components:

- *Mitral annulus:* The ring-like structure to which the mitral valve leaflets attach.
- *Mitral leaflets:* Two leaflets—the anterior mitral leaflet (AML) and the posterior mitral leaflet (PML).
  - AML covers approximately one-third of the circumference of the annulus.
  - PML covers approximately two-thirds of the circumference of the annulus.
  - AML is longer than PML.

- *Chordae tendineae:* Cord-like tendons that connect the leaflets to the papillary muscles.
- *Papillary muscles:* Muscles that anchor the chordae tendineae and help in maintaining valve closure.

*Transthoracic echocardiography (TTE) views for studying MV anatomy and function:* To assess both the anatomy and function of the mitral valve using TTE, the following views are commonly utilized:

- *Parasternal long-axis and short-axis views:*
    - These views provide detailed visualization of the mitral valve anatomy, including the annulus and leaflets.
- *Apical four-chamber and two-chamber views:*
    - These views allow assessment of the mitral valve from different angles, providing insights into leaflet motion, regurgitation severity, and associated chamber dimensions.

By employing these TTE views, clinicians can effectively evaluate the structural integrity and functional dynamics of the mitral valve, aiding in diagnosis and management decisions for patients with MR.

*Two types of MR usually we see:*

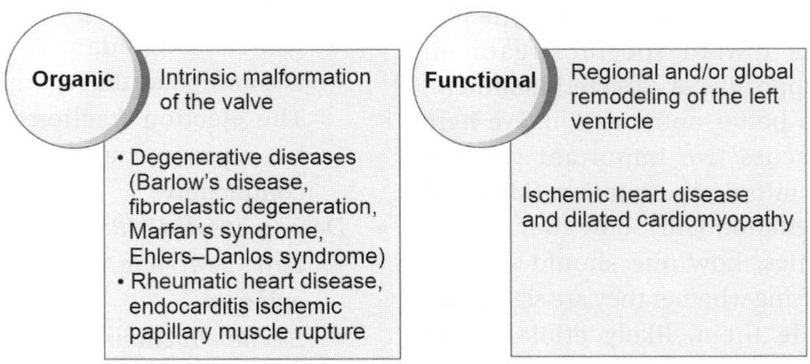


## Carpentier's Classification of Mitral Regurgitation Based on Leaflet Motion

Carpentier's classification categorizes MR based on the motion and pathology of the mitral valve leaflets. Here are the types and their characteristics:

- *Type I: Normal leaflet motion with coaptation defect—*
    - *Cause:* Often secondary to degenerative or ischemic annular dilation, or leaflet perforation (e.g., endocarditis)
    - *Characteristic:* Normal leaflet motion but with inadequate coaptation due to structural defects
- *Type II: Excessive leaflet motion—*
    - *Causes:*
        - *Billowing leaflet:* Mitral leaflet bulges above the annulus toward the left atrium during systole, maintaining coaptation below the annulus.
        - *Floppy valve:* Myxomatous degeneration with thickened, redundant leaflets (>5 mm in diastole) and elongated chordae

- *Prolapse:* Coaptation line is above the annulus (>2 mm), with the leaflet tip directed toward the left ventricle
- *Flail:* Free edge of the leaflet is upturned in the left atrium, with the tip directed toward the left atrium due to chordal rupture
- *Characteristics:* Excessive motion due to conditions like chordal stretching or rupture, papillary muscle rupture, or degenerative disease

- *Type III: Restricted leaflet motion—*
    - *Causes:*
        - *Type IIIa:* Organic causes, primarily rheumatic heart disease, restrict leaflet movement both in systole and diastole.
        - *Type IIIb:* Functional causes, such as ischemic heart disease, result in systolic tethering of leaflets due to papillary muscle displacement or left ventricular dilation, while leaflet motion is normal during diastole.
    - *Characteristics:* Leaflet motion is restricted due to underlying pathologies like rheumatic heart disease, dilated cardiomyopathy, or ischemic cardiomyopathy.

Carpentier's classification helps in understanding the diverse mechanisms leading to MR based on the dynamics of leaflet motion and assists in guiding appropriate treatment strategies, including surgical interventions.

## Consequences of Mitral Regurgitation

- Left ventricular volume overload
- Elevated left ventricular filling pressure
- Pulmonary hypertension
- Tricuspid regurgitation
- Reduced systolic wall stress
- Reduced afterload

## CASE SCENARIO

A 45-year-old male post balloon valvotomy for mitral stenosis of RHD origin 5 years back presented with community-acquired pneumonia leading to acute respiratory distress syndrome (ARDS), managed with lung-protective ventilation and two sessions of proning, before attempting for weaning you are screening cardiac functions as baseline not available because of critical initial condition, founds to have dilated LV with regurgitant jet across mitral valve.

**Q1. How will you assess mitral valve echocardiographically?**

**Ans.** *Various echocardiographic modalities for mitral valve assessment* **(*Table 1*)**.

Watch for eccentric jets where the color Doppler area may underestimate the severity of mitral regurgitation (due to Coanda effect).

### Semiquantitative Assessment of Regurgitant Jet in Mitral Regurgitation

When performing echocardiography to assess mitral regurgitation (MR) semiquantitatively, several key points are considered:

- *Visualization of regurgitant jet:*
    - The regurgitant jet is visualized starting from the mitral valve into the left atrium.
- *Regurgitant jet area:*
    - Represents the spatial area of the jet, which correlates with the velocity of blood regurgitating into the left atrium.
    - Dependent on the pressure gradient between the left ventricle and left atrium.
    - Changes in left ventricular pressure, such as due to hypovolemia or reduced contractility, can falsely reduce the apparent area of the regurgitant jet.

**TABLE 1:** ECHO modalities and findings in MR.

| *ECHO method* | *Potential findings* | *Evaluation* |
|---|---|---|
| 2D imaging | • Mitral valve apparatus abnormalities<br>• Mitral annular calcification<br>• Left atrial dilation<br>• Left ventricle dilation | • Mitral annulus dilation<br>• Interatrial septum bowed to right |
| Color Doppler | Regurgitant flow into left atrium | • Regurgitant flow area<br>• Left atrium area<br>• Vena contracta |
| Pulsed wave Doppler | • Increased E-wave velocity (>1.2 m/s)<br>• Systolic pulmonary venous inflow blunting or reversal | • Mitral valve VTI/LVOT<br>• VTI (NB: as long as no significant aortic regurgitation) |
| Continuous wave Doppler | • Mitral regurgitation jet<br>• Pulmonary hypertension | • Jet density and symmetry<br>• Tricuspid regurgitation |

(LVOT: left ventricular outflow tract; MR: mitral regurgitation; VTI: velocity time integral)

- *Color gain control:*
  - Important for optimizing visualization of the regurgitant jet:
    - *Appropriate gain:* Ensures that the regurgitant jet appears as a distinct color flow without artifactually enlarging or reducing its size.
    - *High gain:* Can overestimate the jet area, showing turbulence in areas with no actual flow.
    - *Low gain:* May underestimate the jet area, failing to show subtle regurgitant jets.
- *Color gain scale adjustment:*
  - Adjust the color gain scale to eliminate color in areas without flow or with low flow (e.g., atrial walls or adjacent to valve structures).
  - Optimal settings typically involve adjusting the gain until only the regurgitant jet is visualized clearly.
  - A color-coded velocity scale of around 50–60 cm/s is recommended to accurately depict the velocity of the regurgitant jet.

These considerations ensure accurate semiquantitative assessment of MR severity using echocardiography, aiding in clinical decision-making regarding management and intervention for patients with MR.

**TABLE 2:** Quantification of MR on the basis of perimeter area.

| | |
|---|---|
| Perimeter area <4 $cm^2$ | Mild |
| Perimeter area >8 $cm^2$ | Severe |

(MR: mitral regurgitation)

**TABLE 3:** Quantification of MR on the basis of ration of regurgitant jet/LA area.

| | |
|---|---|
| <20% | Mild |
| 25–30% | Moderate |
| 30–40% | Moderate-severe |
| >40% | Severe |

(LA: left atrium; MR: mitral regurgitation)

- The perimeter of the regurgitant jet is traced with the cursor and the area is measured **(Table 2)**
- Calculate ratio of area of regurgitant jet/LA area **(Table 3)**

## Quantification Based on Color Doppler

*Mild, moderate, severe:*

- Vena contracta (mm) <3 mild, 3–6.9 moderate, ≥7 severe

*Color Doppler confounders:*

- Geometry of regurgitant orifice
- Multiple jets
- Coanda effect ("wall hugging" jets)
- Driving force (systolic pressure)
- Left atrial (LA) compliance

The proximal portions of the jet (the vena contracta and the flow convergence zone) are more important for the quantification of mitral regurgitation than jet area, length or width **(Fig. 1)**.

Do not base the quantification of mitral regurgitation on a single parameter.

*Indirect signs:*

- Dilated left ventricle
- Hyperdynamic left ventricular function
- Left atrial enlargement
- Interatrial septum bulging (toward RA)

**Q2. What are signs acute MR?**

**Ans.**

- Hyperdynamic left ventricle with a normal size
- Tachycardia
- Abnormal valve morphology (e.g., papillary muscle rupture, flail leaflet)
- Low velocity of the MR signal (shock)
- Triangular-shaped MR spectrum
- Elevated MV inflow velocity

**Q3. Will ECHO can help in differentiating between etiologies of mitral regurgitation?**

**Ans.** Morphology of MV and symmetry of intraventricular septum helps to differentiate etiology **(Flowchart 1)**.

Leaflet adjacent to interventricular septum is anterior mitral leaflet (AML).

The ruptured leaflet always extends behind the nonruptured leaflet to which it frequently lies parallel. This sign may be helpful in cases of subtle chordal rupture.

**Q4. How does the management differ depending on the etiology of MR [if MR is secondary to primary valvular, secondary to ischemic and secondary to hypertrophic obstructive cardiomyopathy (HOCM) associated systolic anterior motion (SAM)]?**

**Ans.** Usual cardiac grid, i.e., hemodynamic goals for MR if 3F—fast, forward, full.

Higher normal heart rate, reduced SVR/afterload, and full ventricle favor reduced regurgitant fraction and favor stable hemodynamics. However if it is secondary

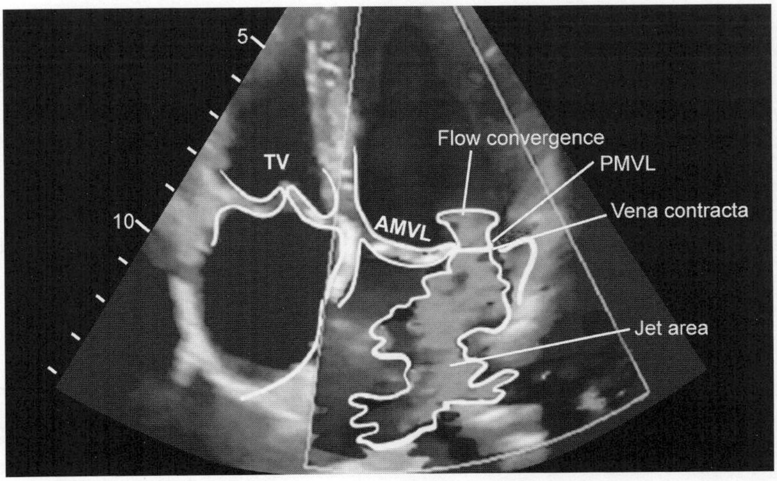


**Fig. 1:** Color Doppler across MV showing flow convergence, vena contracta and jet area. (MV: mitral valve)

**Flowchart 1:** Etiology of MR on basis of echocardiographic findings of mitral valve and interventricular septum.

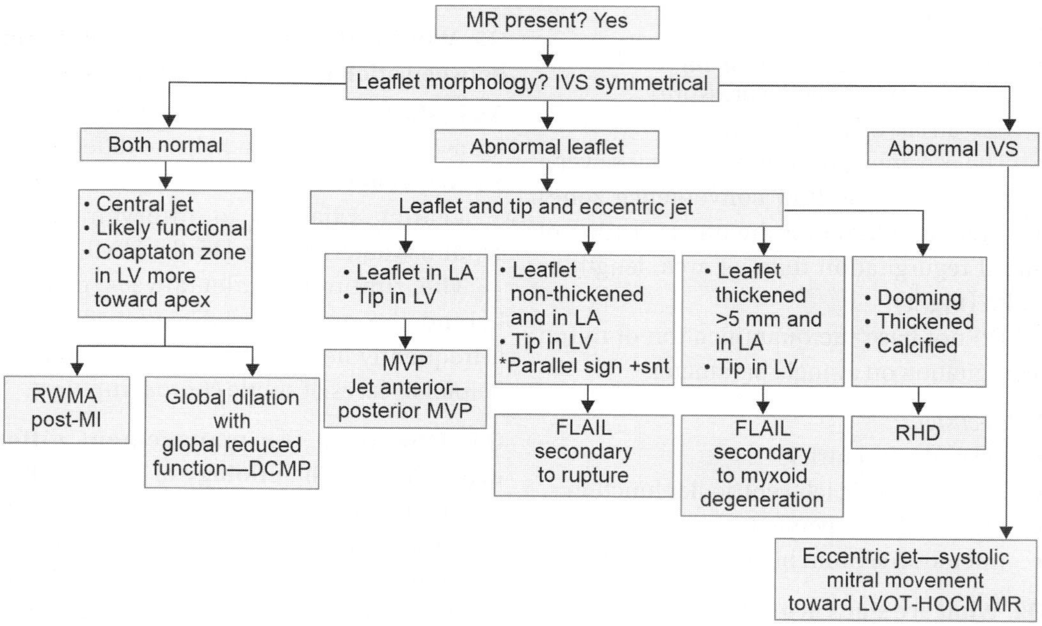


*Note: *Parallel sign—zoomed apical four-chamber view/2D*
(LA: left atrium; LV: left ventricle; LVOT: left ventricular outflow tract; MR: mitral regurgitation; RWMA: regional wall motion abnormalities; HOCM: hypertrophic obstructive cardiomyopathy)

to ischemic out of these heart rate should be low normal to reduce myocardial oxygen demand and if associated with HOCM afterload should be high with low heart rate to reduce dynamic LVOT obstruction.

*PS: In the setting of significant mitral regurgitation, an ejection fraction of 55–60% (which is otherwise considered normal) denotes left ventricular failure.*

## AORTIC REGURGITATION

### Hemodynamic Effect of Aortic Regurgitation

- Left ventricle volume overload
- Dilated left ventricle
- Filling pressure elevated
- Afterload increased

*Quantification of aortic regurgitation should be based on:*

- Aortic regurgitation jet (vena contracta, width, flow convergence)
- Deceleration time or aortic regurgitation spectrum (PHT)
- Retrograde flow in the aorta
- Indirect findings

*Indirect findings in aortic regurgitation:*

- Dilated left ventricle
- Hyperdynamic function
- Eccentric left ventricular hypertrophy
- Slightly enlarged left atrium
- Mitral regurgitation (annular dilatation)
- Diastolic dysfunction

*Concomitant AS and LVH make LV dilatation less prominent. Ventricle compensates more by dilatation than with an increase in ejection fraction.*

## Imaging of Aortic Regurgitation Jet

- Parasternal long axis (PLAX)
- Parasternal short axis (PSAX) (visualize origin of jet)
- Five-chamber view/three-chamber view
- Suprasternal (to determine retrograde flow)

## Aortic Regurgitation: Causes and Echocardiographic Assessment

Aortic regurgitation (AR) typically results from abnormalities of the aortic valve (AV) and/or the aortic root. Here is an overview of the causes and the echocardiographic assessment:

*Causes:*

- *Acute aortic regurgitation:*
  - *Causes:* Usually due to aortic dissection or endocarditis
  - *Endocarditis:* AV endocarditis can lead to perforation or distortion of the cusps, sometimes causing an aortic root abscess that distorts the sinotubular junction.
- *Chronic aortic regurgitation:*
  - *Causes:* Often from calcific degeneration, rheumatic disease, or congenital abnormalities (e.g., bicuspid AV).
  - *Aortic root dilatation:* This includes dilatation of the aortic root components (annulus, Valsalva sinus, sinotubular junction) or of the ascending aorta.
  - *Reduced leaflet overlap:* Chronic regurgitation can lead to reduced leaflet coaptation in diastole, exacerbating the regurgitant flow.

*Echocardiographic evaluation:*

- *2D imaging:*
  - *Purpose:* Look for structural abnormalities of the AV and aorta.
  - *Findings:* Includes bicuspid AV morphology, calcifications, vegetation (indicative of endocarditis), or abscess formation.
- *Color flow Doppler:*
  - *Evaluation of regurgitant jet:*
    - *Parasternal short-axis (PSAX):* Measure the jet area and compare it with the area of the subvalvular left ventricular outflow tract (LVOT) traced in mid diastole.
      - *Interpretation:* A ratio of jet area to LVOT area <25% suggests mild AR, while >60% indicates severe AR.
    - *Parasternal long-axis (PLAX):* Assess the ratio of jet width to LVOT width.
      - *Interpretation:* A ratio ≥65% is indicative of severe AR.

Echocardiography plays a crucial role in assessing the severity and etiology of aortic regurgitation, guiding clinical management decisions and determining the need for intervention based on the severity of regurgitation observed.

Width of the vena contracta—the narrowest portion of the jet located just distal to the regurgitant orifice determines the severity of AR **(Table 4, Fig. 2)**.

## Continuous Wave Doppler—A5C

Pressure half-time (PHT), which is defined as the time required for the pressure gradient

**TABLE 4:** Severity of AR on basis of width of vena contracta.

| | |
|---|---|
| >0.6 cm | Severe AR |
| 0.3–0.6 | Moderate AR |
| <0.3 | Mild AR |

(AR: aortic regurgitation)

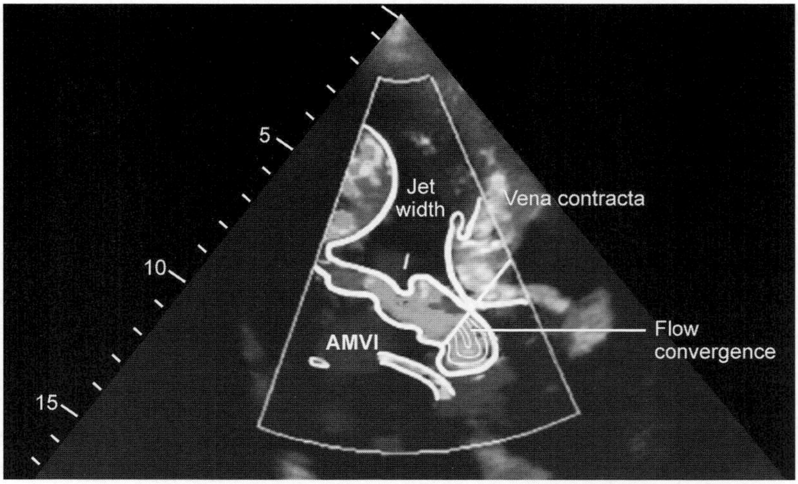


**Fig. 2:** *PLAX*-jet length—if its extends past the level of the papillary muscles. (AMVI: anterior mitral valve leaflet)

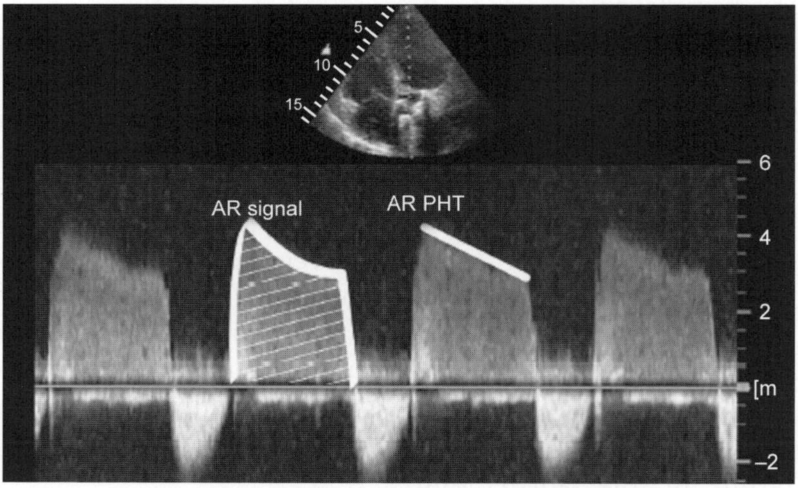


**Fig. 3:** A5C on CW Doppler across AV valve showing PHT on AR signal. (A5C: Apical five-chamber; AV: aortic valve; AR: aortic regurgitation; CW: continuous wave; PHT: Pressure half-time)

across the AV to decrease to half of its maximal value **(Fig. 3)**.

The PHT is inversely proportional to the severity of regurgitation **(Table 5)**.

**TABLE 5:** Severity of AR on the basis of PHT.

| | | |
|---|---|---|
| Pressure half-time (PHT) (m-sec) | <200 | Severe AR |
| | 200–500 | Moderate AR |
| | >500 | Mild AR |

(AR: aortic regurgitation)

*Pitfalls:*
- Complex, eccentric, or multiple jets
- Poor alignment of continuous wave (CW) Doppler with the aortic regurgitation jet
- Calcified valves (it will be difficult to see the proximal flow convergence zone)
- Machine settings (PRF)

*The AR signal should have a velocity above 4.5 m/s. Otherwise the signal quality will be inadequate for assessment of pressure half-time (nonparallel jet alignment).*

## CLINICAL VIGNETTE

A 32-year-old female 24 week pregnant uncomplicated ANC course presented with gradual worsening of dyspnea on exertion, cough with frothy secretions, and increased work of breathing. She denied any significant past cardiac history or any long-term illness during childhood. On auscultation, you hear a diastolic murmur at aortic valve. How will you approach this case?

**Q1. Quantification?**

**Ans.** PSAX/PLAX/A5C (as described above) **(Table 6)**.

**Q2. Acute versus chronic, how ECHO points towards onset?**

**Ans.**

*Echo features of acute aortic regurgitation:*

- Small/slightly dilated left ventricle
- Tachycardia
- "Initially" hyperdynamic left ventricle
- Holodiastolic retrograde flow in the descending aorta
- Short pressure half-time
- Premature mitral valve closure

**Q3. Indication for surgical management?**

**Ans.**

- In symptomatic patients
- In asymptomatic patients with reduced resting LVF (LVEF <50%)
- In patients undergoing CABG or surgery of the ascending aorta, or another valve.
- In asymptomatic patients with severe LV dilatation (left ventricular end diastolic diameter = LVEDD >70 mm, LV end systolic diameter = LVESD >50 mm or LVESD/BSA >25 mm/m$^2$)
- If EF is too poor (<30–35%), candidates for heart transplantation

**TABLE 6:** Quantification AR on basis of Vena contracta, jet width, and PHT.

| | *Mild* | *Moderate* | *Severe* |
|---|---|---|---|
| Vena contracta | <3 mm | 3–6 mm | >6 mm |
| Jet width (% of LVOT) | <25 | 25–65 | >65 |
| PHT | >500 | 200–500 | <200 |

(AR: aortic regurgitation; LVOT: left ventricular outflow tract; PHT: pressure half-time)

**TABLE 7:** Various echocardiographic parameters while evaluating TR.

| *Echocardiography method* | *Potential findings* | *Evaluation* |
|---|---|---|
| 2D imaging | • Tricuspid annular dilation<br>• Right ventricle dilation<br>• Right atrial dilation | Tricuspid valve abnormalities |
| Color Doppler | • Tricuspid regurgitation<br>• Hepatic vein flow toward probe during systole | Regurgitant jet area Vena contracta |
| Pulsed wave Doppler | Hepatic vein flow | Hepatic vein systolic flow reversal |
| Continuous wave Doppler | Tricuspid regurgitation flow | • Density of regurgitation flow<br>• Asymmetrical shape<br>• Systolic pulmonary artery pressures ($4 \times TR_{Vmax}$) |

(TR: tricuspid regurgitation)

## TRICUSPID REGURGITATION

### Echocardiography Findings in Case of Tricuspid Regurgitation (TR) (Table 7)

**Q1. How to assess severity of TR?**

**Ans.** *Severity of TR can be assessed on the basis of jet quantification, shape, and hepatic vein Doppler* **(Table 8; Figs. 4A and B)**.

**TABLE 8:** Assess severity of TR.

| ***Parameters*** | ***Mild*** | ***Moderate*** | ***Severe*** |
|---|---|---|---|
| Regurgitant jet area | Small central | Intermediate | Large central |
| Vena contracta (mm) | Not defined | <7 | >7 |
| TR CWD | Faint | Filled parabolic | Dense asymmetrical |
| Hepatic vein flow | Systolic dominance | Systolic blunting | Systolic reversal |

(TR CWD: tricuspid regurgitation continuous wave Doppler trace)

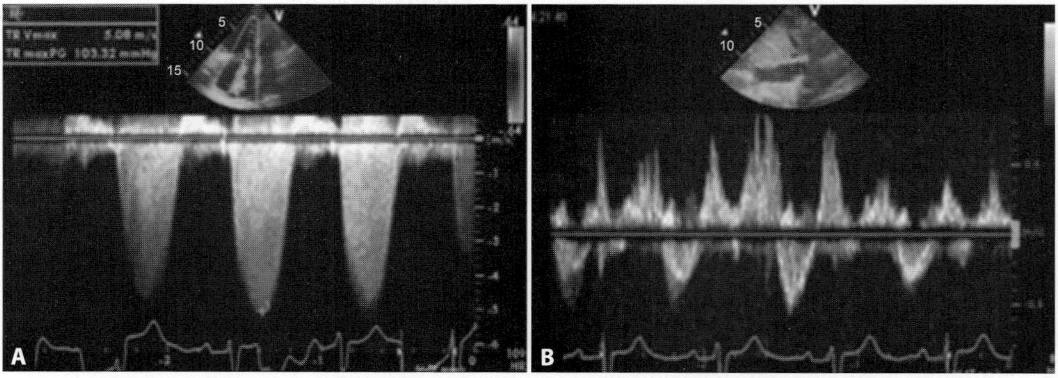


**Figs. 4A and B:** Tricuspid regurgitation assessment: (A) Tricuspid regurgitation continuous wave Doppler trace; (B) Hepatic vein flow (systolic flow reversal).

CHAPTER 12

# Prosthetic Valves

Gourav Mittal, Puneet Khanna

## ECHOCARDIOGRAPHIC EVALUATION OF PROSTHETIC HEART VALVES IN THE INTENSIVE CARE UNIT

When evaluating prosthetic heart valves (PHVs) in the intensive care unit (ICU), echocardiography plays a critical role in assessing valve function and detecting potential complications. Here's a summary of the key components of echocardiographic evaluation:

*Two-dimensional (2D) evaluation of the prosthetic valve:* Visual assessment of the prosthetic valve structure, including leaflet motion, presence of thrombi, and any abnormalities.

- *2D evaluation of cardiac chamber size and function*:
  - Assessment of cardiac chambers (atria and ventricles) to evaluate for dilation or hypertrophy.
  - Measurement of ejection fraction and other parameters to assess cardiac function.
- *Color Doppler examination of regurgitation:*
  - Detection and characterization of regurgitant jets around the prosthetic valve.
  - Helps determine the severity and mechanism (e.g., paravalvular leak) of regurgitation.
- *Continuous-wave (CW) and pulsed-wave (PW) Doppler:*
  - *CW Doppler:* Used to assess high-velocity flow across the valve to detect stenosis or regurgitation.
  - *PW Doppler:* It helps in assessing flow velocities and gradients across the valve, particularly useful in detecting pathologic obstruction (stenosis) or significant regurgitation.
- *Evaluation of prosthesis-patient mismatch (PPM):*
  - PPM refers to situations where the effective orifice area (EOA) of the prosthetic valve is too small relative to the patient's body size, leading to hemodynamic compromise.
  - Echocardiography assesses EOA and calculates the valve area relative to body size, helping identify cases of PPM.
  - Mitral PPM, specifically, may lead to complications such as pulmonary hypertension, especially in patients with poor left ventricular function.
- *Assessment of pathologic obstruction and regurgitation:*
  - Identification of any obstructions or abnormal flows around the prosthetic valve using Doppler techniques.
  - Differentiates between normal and pathologic flow patterns to guide clinical management.

Echocardiographic evaluation of PHV in the ICU is crucial for monitoring postoperative recovery, detecting complications such as valve dysfunction or PPM, and guiding therapeutic interventions to optimize patient outcomes.

## CASE SCENARIO

**Q1. A 55-year-old male with a past history of coronary artery bypass grafting (CABG) mechanical valve MVR done 6 months back on therapeutic anticoagulation has presented with sudden onset breathlessness at rest and circulatory failure. You suspected a stuck valve, how will you perform 2D echocardiography to make a diagnosis?**

**Ans.**

Use fluoroscopy wherever it is available to find out the stuck valve. It is a medical as well as surgical emergency.

*Echocardiography findings:*

- Impaired/stuck leaflet
- Echogenicity in valve region (thrombus?)
- Pathologic flow pattern on color Doppler
- Elevated gradients
- Pressure half-time (mitral valve) on continuous wave Doppler (CWD)

*Quantification of Obstruction* ***(Table 1)***

**TABLE 1:** Various echocardiographic parameters for quantification of prosthetic valve obstruction.

| *Aortic valve* | *Mitral valve* |
|---|---|
| • Morphologic findings<br>• Symptoms<br>• Velocity >3.0 m/s<br>• Doppler velocity index <0.3 (Doppler velocity index = VLVOT/VProsth valve) | • Morphologic findings<br>• Symptoms<br>• Mean gradients (>6–8 mm Hg)<br>• PHT >130 ms |

(PHT: pulmonary hypertension; VLVOT: valsalva left ventricular outflow tract; VProsth: prosthetic valve)

**Q2. What is the differentiation between pannus and thrombus?**

**Ans.**

*Differentiation Pannus Versus Thrombus*

It is important to differentiate between the two as management completely changes the trial of medical vs surgical **(Flowchart 1)**.

Indirect differentiation between pannus and thrombus is discussed in **Table 2.**

**Q3. What are the echocardiographic findings in a bioprosthetic valve?**

**Ans.**

- Thickened calcified leaflets
- Reduced mobility
- Elevated gradients
- Prolonged pressure half-time (mitral prosthesis)
- Turbulent flow
- Dilated left atrium with spontaneous contrast (mitral prosthesis)
- LV dysfunction (eventually)

**Q4. You will make a decision to thrombolysis vs urgent surgery?**

**Ans.**

When faced with prosthetic valve obstruction, whether to proceed with thrombolysis or urgent surgery depends on several critical factors. Here's a structured approach to decision-making:

*Factors Favoring Fibrinolysis*

- *Clinical features:*
  - *High surgical risk:* Patients who are deemed high-risk candidates for surgery due to comorbidities or frailty.
  - *New York Heart Association (NYHA) functional class I to III:* Patients with relatively stable symptoms or mild to moderate functional impairment.
  - *No contraindication to fibrinolysis:* Absence of conditions that would preclude fibrinolytic therapy, such as recent major bleeding.

**Flowchart 1:** Differentiating between pannus and thrombus as a cause of prosthetic valve obstruction.

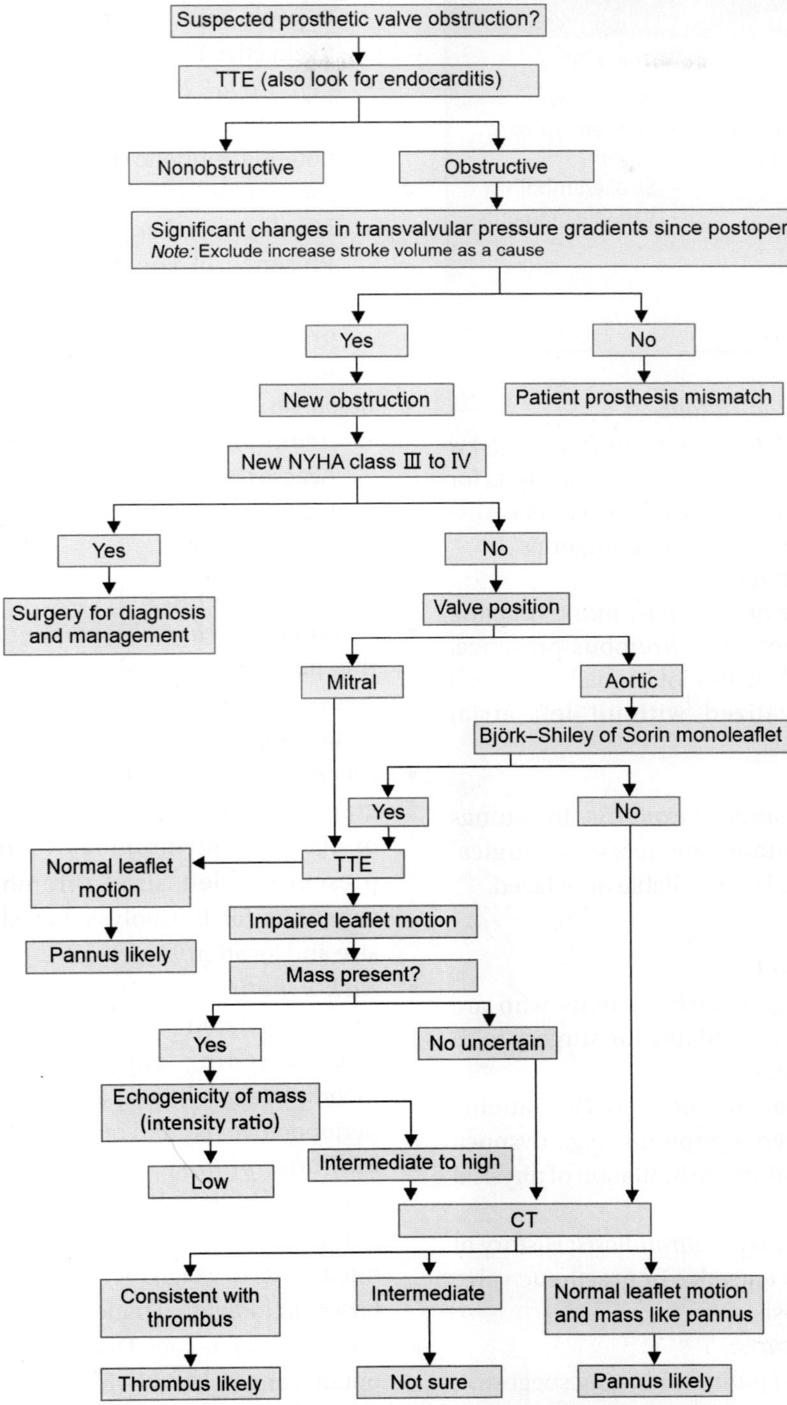


*Note:* Intensity ratio mass/prosthesis; ≤0.45 low, >0.45 high.

(CT: computed tomography; NYHA: New York Heart Association; TTE: transthoracic echocardiogram)

**TABLE 2:** Indirect signs and symptoms differentiating between pannus and thrombus.

| *Pannus* | *Thrombus* |
|---|---|
| • International normalized ratio (INR) in the therapeutic range<br>• Slow onset of symptoms<br>• Higher age of prosthesis<br>• Stable gradients | • INR too low<br>• Sudden symptom onset<br>• Stroke/embolism<br>• Variable gradients |

- *Concurrent indications:*
  - *No need for other cardiac surgery:* Absence of concurrent indications for major cardiac surgery such as CABG and other valve/aortic surgeries.
- *Imaging findings:*
  - *Presence of thrombus mass:* Imaging consistent with thrombus presence, especially if the clot is small ($\leq$0.8 $cm^2$) and localized without left atrial thrombus.
- *Resources:*
  - *Limited surgical expertise:* In settings where immediate access to surgical expertise is unavailable or delayed.

*Factors Favoring Surgery*

- *Clinical features:*
  - *Low surgical risk:* Patients who are suitable candidates for surgery with low perioperative risk.
  - *NYHA functional class IV:* Patients with severe symptoms (e.g., dyspnea at rest and severe limitation of physical activity).
  - *Recurrent valve thrombosis:* History of multiple episodes of prosthetic valve thrombosis.
- *Imaging features:*
  - *Suspected pannus:* Imaging suggestive of pannus formation obstructing the valve.
  - *Large clot (>0.8 $cm^2$):* Presence of a large thrombus that is not amenable to effective fibrinolysis.
  - *Left atrial thrombus:* Presence of thrombus in the left atrium, indicating potential embolic risk.
- *Concurrent indications:*
  - *Need for other cardiac surgery:* Presence of concomitant coronary artery disease necessitating CABG or other structural heart disease requiring surgical intervention.
- *Resources:*
  - *Availability of surgical expertise:* Access to experienced cardiac surgical teams capable of performing urgent valve surgery.

*Decision-making Process*

- *Assessment of clinical condition:* Evaluate the patient's hemodynamic stability, symptoms (NYHA class), and overall clinical status.
- *Imaging evaluation:* Utilize echocardiography to assess the nature and extent of obstruction (thrombus vs. pannus), presence of left atrial thrombus, and suitability for fibrinolysis based on clot size and location.
- *Risk-benefit analysis:* Consider the risks associated with both fibrinolysis (e.g., bleeding complications, and incomplete resolution) and surgery (e.g., perioperative risk and recovery time).
- *Multidisciplinary approach:* Consult with a multidisciplinary team including cardiologists, cardiac surgeons, and intensivists to weigh the risks and benefits based on individual patient factors.
- *Patient preference:* Discuss treatment options and risks with the patient or their surrogate, considering their preferences and values.

Ultimately, the decision between thrombolysis and urgent surgery for prosthetic valve obstruction should be individualized based on these considerations, aiming to optimize patient outcomes and minimize risks.

**Q5. Enlist urgent therapy for stuck valves.**

**Ans.**

When dealing with a stuck prosthetic valve, whether due to thrombosis, pannus formation, or a combination of both, urgent intervention is crucial to manage symptoms and prevent complications. Here is an outline of the urgent therapies based on the underlying pathology:

- *Presumptive thrombosis*:
  - *Indications for urgent intervention:*
    - *NYHA class IV symptoms or hemodynamic instability:* Patients experiencing severe symptoms such as dyspnea at rest, orthopnea, or cardiogenic shock.
    - *Size and mobility of thrombus:* Mobile thrombus ≥0.3 cm in diameter or a large nonmobile thrombus (≥0.8 $cm^2$) on imaging.
  - *Preferred intervention:*
    - *Surgery:* Surgery is typically recommended over fibrinolysis for patients with obstructive left-sided mechanical valve thrombosis. It allows direct visualization and removal of thrombus or pannus, providing immediate relief.
- *Presumptive pannus:*
  - *Indications for urgent intervention:*
    - *Moderately to severely symptomatic obstruction:* Patients with symptoms suggestive of valve obstruction due to pannus formation.
  - *Treatment options:*
    - *Surgery:* Surgical intervention is the preferred approach for patients with symptomatic pannus obstructing the valve. It allows for definitive management by removing or correcting the obstructing tissue.
    - *Palliative care:* In cases where surgical intervention is not feasible or appropriate due to patient factors or advanced disease, palliative measures may be considered to alleviate symptoms and improve comfort.
- *Presumptive thrombosis plus pannus*:
  - *Indications for urgent intervention:*
    - *Moderately to severely symptomatic obstruction with mixed etiology:* Patients presenting with symptoms suggestive of obstruction from both thrombus and pannus.
  - *Treatment options:*
    - *Surgery:* Surgery remains the preferred option due to the complexity of the obstruction involving both thrombus and pannus. It allows for comprehensive management by addressing both components directly.
    - *Fibrinolysis:* Fibrinolytic therapy may be considered in hemodynamically stable patients with clear evidence of predominant thrombus and where surgery is not immediately available or feasible. However, its efficacy in resolving combined thrombotic and pannus obstructions is limited.

CHAPTER 13

# Pericardial Disease (Effusion, Tamponade, and Tamponade Physiology)

Gourav Mittal

## INTRODUCTION

A pericardial effusion is commonly detected using both transthoracic echocardiography (TTE) and transesophageal echocardiography (TEE). While most pericardial effusions are small and of no clinical consequence, larger effusions necessitate further evaluation to determine their etiology and assess for hemodynamic consequences, such as pericardial tamponade.

## ROLE OF ECHOCARDIOGRAPHY

- *Detection and characterization of pericardial effusion:*
  - Echocardiography can identify the presence and size of pericardial effusion.
  - It helps in characterizing the effusion (e.g., loculated vs. free-flowing, echogenicity indicating the presence of blood or pus).
- *Identifying findings consistent with tamponade:*
  - Echocardiographic signs of tamponade include:
    - Right atrial and right ventricular diastolic collapse
    - Plethoric inferior vena cava without respiratory variation
    - Exaggerated respiratory variation in mitral and tricuspid inflow velocities (pulsus paradoxus)
- *Guiding pericardiocentesis:*
  - Echocardiography is invaluable for guiding the needle during pericardiocentesis to ensure accurate and safe removal of pericardial fluid.
  - It helps in identifying the optimal site for puncture and in monitoring the procedure to avoid complications.

## WHAT IS IMPORTANCE OF PERICARDIUM IN HEALTHY MAN?

- It limits the distension of myocardium.
- It facilitates interaction and coupling of the ventricles/atria.
- It also facilitates twist and torsion of heart.
- It contains fluid whose normal quantity is <50 mL.

## BRIEF ABOUT TYPES OF PERICARDIAL EFFUSION ALONG WITH POSSIBLE ETIOLOGY?

**Table 1** shows the types and possible etiology of pericardial effusion.

## ECHOCARDIOGRAPHIC DIAGNOSIS OF PERICARDIAL EFFUSION

- *Identifying pericardial effusion:*
  - *Echo-free space:* Measure the echo-free space surrounding the epicardium

**TABLE 1:** Types and possible etiology of pericardial effusion.

| ***Transudative*** | ***Exudative*** | ***Hemorrhagic*** | ***Malignant*** |
|---|---|---|---|
| Congestive heart failure, myxedema, nephrotic syndrome | Tuberculosis, spread from empyema | Trauma, rupture of aneurysms, malignant effusion, iatrogenic | Often hemorrhagic |

during end-diastole. This space indicates the presence of pericardial fluid.

- *Multiple views:* Use various echocardiographic views, especially subcostal views, to obtain a comprehensive assessment.
- *Atypical views:* Employ atypical views to visualize areas around the right ventricle, which can help identify fluid in less accessible areas.

- *Quantifying pericardial effusion:*
    - *Detection threshold:* Pericardial fluid is typically detectable on echocardiography when it exceeds 15–35 mL, as it causes separation of the pericardial layers.
- *Follow-up:*
    - *Consistent views:* To monitor pericardial effusion, use the same echocardiographic views as initially used for diagnosis.
    - *Measurement consistency:* Measure the effusion in the same region each time to ensure accurate comparison.
    - *Visual assessment:* Regularly assess the pericardial effusion visually to observe changes in the amount of fluid over time.

## QUANTIFICATION OF PERICARDIAL EFFUSION BY ECHOCARDIOGRAPHY

- *Small effusion:*
    - *Distance between layers:* Less than 1 mm
    - *Volume:* Approximately 300 mL

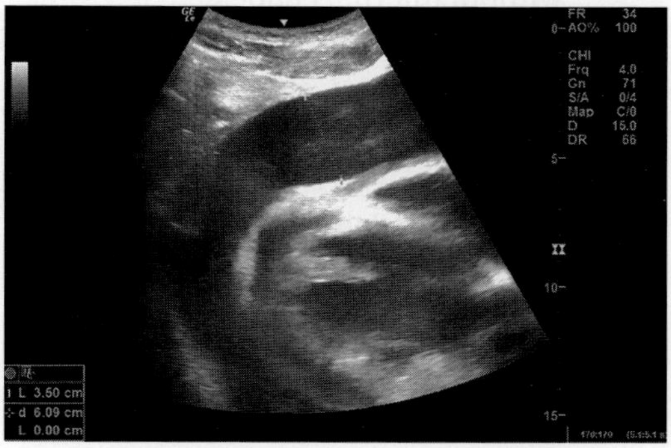

**Fig. 1:** Very large pericardial effusion.

- *Moderate effusion:*
    - *Distance between layers:* 10–20 mm
    - *Volume:* Approximately 500–700 mL
- *Large effusion:*
    - *Distance between layers:* Greater than 20 mm
    - *Volume:* More than 700 mL
- *Very large effusion* **(*Fig. 1*)**:
    - *Distance between layers:* Greater than 30 mm
    - *Additional feature:* Presence of constriction sign

## HOW AMOUNT AND ECHO CHARACTERISTICS OF EFFUSION HELPS IN NARROW DOWN DIFFERENTIALS?

- *Causes of large effusions usually:* Neoplastic, uremic, TB, and myxedema
- *Causes of regional effusions:* Postoperative, trauma, and purulent

## CHARACTERISTICS OF PERICARDIAL EFFUSION ON ECHOCARDIOGRAPHY

- *Anechoic effusion:*
  - Likely *transudate*
  - Appears as a simple, clear fluid without internal echoes
- *Increased echogenicity, stranding, septations, pericardial thickening, and/or masses:*
  - Associated with *exudative effusions*
  - Often related to underlying conditions such as *infection* or *malignancy*
  - These features suggest a more complex fluid composition and may indicate additional pathology

## HOW IS ECHO HELPFUL IN MANAGING PERICARDIAL EFFUSION?

*It is helpful in following way:*

- Establish the diagnosis
- Help to find its cause
- Hemodynamic importance
- Direct pericardiocentesis

## DIFFERENTIAL DIAGNOSIS OF ECHO FREE SURROUNDINGS OF EPICARDIUM?

- *Pleural effusion:*
  - *Location:* Posterior to the descending aorta.
  - *Identification:* Distinguishing pleural effusion from pericardial effusion can be done by noting the location relative to the descending aorta.
- *Epicardial fat:*
  - *Characteristics:*
    - Follows the normal motion of the pericardium.
    - Often associated with abdominal fat.
    - Not completely echo-free; appears as low-intensity echoes.
    - Absent above the right atrium, but usually prominent in the atrioventricular groove and around the atrial appendages.
- *Pericardial cyst:*
  - *Characteristics:* A well-defined, often thin-walled, fluid-filled sac located within the pericardial space. It usually has a uniform echogenicity and does not change with respiration.
- *Ascites:*
  - *Location:* Fluid in the peritoneal cavity, which can sometimes extend into the pericardial space.
  - *Identification:* Differentiation can be made based on the location of the fluid and its relationship to other structures. Ascitic fluid is usually in the abdominal cavity rather than the pericardial space.

*Key differentiators:*

- *Pericardial effusion:* Anterior to the descending aorta
- *Pleural effusion:* Posterior to the descending aorta

## WHAT ARE THE BASICS TERMINOLOGY RELATED TO PERICARDIAL EFFUSION ONE SHOULD KNOW?

- *Tamponade:* Intrapericardial fluid
- *Constriction:* "Stiff" pericardial sac
- *Effusive constrictive:* "Stiff" pericardial sac + fluid

*Echocardiographic signs of cardiac tamponade **(Table 2)**:*

**TABLE 2:** Various echocardiographic features and their sensitivity and specificity for diagnosing cardiac tamponade.

| ***Echocardiographic feature*** | ***Sensitivity*** | ***Specificity*** |
|---|---|---|
| Large pericardial effusion with swinging heart | NA | NA |
| Diastolic collapse of the right atrium (RA) | 50–100% | 33–100% |
| Duration of diastolic collapse of the RA as ratio on the cardiac cycle length >0.34 | >90% | 100% |
| Diastolic collapse of the right ventricle | 48–100% | 72–100% |
| Respiratory changes of the mitral E velocity >25%, tricuspid E velocity >40% | NA | NA |
| Inferior vena cava plethora (dilatation >20 mm and <50% reduction of diameter with respiratory phases) | 97% | 40% |

(NA: not available)

*Chamber collapse in cardiac tamponade:*

- *General principle:*
    - Lower pressure cardiac chambers (atria) collapse before higher pressure chambers (ventricles)
    - The compressive effect is more evident during the phase of the cardiac cycle when the filling pressure within a cavity is lower—systole for the atria and diastole for the ventricles
- *Right atrial chamber collapse (inversion):*
    - *Onset:* Right atrial collapse typically begins in late diastole.
    - *Clinical correlation:* This collapse often precedes more obvious clinical signs of cardiac tamponade.
    - *Sensitivity and specificity:*
        - The sign is sensitive but not highly specific for cardiac tamponade.
        - Specificity improves if the duration of right atrial collapse exceeds 30% of the cardiac cycle.

*Right ventricular chamber collapse (inversion):*

- *Onset and timing:* Right ventricular wall inversion typically occurs in early diastole, when intracavitary RV pressure and volume are at their lowest.
- *Progression:* As the hemodynamics of tamponade worsen, right ventricular wall inversion extends further into diastole, resulting in a longer duration of collapse.
- *Echocardiographic findings:*
    - This finding is often best visualized in the parasternal long-axis view.
    - Look for transient "dimpling" of the right ventricular outflow tract anterior wall, particularly noted when the mitral valve opens.

*Left atrial and left ventricular chamber compression:*

- *Postcardiac surgery:*
    - Left atrial and left ventricular chamber compression is primarily associated with loculated collections following cardiac surgery.
- *Severe pulmonary hypertension:*
    - Although rare, circumferential pericardial effusion can lead to left ventricular diastolic compression in the context of severe pulmonary hypertension.

*Large left pleural effusions and tamponade physiology:*

- *Tamponade physiology:* Large left pleural effusions can occasionally mimic tamponade physiology, sometimes showing echocardiographic signs such as right ventricular diastolic collapse.
- *Differentiation challenges:* In these cases, pericardial effusion is often present, making it challenging to determine which fluid collection is more significant.
- *Management approach:* Clinical practice generally favors initially draining the more accessible pleural fluid. After this, both clinical assessment and echocardiography are used to re-evaluate the situation and determine the need for further intervention.

## CLINICAL VIGNETTE

A 50-year-old male, chronic smoker, known case of carcinoma lung on chemotherapy, bedridden at home, presented to emergency with chief complaint of breathlessness, dry cough, dizziness, decreased urine output. On initial evaluation, his temperature was 98°F, HR 120 bpm, BP 74/46 mm Hg, and oxygen saturation ($SpO_2$) 86% on room air. ECG shows low-voltage QRS complexes with electrical alternans. On auscultation, heart sounds not clearly audible. You are suspecting pericardial effusion/tamponade.

**Q1. How you will confirm the diagnosis, what is tamponade physiology on 2D echocardiography?**

**Ans.** *Important note on pericardial tamponade diagnosis:*

- *Echocardiographic findings:* No single echocardiographic finding is diagnostic of pericardial tamponade.
- *Diagnosis:*
  - The diagnosis of pericardial tamponade requires clinical evidence of hemodynamic compromise.
  - Echocardiography supports the diagnosis by identifying signs of tamponade but cannot establish it independently.

*View needed:* Parasternal long axis (PLAX)–RV collapse

- *Pericardial effusion presence:* On echo, a pericardial effusion appears as an anechoic space between the heart and pericardial sac. The acuity of the pericardial effusion is more important than the size of the effusion.
  With larger pericardial effusions swaying of the heart is often present.
- *Right ventricular (RV) diastolic collapse* ***(Fig. 2)***:
  - RV collapse during diastole is specific for cardiac tamponade
  - 2D assessment—subcostal view
    Look for RV-free wall collapse while the tricuspid valve is open. Watch as the ventricle is filling. Look for an indent anywhere in the free wall caused by the effusion.

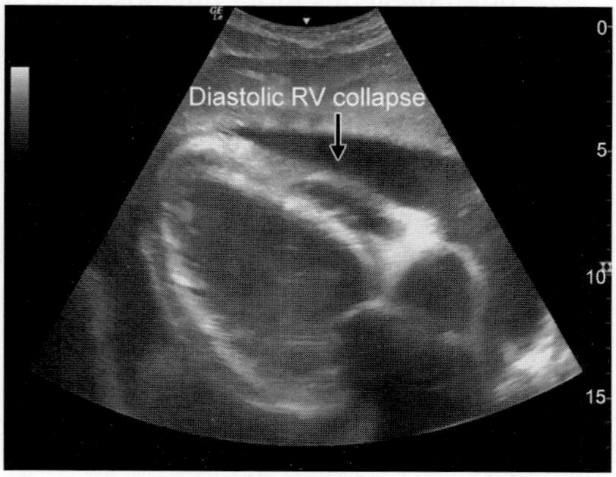


**Fig. 2:** Large pericardial effusion with diastolic RV collapse. (RV: right ventricular)

- *M-mode assessment—PLAX view:*
    - Place the cursor over the RV and mitral valve. Evaluate the M-mode tracing to see if the RV collapse occurs as the mitral valve is open.
    - *Alternative method:* Apply ECG leads and look for collapse in diastole: between the T and QRS waves. Early collapse will appear just before or right on the QRS.
- *Right atrial (RA) collapse in systole:*
    - RA collapse during systole is an early sign of cardiac tamponade.
    - Subcostal/A4C view scroll carefully through the 2D clip, and look for right atrial collapse while the tricuspid valve is closed.
- *Distended inferior vena cava (IVC):* Due to elevated right atrial pressure, the IVC becomes plethoric with minimal respiratory variation.
    - However, this is a common finding in mechanically ventilated patients and needs to be taken in clinical context.
- *Respiratory variation of the mitral valve (MV) and tricuspid valve (TV) inflow patterns:*
    - Least sensitive sign for tamponade
    - Ideally a respiratory lead and ECG leads are applied.
    - In the apical 4 chamber (AP4), place the pulse wave Doppler marker just distal to the mitral valve or tricuspid valve.
    - Decrease the sweep speed to around 25 mm/s to see more beats on one screen.
    - Measure velocity max and velocity min with respiration (change/max).
    - A 25% decrease in the MV inflow velocities correlates with tamponade.
    - A 40% decrease in TV inflow velocities correlates with tamponade.
    - It is not valid in atrial fibrillation and other arrhythmias.

*PS:* Both RA and RV compressions are reduced when right-sided pressures are increased. The presence of RV hypertrophy reduces compression effect, and the volume status of the patient may influence the degree of compression.

**Q2. How does echo help you manage this case?**

**Ans.**

- *Preferred method for guidance:* Echocardiography is the preferred imaging modality for guiding pericardiocentesis due to its ability to provide real-time visualization.
- *Scanning and preparation:*
    - *Scanning:* The patient is examined from multiple views (parasternal, apical, and subcostal) to identify the safest site, angle, and depth for needle insertion.
    - *Site marking:* The puncture site is marked, and measurements are taken to ensure a safe distance (>10 mm) for needle insertion.
    - *Angle determination:* The optimal angle for needle insertion is determined before sterile skin preparation.
- *Confirmation and procedure setup:*
    - *Preprocedure confirmation:* After sterile preparation and equipment setup (including the probe in a sterile sheath), the operator confirms the site, angle, and depth for needle insertion with a repeat scan.
    - *Real-time guidance:* While real-time guidance during the actual puncture is not always necessary, it helps ensure accurate needle tip positioning.

**Q3. Discuss the timeline of complications after MI and their ECHO characteristics.**

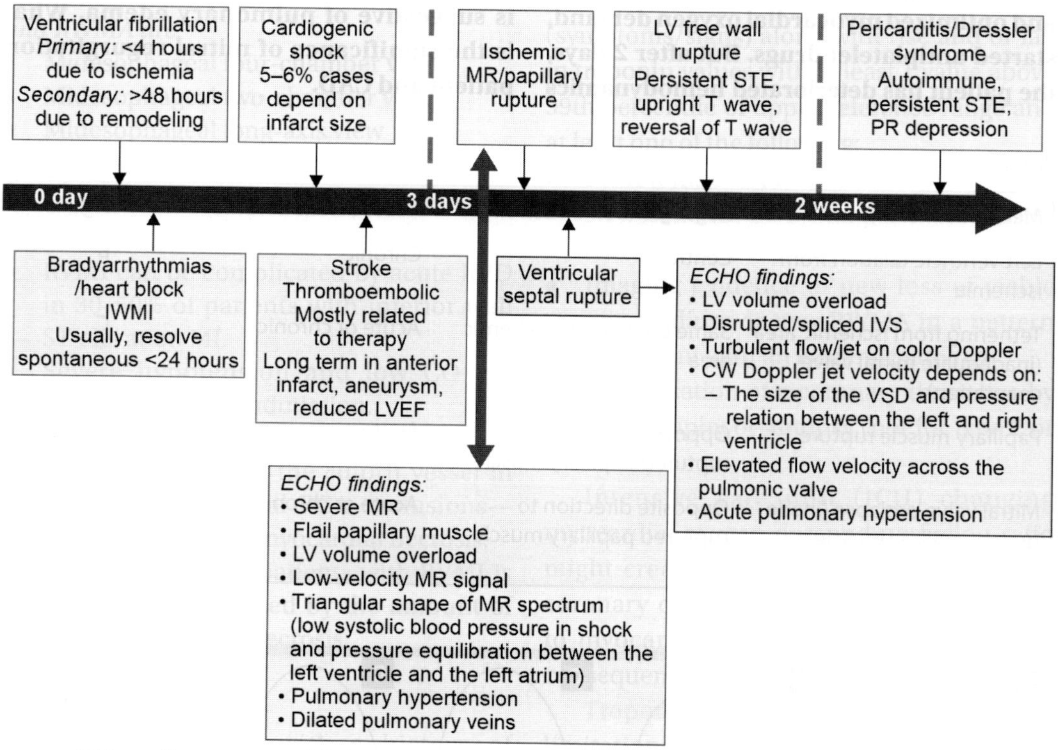


(CW: continuous wave; IVS: intervening sequence; IWMI: inferior wall myocardial infarction; LVEF: left ventricular ejection fraction; STE: ST-segment elevation; VSD: ventricular septal defect)

## ASSESSMENT OF MYOCARDIAL ISCHEMIA AND VIABILITY USING TISSUE DOPPLER AND DEFORMATION IMAGING

Tissue Doppler imaging (TDI) and strain rate imaging are indeed valuable tools in ECHO for assessing myocardial function. They provide quantitative data that can complement traditional ECHO assessments, offering insights into myocardial mechanics and contractile function.

- *TDI:*
    - TDI utilizes Doppler principles to measure the velocity of myocardial tissue motion. By placing the Doppler sample volume on the myocardium, TDI can measure velocities along the longitudinal, radial, and circumferential axes of the heart. This allows for the assessment of regional and global myocardial function.
    - TDI is particularly useful for detecting abnormalities in myocardial contraction and relaxation, making it a valuable tool in diagnosing various cardiac conditions, including myocardial ischemia, cardiomyopathies, and heart failure.
- *Strain rate imaging:*
    - Strain rate imaging is a technique that measures the rate of deformation of myocardial tissue. It provides information about the velocity

gradient within the myocardium, indicating how quickly the tissue is stretching or contracting.

- By quantifying the rate of myocardial deformation, strain rate imaging can detect subtle changes in myocardial function that may not be evident with traditional ECHO measures.
- Strain rate imaging is particularly useful for assessing myocardial mechanics, identifying regions of abnormal contractility, and evaluating the effects of ischemia or fibrosis on cardiac function.
- Strain and strain rate imaging have been shown to be able to differentiate between transmural and nontransmural infarcts.
- Patients with transmural infarction were shown to have significantly lower circumferential and longitudinal strain and strain rates compared with those with subendocardial infarction, with no significant differences in radial strain.
- In MI, transmural extension of scar distribution in the infarct zone is proportionally related to the reduction in systolic function measured by the radial transmural velocity gradient or by strain rate imaging.
- Measurement of both systolic and postsystolic deformation both at rest and during a graded dobutamine infusion may help distinguish between transmural and nontransmural infarcts.

CHAPTER 15

# Infective Endocarditis

Gourav Mittal

## INDICATIONS FOR TRANSESOPHAGEAL ECHOCARDIOGRAPHY IN SUSPECTED ENDOCARDITIS

Transesophageal echocardiography (TOE) plays a crucial role in the diagnosis and management of infective endocarditis (IE), especially in cases where a more detailed assessment is necessary beyond transthoracic echocardiography (TTE). Following are the key indications for performing TOE in suspected endocarditis:

- *Negative or inconclusive TTE:* TOE should be performed if there is clinical suspicion of endocarditis despite a negative or suboptimal quality TTE.
- *Prosthetic valve or intracardiac device:* TOE is recommended as a routine examination in suspected endocarditis involving prosthetic valves or intracardiac devices due to the higher likelihood of complications and the potential limitations of TTE in visualizing these areas.
- *Complications assessment:* Following a positive TTE, TOE is indicated to assess for local complications such as abscess formation, valve perforation, or other intracardiac pathology that may require more precise visualization than TTE can provide.
- *Isolated right-sided native valve endocarditis (with good-quality TTE):* In cases of isolated right-sided native valve endocarditis where the TTE quality is adequate and there is no suspicion of local complications, TOE may not be routinely necessary. However, clinical judgment should guide this decision.

## CLINICAL VIGNETTE

A 20-year-old male, a chronic intravenous (IV) drug abuser presented with long-standing fever along with intermittent chest pain and dyspnea on exertion. He denied any history of pain abdomen, burning micturition, and cough with expectoration. On examination, peripheries were warm with a bounding pulse and vitals showed tachycardia, tachypnea, and hypotension. Fluid resuscitation started along with suspicion of IE was there; a two-dimensional (2D) echo was ordered.

**Q1. Discuss risk factors and describe findings in a case of IE on echocardiography (ECHO).**

**Ans.** Various risk factors are there which can predispose to IE including cardiac and noncardiac **(Table 1)**.

*ECHO:* The sensitivity of TTE for identifying endocarditis is relatively low (55% for native valves and lower still for prosthetic valves). Therefore, if TTE is inconclusive and clinical suspicion is high, the patient should undergo TOE **(Flowchart 1)**.

**TABLE 1:** Various cardiac and noncardiac risk factors for development of IE.

| ***Cardiac risk factors*** | ***Noncardiac risk factors*** |
|---|---|
| • Bicuspid aortic valve<br>• Mitral valve prolapse<br>• Rheumatic valve disease<br>• Congenital heart disease<br>• Prior infective endocarditis<br>• Implanted cardiac devices<br>• Prosthetic heart valves | • IV drug use<br>• Long-term hemodialysis<br>• Chronic liver disease<br>• Malignancy<br>• Advanced age<br>• Corticosteroid use<br>• Poorly controlled diabetes mellitus<br>• Long-term venous access device<br>• Immunocompromised state |

**Flowchart 1:** How to proceed with ECHO in suspected cases of IE.

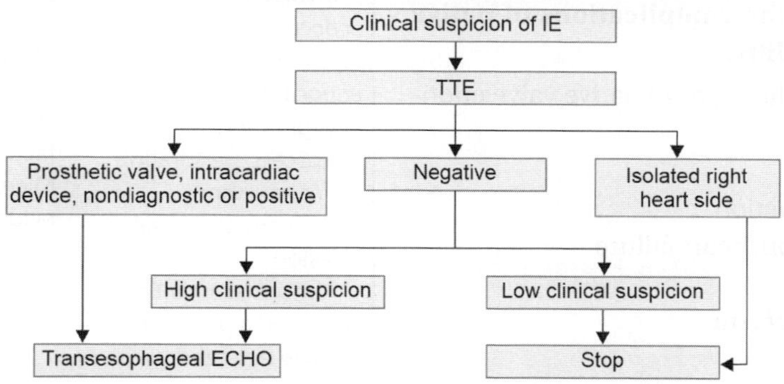


*Views:* Parasternal long axis (PLAX), parasternal short axis (PSAX), apical 4 chamber (A4C), apical 2 chamber (A2C)—look for valves thickening; mobile structures attach to them.

## Q2. Algorithm combing ECHO, modified Duke, and newer modalities in diagnosis of IE?

**Flowchart 2:** Combining dukes, ECHO, and advanced modalities for diagnosing IE.

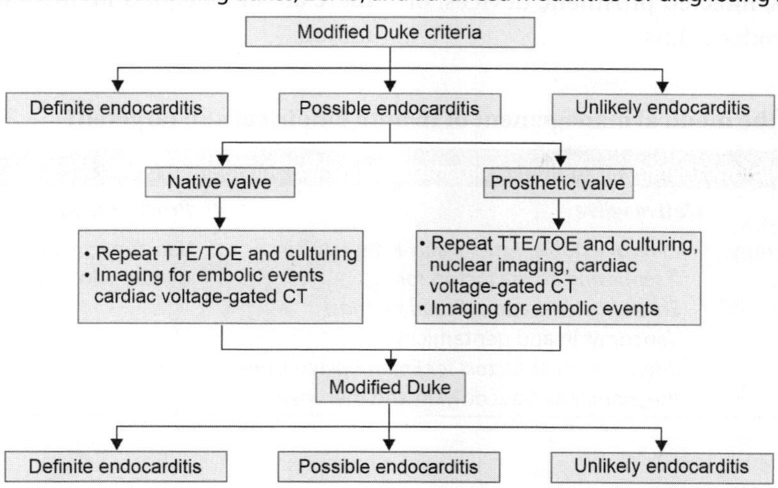

**Q3. In ECHO, what else one should look for in case of IE?**

**Ans.** One should look for:

- Involvement of other valves
- Regurgitations and resulting volume overload
- Myocardial function (right + left)
- Pericardial/pleural effusion
- Valve obstruction (large vegetation—rare)
- Coronary embolization of vegetation leading to wall motion abnormalities (rare)

**Q4: What are the complications of native valve endocarditis?**

**Ans.** The complications of native valve endocarditis are:

- Embolism
- Valve destruction
- Regurgitation/heart failure
- Abscess
- Pseudoaneurysm
- Perforation
- Fistula
- Mycotic aneurysm

**Q5. What are the criteria to diagnose IE?**

**Ans.** Diagnosis of endocarditis is made using the modified Duke criteria **(Flowchart 1)**. However, this approach has low sensitivity and may not account for culture-negative endocarditis, infected prosthetic devices, or right-sided endocarditis.

Clinical suspicion of endocarditis should trigger blood culture sampling and ECHO.

| *Major* | *Minor* |
|---|---|
| *Positive blood cultures:*<br>• Typical organisms from two separate samples<br>• Persistently positive blood cultures with typical organisms<br>• Evidence of endocardial involvement<br>*Echocardiographic or CT features for endocarditis:*<br>• Vegetation<br>• Abscess, perforation or aneurysm<br>• New prosthetic valve lesion<br>• Abnormal activity around a prosthetic valve detected by CT imaging<br>• Paravalvular lesions detected by cardiac CT | • Predisposing risk factor<br>• Fever >38°C<br>• *Vascular phenomena:* Arterial emboli, splenic infarction, mycotic aneurysms, intracranial hemorrhage, Janeway lesions<br>• *Immunological phenomena:* Osler's nodes, Roth's spots, positive rheumatoid factor<br>• Microbiological evidence that is not in keeping with major criteria |

Endocarditis is likely when there are two major, one major and three minor, or five minor criteria. Endocarditis is possible when there are one major and one minor or three minor.

**Q6. What is the medical management of IE both empirical and targeted?**

**TABLE 2:** Antibiotic therapy according to organism suspected and identified.

| | *Native valve* | *Prosthetic valve* |
|---|---|---|
| Empirical therapy | • *Clinically stable:* Amoxicillin + gentamicin<br>• *If septic and no risk factors for Enterobacteriaceae or Pseudomonas*: Vancomycin and gentamicin<br>• *If septic and risk factors for Enterobacteriaceae or Pseudomonas:* Vancomycin and meropenem | Vancomycin, rifampicin and gentamicin |

*Contd...*

*Contd...*

| | ***Native valve*** | ***Prosthetic valve*** |
|---|---|---|
| *Staphylococcus endocarditis* | • Flucloxacillin for MSSA<br>• Vancomycin and rifampicin for MRSA, vancomycin-susceptible and rifampicin susceptible<br>• Daptomycin and rifampicin or gentamicin MRSA, VRSA, daptomycin-susceptible, or patient unable to tolerate vancomycin | • Flucloxacillin and rifampicin and gentamicin for MSSA, rifampicin-susceptible<br>• Vancomycin and rifampicin and gentamicin for MRSA, VSSA, or penicillin allergy<br>• Daptomycin and rifampicin and gentamicin for MRSA, VRSA and daptomycin-susceptible or patient unable to tolerate vancomycin |
| *Streptococcal endocarditis* | Benzylpenicillin + gentamicin<br>Vancomycin + gentamicin or teicoplanin + gentamicin if penicillin allergy | |
| *Enterococcal endocarditis* | • Amoxicillin or benzylpenicillin + gentamicin<br>• Vancomycin and gentamicin if penicillin allergy<br>• Teicoplanin and gentamicin if renal impairment | |
| HACEK endocarditis | • Amoxicillin and gentamicin for amoxicillin-sensitive and beta-lactamase-negative organisms<br>• Ceftriaxone and gentamicin for amoxicillin-resistant and beta-lactamase-positive organisms or penicillin allergy | |
| *Bartonella endocarditis* | • Amoxicillin and gentamicin<br>• Doxycycline and gentamicin if penicillin allergy | |
| Gram-negative endocarditis | Changing resistance patterns mean that recommendations may vary between amoxicillin, cephalosporin or meropenem together with gentamicin | |
| Fungal endocarditis | • Caspofungin or amphotericin B and flucytosine for *Candida*<br>• Voriconazole or amphotericin B and flucytosine for *Aspergillus* | |

(HACEK: *Haemophilus*, *Aggregatibacter*, *Cardiobacterium*, *Eikenella*, and *Kingella*; MRSA: methicillin-resistant *Staphylococcus aureus*; MSSA: methicillin-susceptible *Staphylococcus aureus*; VRSA: vancomycin-resistant *Staphylococcus aureus*)

## Q7. What are the indications for surgical management?

**TABLE 3:** Indication for surgery in patients with IE.

| ***Recommendations*** | ***COR*** | ***LOE*** |
|---|---|---|
| ***What are the indications for surgery in patients with IE?*** | | |
| Patients with IE who present with valve dysfunction resulting in symptoms of heart failure—independent of completion of antibiotics course | I | B |
| Patients with left-sided IE caused by *S. aureus*, fungal, or other highly resistant microorganisms—independent of completion of antibiotics course | I | B |
| Patients with IE complicated by heart block, annular or aortic abscess, or destructive penetrating lesions—independent of completion of antibiotics course | I | B |
| Patients with evidence of persistent infection as manifested by persistent bacteremia or fever lasting longer than 5–7 days after initiation of appropriate antimicrobial therapy | I | B |

*Contd...*

*Contd...*

| *Recommendations* | *COR* | *LOE* |
|---|---|---|
| Surgery is recommended for patients with PVE and relapsing infection (defined as recurrence of bacteremia after a complete course of appropriate antibiotics and subsequently negative blood cultures) without other identifiable sources for portal of infection | IIa | C |
| Is reasonable in patients with IE who present with recurrent emboli and persistent vegetations despite appropriate antibiotic therapy | IIa | B |
| Urgent or even emergency surgery may be considered in patients with NVE or PVE who exhibit mobile vegetations >10 mm in length with clinical evidence of embolic phenomena despite appropriate antimicrobial treatment | IIb | B |
| In patients with right-sided IE, surgery should be considered for NVE or PVE when large vegetations are present and there is evidence of persistent infection manifested by persistent bacteremia or fevers lasting longer than 5–7 days after initiation of appropriate antimicrobial therapy, or in those with evidence of septic pulmonary embolism | IIb | B |
| ***When should the patient undergo operation?*** | | |
| Once an indication for surgery is established, the patient should be operated on within days | I | B |
| Earlier surgery (emergency or within 48 hours) is reasonable for patients with large mobile vegetations at imminent risk of embolism | IIa | B |
| In patients with stroke and neurologic deficits, timing is decided by weighing the need for cardiac surgery against the risk of expanding the stroke or provoking intracranial bleeding during the operation | IIa | B |

(NVE: native valve endocarditis; *S. aureus*: *Staphylococcus* aureus; PVE: prosthetic valve endocarditis)

**Q8. What are the types of noninfective/abacterial endocarditis? Describe ECHO findings associated with them.**

**Ans.** *The types of noninfective/abacterial endocarditis:*

- Marantic endocarditis
- Hypercoagulable state
- Libman–Sacks endocarditis
- Antiphospholipid syndrome

*The ECHO findings are:*

- Valve thickening
- Mild or moderate regurgitation
- Small vegetations
- Pericardial effusion

**Q9. What are the ECHO findings of poor outcomes in IE.**

**Ans.** Echocardiography plays a pivotal role in assessing the severity and complications of IE, helping clinicians predict outcomes and guide management. Following are some key echocardiographic findings associated with poor outcomes in IE:

- *Periannular complications:* These include abscess formation, fistulae, pseudoaneurysms, or severe paravalvular leakage, which indicate extensive tissue involvement and potential for worsening infection or hemodynamic instability.
- *Severe left-sided valve regurgitation:* Significant regurgitation, whether aortic or mitral, reflects extensive valve damage and can lead to heart failure or exacerbate existing hemodynamic compromise.
- *Low left ventricular ejection fraction (LVEF):* A reduced LVEF indicates impaired cardiac function, often exacerbated by severe valve regurgitation or myocardial involvement due to IE.
- *Pulmonary hypertension:* Elevated pulmonary pressures suggest right heart

strain due to severe left-sided valve disease or associated complications such as pulmonary emboli or abscesses.

- *Large vegetation (>10 mm):* Larger vegetations are associated with an increased risk of embolization, persistent infection despite therapy, and higher mortality rates.
- *Severe prosthetic valve dysfunction:* Dysfunction such as prosthetic valve obstruction or severe regurgitation indicates failure of the prosthetic valve due to IE, often requiring urgent intervention.
- *Premature mitral valve closure and elevated diastolic pressures:* These signs indicate elevated left atrial pressures due to severe mitral valve regurgitation or other obstructive lesions, contributing to heart failure symptoms and poor outcomes.

*Clinical implications:* Identifying these echocardiographic findings in patients with IE is crucial for risk stratification, therapeutic decision-making, and predicting clinical outcomes. Close monitoring and timely intervention are essential to mitigate the risks associated with these poor prognostic indicators and improve patient outcomes in IE.

**Q10. What is the differential diagnosis of a cardiac infective vegetation noted on echocardiography.**

**Ans.** When evaluating cardiac vegetation, several differential diagnoses should be considered based on clinical context, echocardiographic findings, and patient history. Following are the main differential diagnoses for infective vegetation:

- *Thrombi:* They can form on damaged or prosthetic heart valves, resembling infective vegetation. However, they lack the inflammatory component seen in IE.
- *Chordal rupture:* Chordal rupture can lead to mobile echogenic structures resembling vegetations, especially in the context of mitral valve pathology.
- *Valve fibroelastoma:* Fibroelastomas are rare, benign tumors attached to cardiac valves. They can mimic vegetation on ECHO due to their mobile nature.
- *Myxomatous valve disease:* Myxomatous degeneration of heart valves, such as seen in mitral valve prolapse, can sometimes present with thickened valve leaflets or redundant tissue that may resemble vegetations.
- *Strands:* Strands or fibrinous strands can be present in the heart, particularly in the setting of previous cardiac surgery or inflammation and may appear similar to vegetation.
- *Libman-Sacks lesions (lupus):* In systemic lupus erythematosus (SLE), Libman-Sacks endocarditis can occur, characterized by sterile vegetations on the cardiac valves, often affecting the mitral and aortic valves.
- *Marantic vegetation:* Also known as nonbacterial thrombotic endocarditis (NBTE), marantic vegetations are sterile, fibrin-rich deposits that occur in hypercoagulable states or chronic wasting illnesses, such as malignancies. They can resemble infective vegetation but lack the inflammatory changes.

*Clinical considerations:* Distinguishing between infective vegetation and its differential diagnoses is critical for appropriate management and treatment decisions. ECHO, clinical history (including risk factors for infection and thrombosis), and sometimes histopathological examination are essential in making an accurate diagnosis and guiding therapy in suspected cases of IE.

CHAPTER 16

# Pulmonary Embolism and Deep Vein Thrombosis

*Gourav Mittal, Puneet Khanna*

## INTRODUCTION

In the absence of hypotension or shock, the diagnostic algorithm for patients with suspected pulmonary embolism (PE) relies on D-dimer and CT angiography but not on echocardiography.

In the presence of hypotension or shock, if CT angiography cannot be performed immediately or if the patient is too unstable, echocardiography should be performed straightway to look for right ventricular (RV) dysfunction (RVD).

## KEY POINTS

- Echo RVD is present in 30–56% of normotensive patients with PE.
- All-cause 30-day mortality rate is 5.4–10%, and inhospital mortality rate directly attributed to PE was 1.1–3.3%.
- Cardiogenic shock occurs in ~5% of acute PE cases with a 90-day mortality rate >50%.
- RV cannot acutely overcome a systolic pulmonary artery pressure (PAP) >50 mm Hg.
- Conversely, acute-on-chronic RV failure (RVF) can tolerate significantly higher PAP.

## CLINICAL VIGNETTE

A 30-year-old female presented to emergency with sudden-onset shortness of breath and circulatory failure. She does not have comorbidity but has been on oral contraceptive pills (OCP) for gynecological issues for 3 months. She had a history of leg swelling and leg pain for the last 2 days and partially relived on over-the-counter (OTC) medications. On examination, she is drowsy, has tachycardia with high oxygen requirement, and is on high doses of vasopressors. You suspected PE, but she is too unstable to be shifted for computed tomography pulmonary angiogram (CTPA).

**Q1. How does a two-dimensional (2D) echo help to make a diagnosis certain?**

**Ans.** Background of OCP intake, leg swelling with acute presentation, along with hemodynamic instability D/D must include PE. However, without CTPA, ruling in PE is difficult, but for CTPA, transport is needed which is often not feasible due to hemodynamic instability. Ruling out PE or making diagnosis is important as directed treatment can change outcomes drastically.

Transthoracic echocardiogram (TTE) can help support the diagnosis of PE and can aid in further risk stratification of PE. RV pressure overload and dysfunction caused by acute pulmonary emboli can be detected by echocardiogram. There are multiple echocardiographic parameters that can be found in the presence of acute PE, none of which are completely reliable in diagnosing

PE. Pretest probability (scoring), often needed because certain signs of RV dysfunction, can also be present in the absence of PE and because of other cardiopulmonary diseases. With a sensitivity of approximately 50% and a negative predictive value of 40–50%, a negative echocardiogram does not completely rule out a PE.

In hemodynamically stable patients,

- Echocardiogram to rule out other causes of shortness of breath
- With elevated troponins, an echocardiogram without RVD intermediate-low risk—warrants only anticoagulation compared with patients with RVD (intermediate-high risk) who are at higher risk of hemodynamic decompensation.

Echocardiogram to rule out other causes of shock such as pericardial tamponade, systolic left ventricular (LV) failure, acute severe valvular dysfunction, or aortic dissection.

In suspected PE and high pretest probability, echo findings can also be useful to identify certain findings of RVD **(Fig. 1)** and shortened pulmonary acceleration time **(Fig. 2)** that can warrant emergency reperfusion or pulmonary artery debulking therapies.

*Classical signs on echo suggestive of PE are:*

- Increased right ventricle: Left ventricle size ratio (EDD ratio >0.9/EDA ratio >0.6)

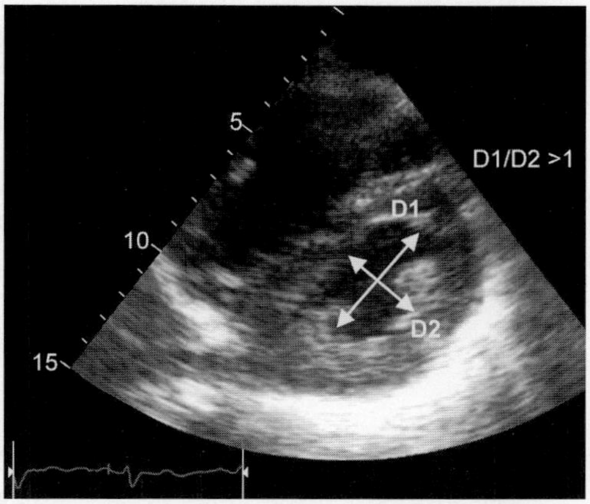


**Fig. 1:** D-shape—measurement of the eccentricity index (D1/D2). Normal value ≤1 and in ACP >1.

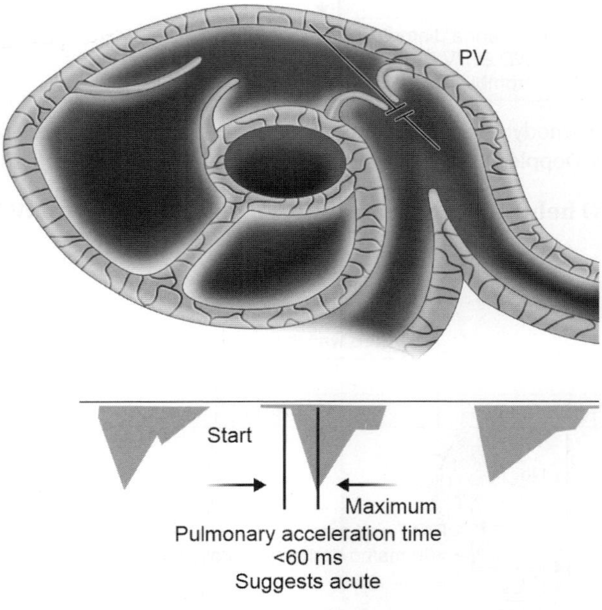


**Fig. 2:** Pulmonary flow acceleration time measurement.

- Abnormal septal motion (D-shaped LV)
- McConnell's sign
- Tricuspid regurgitation (usually <3.4 m/s)
- Elevated pulmonary artery systolic pressure (not >60 mm Hg)
- Decreased tricuspid annular plane systolic excursion (<16 mm)
- Decreased S', pulmonary artery mid-systolic notching (<10 cm/s)
- 60/60 sign

**Q2. What is the algorithm for interpreting the above signs and PE as a likely cause of hemodynamic instability?**

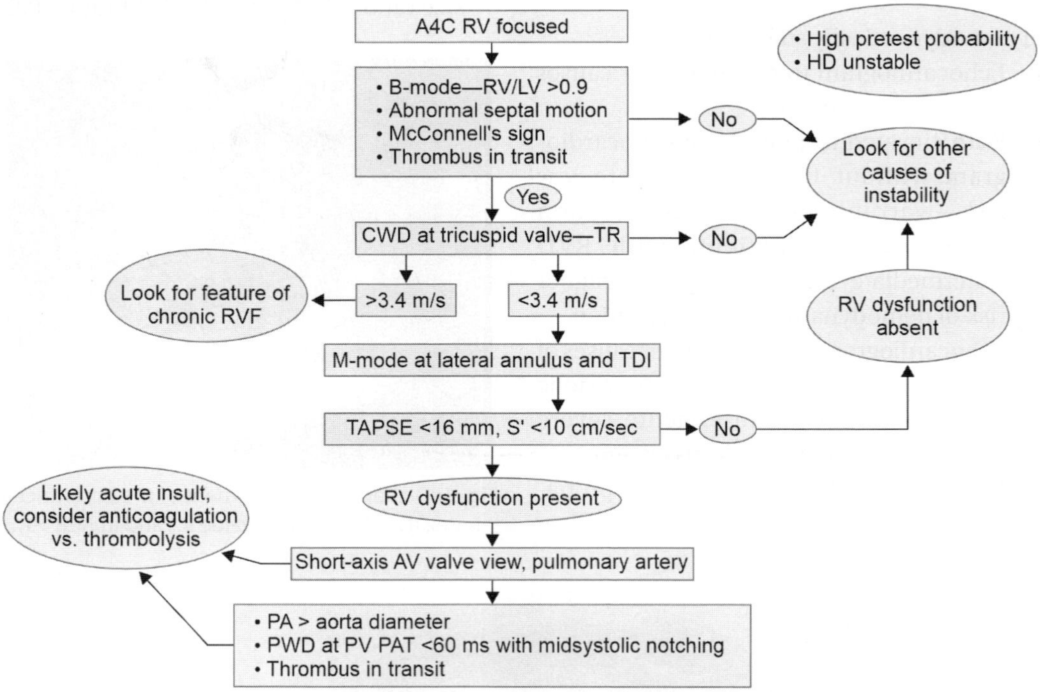


(AV: arteriovenous; HD: hemodynamic; PA: pulmonary artery; PAT: pulmonary acceleration time; PV: pulmonic valve; PWD: pulsed wave Doppler; TAPSE: tricuspid annular plane systolic excursion; TR: tricuspid regurgitation)

**Q3. How does ECHO help you to differentiate whether an insult to RV is acute or chronic?**

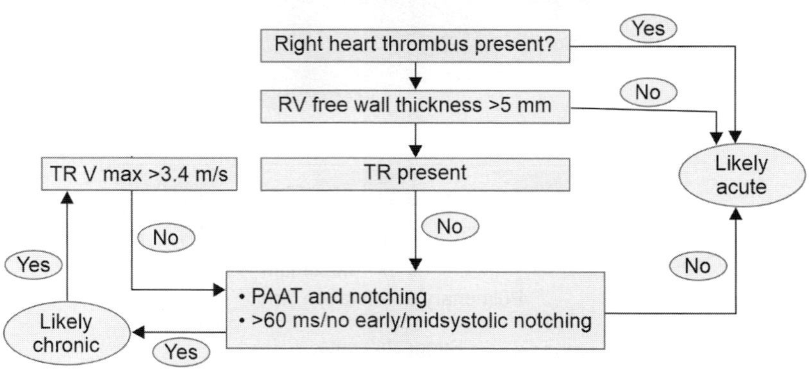


(PAAT: pulmonary artery acceleration time)

**Q4. Brief about RVF therapies and likely effect on overall circulation.**

**Ans.** Various therapies and impact on circulation.

| | *Cardiac index* | *PVR* | *SVR* | *RV/PA coupling* | *RV ischemia* | *Remarks* |
|---|---|---|---|---|---|---|
| Volume depletion | ↑ | – | – | ↑ | ↓ | Improve end-organ function, RV/LV interference and TR (RAP 8–12 mm Hg) |
| Norepinephrine | ↑ | ↑ | ↑↑ | ↑ | ↓ | First line |
| Low-dose vasopressin | ↑ | ↓ | ↑↑ | ↑ | ↓ | PA vasodilator at low dose |
| Dobutamine | ↑ | ↓ | ↓ | ↑ | ↑ | Triggers arrhythmias and favors hypotension |
| PDE3 inhibitor | ↑ | ↓ | ↓ | ↑ | ↑ | Hypotension |
| Levosimendan | ↑ | ↓ | ↓ | ↑ | ↓ | Hypotension |

(PDE3: phosphodiesterase III; PVR: pulmonary vascular resistance; RAP: right atrial pressure; SVR: systemic vascular resistance)

**Q5. What is deep vein thrombosis (DVT) assessment (various methods)?**

**Ans.**

- Venous ultrasonogram (USG)
- Technically difficult—venography
- Two techniques
- Compression USG (CUS)
- Duplex USG—radiologist

**Q6. What is the CUS (technique)?**

**Ans.**

1. Compressing the vessel
2. Gentle pressure

**Q7. How to confirm?**

**Ans.**

- CUS + pretest probability scores + D-dimer
- Pretest probability scores—Wells score
- High (3–8), moderate (1–2), and low (–2 to 0)
- D-dimer-fibrin degradation product (FDP)—acute DVT

**Q8. How to scan?**

**Ans.** Lower limb scan with linear high-resolution transducer probe at different positions **(Fig. 3)**

**Q9. Enumerate false positives in DVT.**

**Ans.**

- Baker's cyst
- Lymph node
- Groin hematoma
- Superficial thrombophlebitis
- Pseudoaneurysm

**Q10. Patient is having lower limb swelling as well as risk factors for DVT. What is the role of point-of-care ultrasound (POCUS) in DVT diagnosis?**

**Ans.** Compression ultrasound of lower limbs helps in identifying the presence of thrombus in lower limbs. Patent veins are fully compressible under light pressure applied with the transducer, with the visible lumen completely disappearing as the opposing venous walls come into full contact **(Fig. 4)**. Inability to completely compress the venous lumen is the main criterion for the diagnosis of DVT. The amount of pressure required has to be lower than the pressure required to collapse the artery.

*Common Femoral Vein*

Compression is done from above the inguinal ligament every 1–2 cm, crossing the inguinal

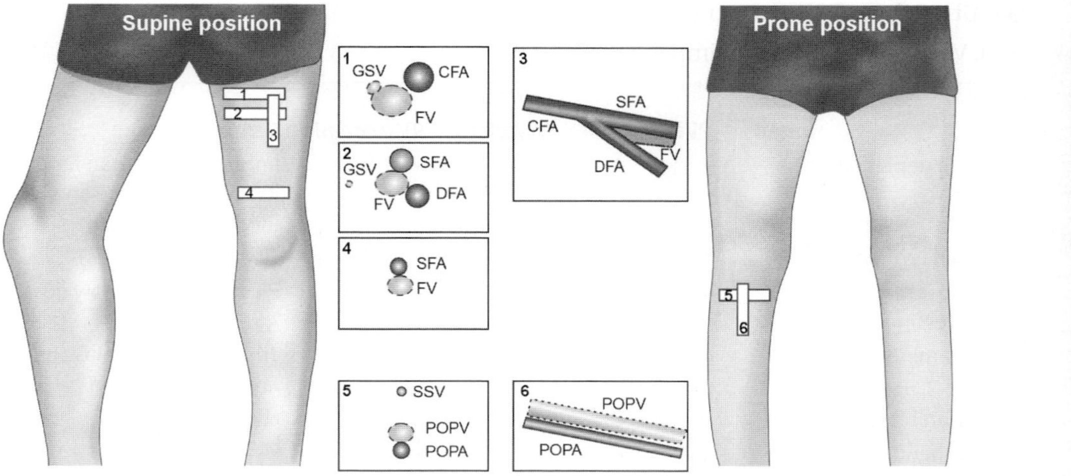


**Fig. 3:** Transducer positions on the leg. (CFA: common femoral artery; DFA: deep femoral artery; FV: femoral vein; GSV: great saphenous vein; POPA: popliteal artery; POPV: popliteal vein; SFA: superficial femoral artery; SSV: superficial saphenous vein)

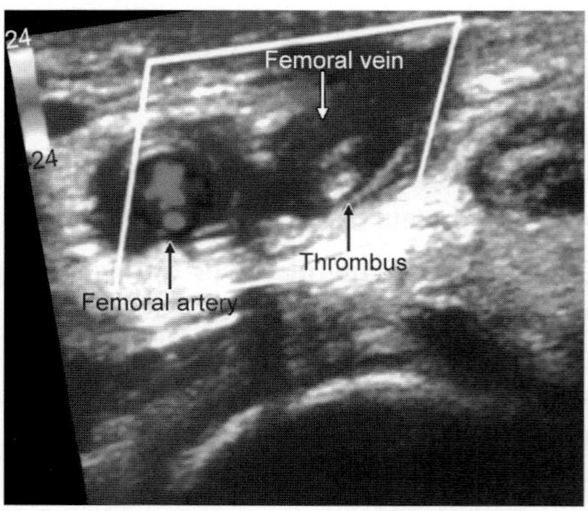


**Fig. 4:** Visualizing thrombus occluding femoral vein on light compression.

ligament to the proximal common femoral vein. Then the superomedial entrance of the greater saphenous vein is compressed moving over the lateral perforator-common femoral vein junctions, ending at the branch of the common femoral—deep femoral vein.

*Popliteal Vein*

The knee is flexed approximately 45° and externally rotated, with the transducer placed transversely over the middle fossa. The paired popliteal artery and vein are located in a central position, with vein typically overlying the artery.

CHAPTER 17

# Cardiomyopathies

*Gourav Mittal, Puneet Khanna*

## INTRODUCTION

Cardiomyopathy is the disease of the myocardium resulting in cardiac dysfunction.

## CLASSIFICATION

*As per classification:*

- Hypertrophic
- Dilated
- Restrictive
- Arrhythmogenic right ventricular (RV) cardiomyopathies
- Isolated noncompaction of the ventricular myocardium

Brief echocardiographic differences among the above-mentioned cardiomyopathies denote.

| ECHO | HCM | DCMP | RCMP | Amyloid | Arrhythmogenic RV | Isolated noncompaction |
|---|---|---|---|---|---|---|
| LVEDD | N →↓ | ↑ | N | ± | N | N →↑ |
| Atrial size | ↑ | ↑ | N ↑ | ↑ | N | N →↑ |
| LV wall thickness | ↑ | N | N ↑ | ↑ | N | N → focal ↑ |
| LVEF | N →↑ | ↓ | N →↓ | N →↓ | N | N →↓ |
| RV function | N | N→↓ | N | N →↓ | ↓ | N →↓ |

(DCMP: dilated cardiomyopathy; ECHO: echocardiography; HCM: hypertrophic cardiomyopathy; LV: left ventricular; LVEDD: LV end-diastolic diameter; LVEF: LV ejection fraction; RCMP: restrictive cardiomyopathy)

## Dilated Cardiomyopathy

- Primary myocardial disease
- Often leads to reduced LV systolic function and LV dilatation
- Absence of coronary and valvular heart disease

*Note:* Ischemic cardiomyopathy looks similar to DCMP but by its definition, it is not a form of DCMP.

### *Common Causes*

- Genetic
- Congenital
- Infections
- Drug and alcohol abuse
- Certain cancer medications
- Exposure to toxins

## CLINICAL VIGNETTE

A 56-year-old male, chronic alcoholic, no known comorbidity has presented with worsening breathlessness, peripheral lower limb edema, cold peripheries, and altered mental status. On arrival, he was hypotensive despite resuscitation. Thiamine was administered lactate started increasing.

A lung ultrasonogram (USG) showed a B7 profile bilaterally. He was started on vasopressors and noninvasive ventilation (NIV) support. The resident does a screening echocardiogram (ECHO) and he suspected of alcohol-induced DCMP, since all chambers are dilated.

**Q1. How do you diagnose a case of DCMP: on echocardiography?**

**Ans.**

*ECHO findings:*

- *Two-dimensional (2D) ECHO:*
  - *Initial evaluation:* Left ventricular ejection fraction (LVEF) and fractional shortening (FS) calculation
    - Parasternal long-axis (PLAX) view, LVEF < 40%, and FS < 25%

*American Society of Echocardiography recommendations:*

*Apical four-chamber (A4C) view:*

- LVEDD index above 100 mL/m$^2$ (male upper limit 74 mL/m$^2$ and female 61 mL/m$^2$ in women)
- The end-systolic volume index of the LV >35 mL/m$^2$ is correlated with an unfavorable outcome.
- Left atrial volume index (LAVi) >50 mL/m$^2$ is a characteristic echocardiographic aspect of DCM.
- RV function check is mandatory as the prognosis is considerably worse when there is RV dilatation and/or RV systolic dysfunction.

*Doppler ECHO:* Color Doppler and continuous wave Doppler (CWD) and A4C across mitral valve:

- Presence of mitral regurgitation (MR) (abnormal leaflet tethering mandated by the change in LV shape from ellipsoid to spherical)
- Diastolic dysfunction (deceleration time ≤115 ms, and E/A ratio >1 is a powerful, independent predictor of mortality or the need for transplantation among patients with heart failure)

**Q2. What are the signs of advanced DCMP?**

**Ans.** The signs of *advanced DCMP are:*

- Low cardiac output [LV outflow tract (LVOT) velocity <0.5 m/s]
- Very low ejection fraction
- Atrial size (large atria in more advanced forms)
- Significant MR
- Diastolic function/filling pressure (restrictive pattern)
- Severe pulmonary hypertension and tricuspid regurgitation (TR)
- Poor RV function
- Pleural effusion

Right ventricular failure dysfunction correlates with an outcome better as compared to LV dysfunction.

**Q3. Although it looks similar, how can you differentiate ischemic cardiomyopathy from DCMP?**

**Ans.** Thin, scarred walls with ventricular distortion and clearly segmental myocardial dysfunction

## Takotsubo Cardiomyopathy

- Takotsubo cardiomyopathy is also known as stress-induced cardiomyopathy.
- More often seen in women
- *ECHO features (A4C view):*
  - Segmental wall motion abnormalities (in particular, apical ballooning)
  - Hyperdynamic basal segments which may lead to LVOT obstruction
  - RV involvement
- Usually, coronary angiogram is normal.
- ECHO findings are reversible once the stress has been taken care of.

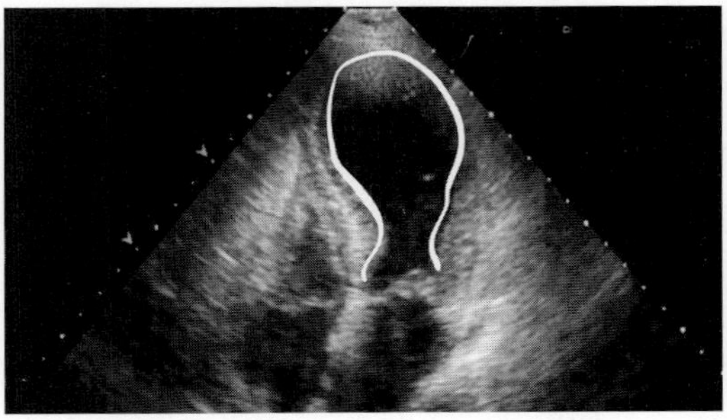

## CLINICAL VIGNETTE

65-year-old female, with no known case comorbidities, lost her husband 1 year ago. She has presented with chest pain and sudden-onset dyspnea. Electrocardiogram (ECG) changes were nonspecific. Deep vein thrombosis (DVT) screen and d dimers were negative. You suspect stress cardiomyopathy.

**Q1. Diagnostic criteria for stress cardio-myopathy.**

**Ans.** Mayo Clinic diagnostic criteria:

- Transient LV systolic dysfunction in form of hypokinesis, akinesis, or dyskinesis.
- Regional wall motion abnormality (RWMA) beyond single epicardial vascular territory.
- Assence of obstructive CAD or acute plaque rupture on coronary angiogram
- New ECG abnormalities (either ST-segment elevation and/or T wave inversion) or modest elevation in cardiac biomarkers
- Absence of pheochromocytoma or myocarditis

**Q2. What are the various variants of wall motion abnormality of LV seen in stress cardiomyopathy?**

**Ans.**

*Apical type:* Systolic apical ballooning of the LV, reflecting depressed mid and apical segments and often hyperkinesia of the basal walls. It is present in 81.7% of patients.

*Less common (atypical) variants:*

- *Midventricular type:* Hypokinesis is restricted to the midventricle with relative sparing of the apex. It is present in 14.6%.
- *Basal type:* Hypokinesis of the base with sparing of the midventricle and apex (reverse or inverted Takotsubo). It is present in 2.2%.
- *Focal type:* Isolated segment (most commonly the anterolateral segment) of the LV
- *Global type:* Rarely do patients have global hypokinesis.

**Q3. How does ECHO help in managing apart from diagnosing stress cardiomyopathy?**

**Ans.** A major key factor is the presence of LVOT obstruction. ECHO helps us to rule out this (discussed in HCM).

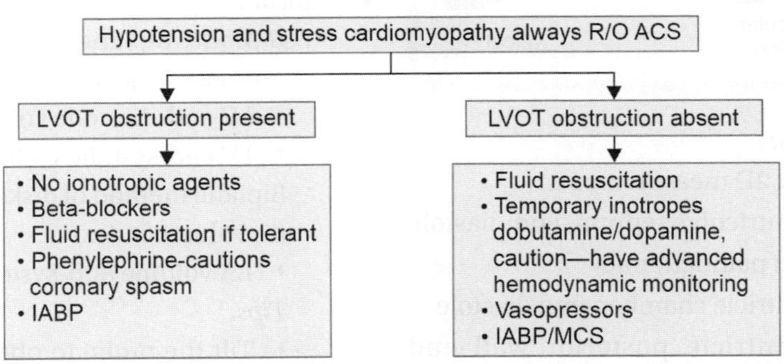


(ACS: acute coronary syndrome; IABP: intra-aortic balloon pump; MCS: mechanical circulatory support)

## Hypertrophic Cardiomyopathy

### *When should one Consider HCM?*

- Presence of unexplained left ventricular hypertrophy (>15 mm)
- Presence of LVOT/LV gradients
- LV cavity—spade shaped
- LV myocardium speckled appearance
- Presence of asymmetrical LV hypertrophy
- Turbulence on color Doppler in LVOT

### *Types of HCM*

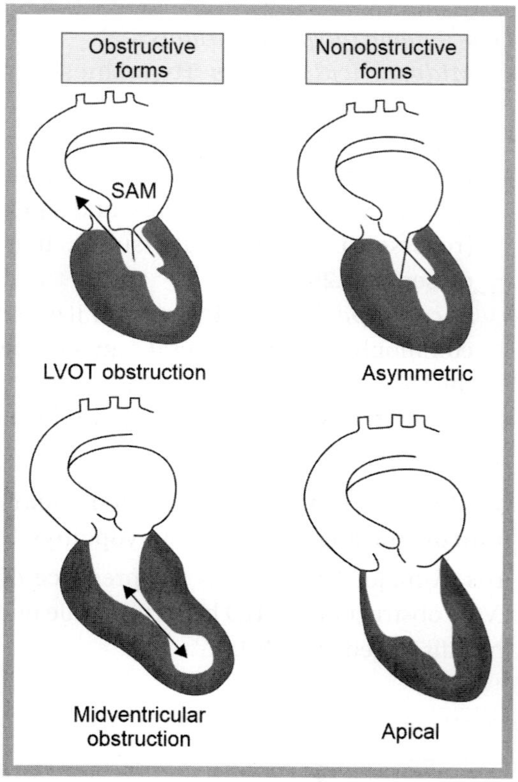


*ECHO findings:*

- *PLAX view:* 2D measurements:
  - Interventricular septum-end diastole >15 mm pathognomic
  - Left ventricle chamber-end diastole
  - Left ventricle posterior wall-end diastole

  *Tips:* Be sure to measure only compacted myocardium and exclude RV structures.

  *Evaluate for SAM:*
  - Evaluate mitral valve (MV) leaflet tips throughout the cardiac cycle
  - M-mode will assist with evaluating the timing of SAM.

  *Tips:*
  - Scroll slowly through the image to define the degree of SAM.
  - SAM with septal contact is considered severe.
  - *Color Doppler:* Evaluate for MR.

    *Tips:*
    - MR is typically posteriorly directed when related to SAM.
    - If MR is anteriorly directed, evaluate closely for intrinsic valve disease.
- *Parasternal short-axis (PSAX) view*:
  - Evaluate for SAM.
  - Measure septal wall thickness on 2D measurement:
    - Interventricular septum—end diastole

    *Tips*:
    - Cross-reference measurements with PLAX views
    - Excellent view to differentiate RV structures from compacted myocardium
- *Apical view:*
  - *B-Mode:* Biplane method of disks for estimating ejection fraction
    - LV end-diastolic volume
    - LV end-systolic volume

    Biplane method of disks for estimating LA volume index
    - LA volume end-systole

    *Tips:*
    - Tilt the probe to obtain the largest LA volume view.

- *Color Doppler:* Define the level of obstruction with color Doppler.
  *Tips:*
  - Set region of interest (ROI) to cover the entire LV from apex to the aortic valve to define the location of obstruction.
  - Compare the B-mode and color Doppler image simultaneously to define the location of obstruction
- *Pulse wave Doppler (PWD):* Define the level of obstruction with PWD.
  *Tip:* Sequential PWD mapping of the LV from apex to atrioventricular (AV) valve.
- *CWD:*
  - Measure peak dynamic gradient. Label appropriately. For example, if the gradient is across the LVOT, label it as "resting LVOT gradient."
  - Measure peak velocity to determine the presence of obstruction and grade severity.

  *Tip:* MR signal can contaminate the LVOT flow acceleration. Move the transducer more laterally and angulate the probe to align through the LVOT and aorta, avoiding the LA.

## CLINICAL VIGNETTE

A 60-year-old male with a history of occasional chest pain was posted for elective unilateral total knee replacement (TKR). His preoperative ECG was unremarkable. He required vasopressors for post spinal hypotension. He was shifted to ICU on norepinephrine infusion, but the intensivist noticed some systolic murmur in the mitral area and noticed worsening hemodynamics with tachycardia. He suspected SAM with HOCM causing LVOT obstruction.

**Q1. Describe the approach to managing patients with HCM with LVOT obstruction.**

**Ans.** In patients with HCM, obstruction is defined as evidence of an LVOT gradient ≥30 mm Hg and systolic anterior motion of the mitral valve at rest or with exercise.

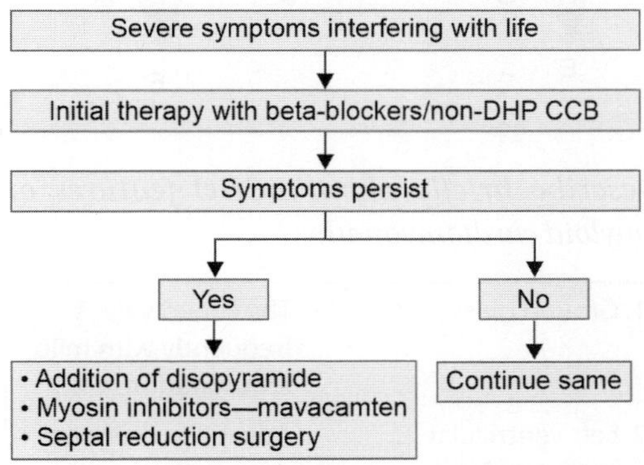


(CCB: calcium channel blockers; DHP: dihydropyridine)

## Restrictive Cardiomyopathy

*Definition:* Idiopathic, usually infiltrative disorder, primarily affecting diastolic function with involvement of either LV and or RV.

*Causes:* Amyloidosis, idiopathic, sarcoid heart disease, endomyocardial fibrosis, radiation, chemotherapy, carcinoid, and hemochromatosis

*ECHO findings*

- Left ventricular hypertrophy (LVH)
- Biatrial enlargement
- Normal LV volume
- Normal LVEF
- Expanded LA appendage
- Dilated inferior vena cava (IVC) and pulmonic veins
- Presence of TR

*How to differentiate between restrictive and constrictive?*

- A4C—MV inflow PWD and TDI
- The E' wave is preserved/exaggerated in constrictive pericarditis.

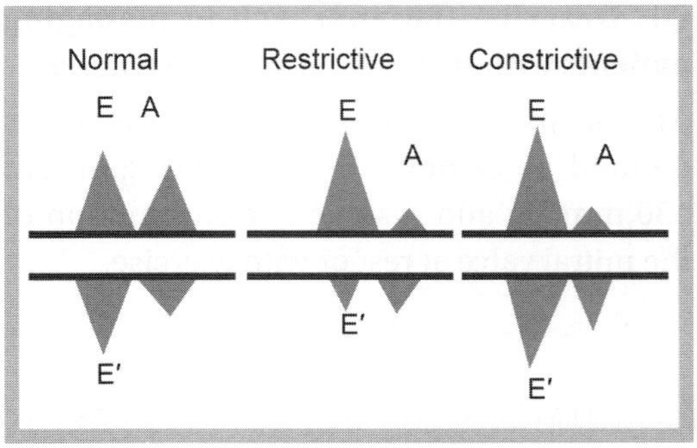


*Describe briefly about ECHO features of amyloid cardiomyopathy.*

| | |
|---|---|
| 1. Ground glass pattern | • Thickened valves frequently with mild regurgitations |
| 2. Left ventricular hypertrophy | • Advanced diastolic dysfunction |
| 3. Atrial enlargement | • Pericardial/pleural effusion |
| 4. Thickened interatrial septum | • "Apical sparing pattern" of longitudinal strain |
| 5. Systolic dysfunction (end stage) | • Right heart involvement |

## Septic Cardiomyopathy

*Five hemodynamic profiles observed in septic cardiomyopathy*

| Function | Pathophysiology | EF | CO |
|---|---|---|---|
| LV systolic dysfunction | • Reduced contractility/ increase LVESV<br>• EF may appear normal falsely (very low SVR)<br>• LV dilation may occur | ↓/– | ↓ |
| LV hyperdynamic function | • Hyperdynamic contractility<br>• Pseudohypertrophy of LV<br>• If preload is normal—CO elevated<br>• Reduced LVESV | ↑ | ↑/↓ |
| Dynamic LVOT obstruction | • Anterior movement of mitral valve against IVS<br>• Severely reduced CO | ↑ | ↓ |
| LV diastolic | • Impaired relaxation<br>• Reduced LVEDV | ↓/– | ↓ |
| RV dysfunction | • Reduced contractility of RV, increased RVESV<br>• RV dilation reduces LV filling<br>• Reduced LVEDV and reduced CO<br>• LV dysfunction may co-occur | ↑/↓ | ↓ |

(EDV: end-diastolic volume; ESV: end-systolic volume; IVS: interventricular septum; SVR: systemic vascular resistance)

## CLINICAL VIGNETTE

A 34-year-old female presented with altered mental status with circulatory failure. She had a history of recurrent urinary tract infection (UTI) and complained of decreasing urine output, burning micturition, and high-grade fever for the last 4 days. She was admitted in ICU in view of persistent hypotension. Baseline ECHO was normal and was managed with intravenous (IV) antibiotics and vasopressors. Though she responded to treatment she had persistent tachycardia along with a low-dose vasopressor requirement.

**Q1. If you suspect sepsis-related cardiomyopathy, how will you proceed with ECHO to diagnose?**

**Ans.**

- Decreased cardiac output [A5C—LVOT velocity time integral (VTI)]
- LV dysfunction (A4C LVEF <45%, TDI MV S' <7.5 cm/s, global longitudinal stain <20%)
- RV dysfunction (A4C RV/LV >0.6, tricuspid annular plane systolic excursion (TAPSE) <16 mm, RV fractional area change <35%)
- LV diastolic dysfunction (A4C, PWD, TDI, lateral E' <7 cm/s, septal <10 cm/s, lateral E/E' >13, septal >15)

**Q2. Describe in brief potential therapeutics while managing septic cardiomyopathy.**

**Ans.**

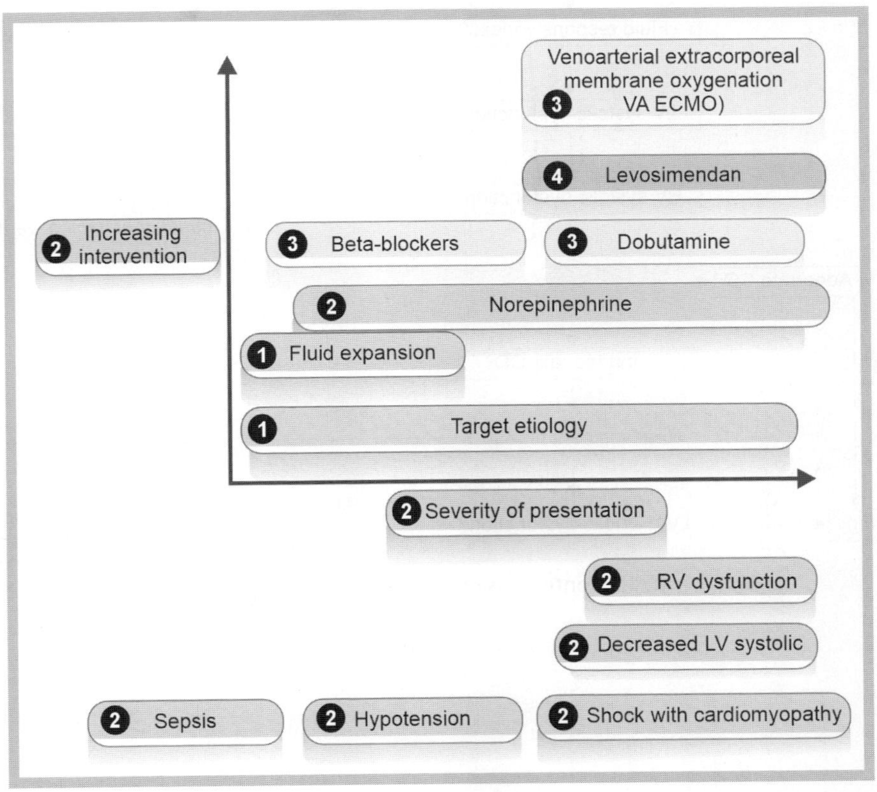


| | |
|---|---|
| ❶ | Strong recommendations, strong quality of evidence |
| ❷ | Strong recommendations, moderate quality of evidence |
| ❸ | Weak recommendations requiring confirmation in prospective clinical trials |
| ❹ | Which should not be used due to weak recommendations, low quality of evidence |

*Note:* Beta-blockers could be discussed in patients with tachycardia with diastolic dysfunction but are not recommended in cases of systolic dysfunction or cardiogenic shock.

# ECHO APPROACH TO PATIENT IN SEPSIS

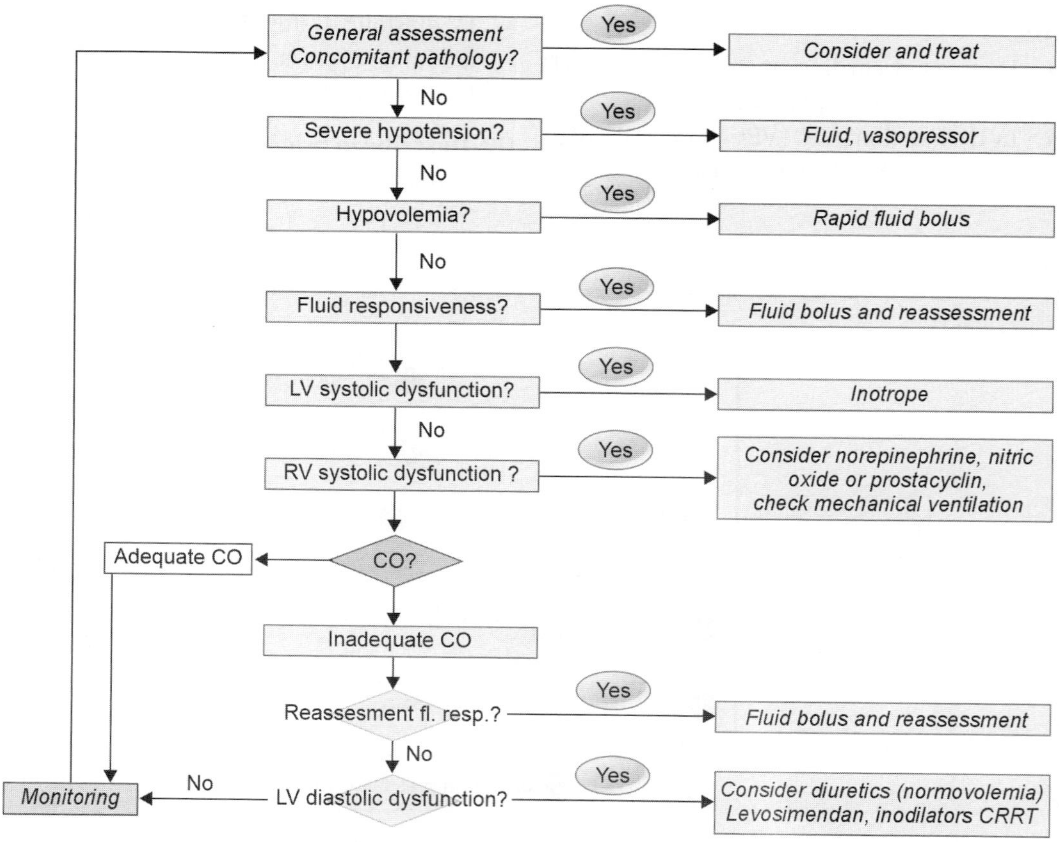


(CRRT: continuous renal replacement therapy)

CHAPTER 18

# Echocardiography for Aorta: Differentiation between Dissection and Disruption

*Gourav Mittal, Puneet Khanna*

## ACUTE AORTIC SYNDROME

Acute aortic syndrome is an umbrella term for various acute life-threatening aortic conditions comprised of aortic dissection, intramural hematoma, penetrating atherosclerotic ulcer, and thoracic aortic aneurysm rupture, excluding traumatic entities.

Comparing and contrasting modalities for aortic imaging.

| *Parameters* | *CT* | *MRI* | *TTE* | *TOE* | *US (Abdo)* |
|---|---|---|---|---|---|
| Availability | +++ | ++ | +++ | ++ | +++ |
| Portability | – | – | +++ | +++ | +++ |
| Speed of acquisition | +++ | + | ++ | ++ | ++ |
| Special resolution | +++ | ++ | ++ | +++ | ++ |
| Temporal resolution | + | ++ | +++ | +++ | +++ |
| 3D data | +++ | ++ | + | + | + |
| Arch branch vessel evaluation | +++ | +++ | ++ | + | NA |
| Valve and ventricular function | + | ++ | +++ | +++ | NA |

(3D: three dimensional; Abdo: abdomen; CT: computed tomography; MRI: magnetic resonance imaging; NA: not applicable; TOE: transesophageal echocardiogram; TTE: transthoracic echocardiogram; US: ultrasound)
+++ Excellent results; ++ good results; + fair results; and – not available

## BRIEF PRESENTATION OF ACUTE AORTIC SYNDROME

Chest pain is usually sudden in onset and of sharp, tearing, or ripping quality with maximal severity at onset. Starting from chest, it can radiate to the back or the abdomen. Sometimes, presentation is with complications such as ischemic stroke, acute coronary syndrome (ACS), mesenteric ischemia, or mimic kidney stone.

On examination, absent upper extremity or carotid pulse or large discrepancy in systolic blood pressure (SBP) between extremities usually point toward acute aortic syndrome (AAS). Aortic regurgitation often leads to new diastolic murmur. Neurological presentation such as stroke, altered mental status, Horner syndrome, paraplegia (spinal cord ischemia), or hoarseness (vocal cord paralysis) are often seen in up to 30% of cases.

Echocardiogram (ECHO) view useful for evaluation of aorta and its segment.

| ***ECHO View*** | ***Aorta Visualize*** |
|---|---|
| ***Transthoracic ECHO*** | |
| • Parasternal long + short axis<br>• Apical four chamber<br>• Apical two chamber<br>• Suprasternal<br>• Subcostal | • Ascending + descending thoracic<br>• Descending thoracic<br>• Descending thoracic<br>• Arch, descending + ascending thoracic<br>• Abdominal (+ascending thoracic) |
| ***Transesophageal ECHO*** | |
| • Upper esophageal<br>• long + short axis<br>• Aortic (long + short axis) | • Ascending thoracic<br>• Descending thoracic + arch |

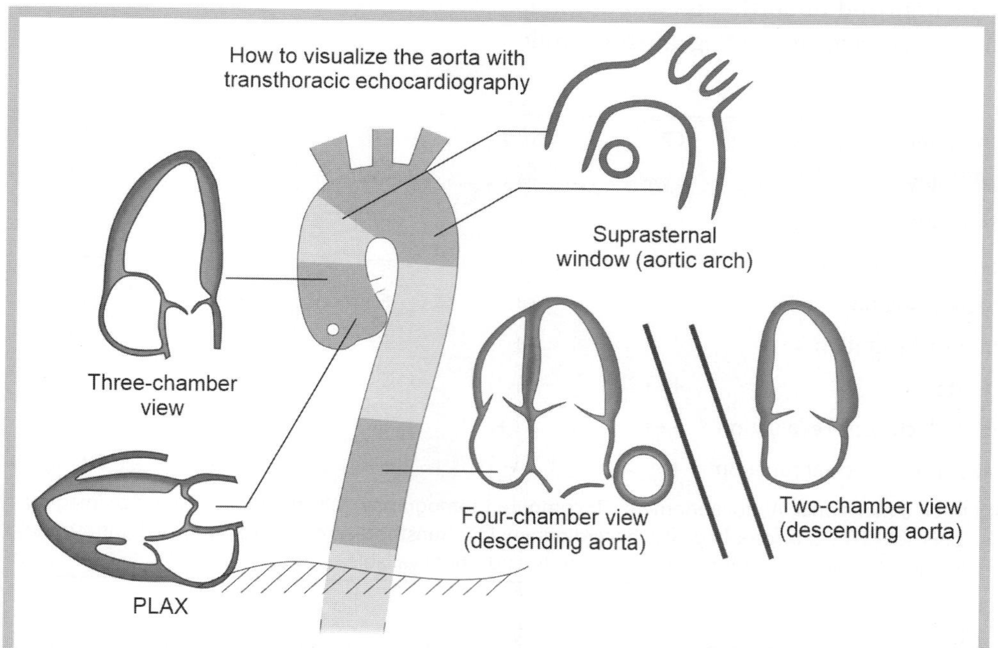


Modified parasternal long axis (PLAX) (1 intercostal space cranial) to visualize more of ascending aorta.

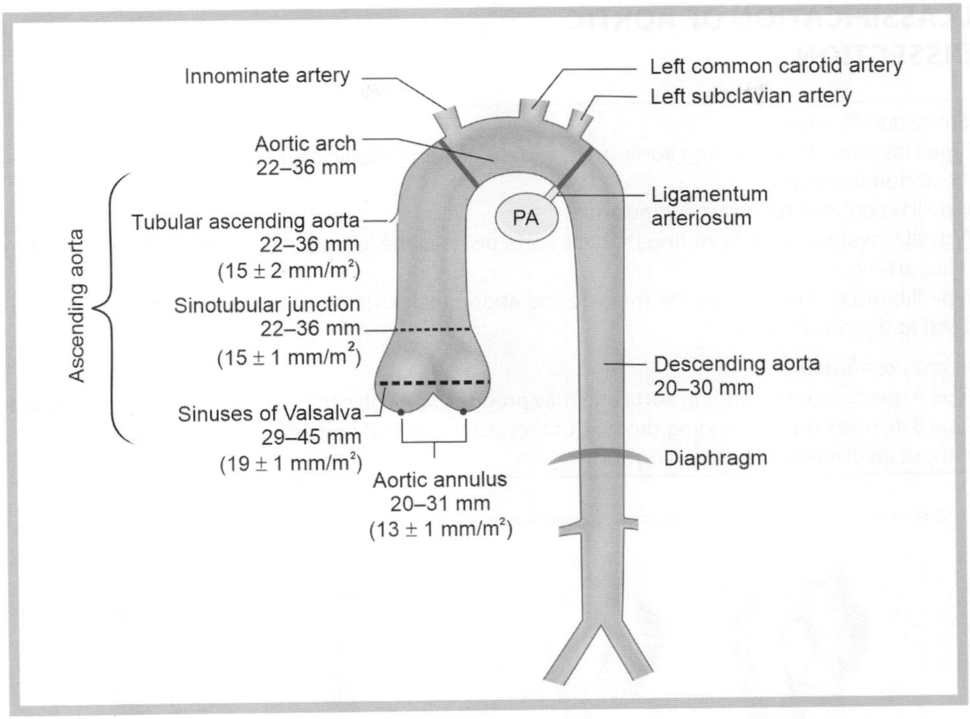


Normal size of aorta and root for reference.

## USEFULNESS OF ECHO IN ACUTE AORTIC PATHOLOGIES

- Intimal flap separating the true and false lumens (diagnostic finding)
- Distinction between true and false lumen using color-flow mapping
- Aortic valve regurgitation resulting from aortic dissection and its mechanism

## PITFALLS OF TRANSTHORACIC ECHOCARDIOGRAM/ TRANSESOPHAGEAL ECHOCARDIOGRAM

- Transthoracic echocardiogram (TTE) usually has low-sensitivity diagnosis of aortic lumen dissection but still does well in case of Stanford A.
- Artifacts while performing TOE kept in mind—in case of true dissection, echo intensity remains constant through its course and mobility will be random while in case of artifacts, echo intensity reduces from origin to distant, and echo will be rigid and fixed.
- Even with transesophageal echocardiogram (TOE), visualization of the distal ascending aorta and proximal arch is difficult because of interposition of trachea and the main bronchus.
- While performing TOE, one should consider contraindications such as esophageal and cervical spine disease and also rare complications (aspiration, hematemesis, arrhythmias, esophageal perforation, and laryngospasm).

## CLASSIFICATION OF AORTIC DISSECTION

*DeBakey classification:*

- Type I involves the ascending aorta, arch, and descending thoracic aorta and may progress to involve the abdominal aorta
- Type II is confined to the ascending aorta
- Type IIIa involves the descending thoracic aorta distal to the left subclavian artery and proximal to the celiac artery
- Type IIIb dissection involves the thoracic and abdominal aorta distal to the left subclavian artery and distal to the celiac artery

*Stanford classification:*

- Type A involves the ascending aorta and may progress to involve the arch and thoracoabdominal aorta
- Type B involves the descending thoracic or thoracoabdominal aorta distal to the left subclavian artery without involvement of ascending aorta

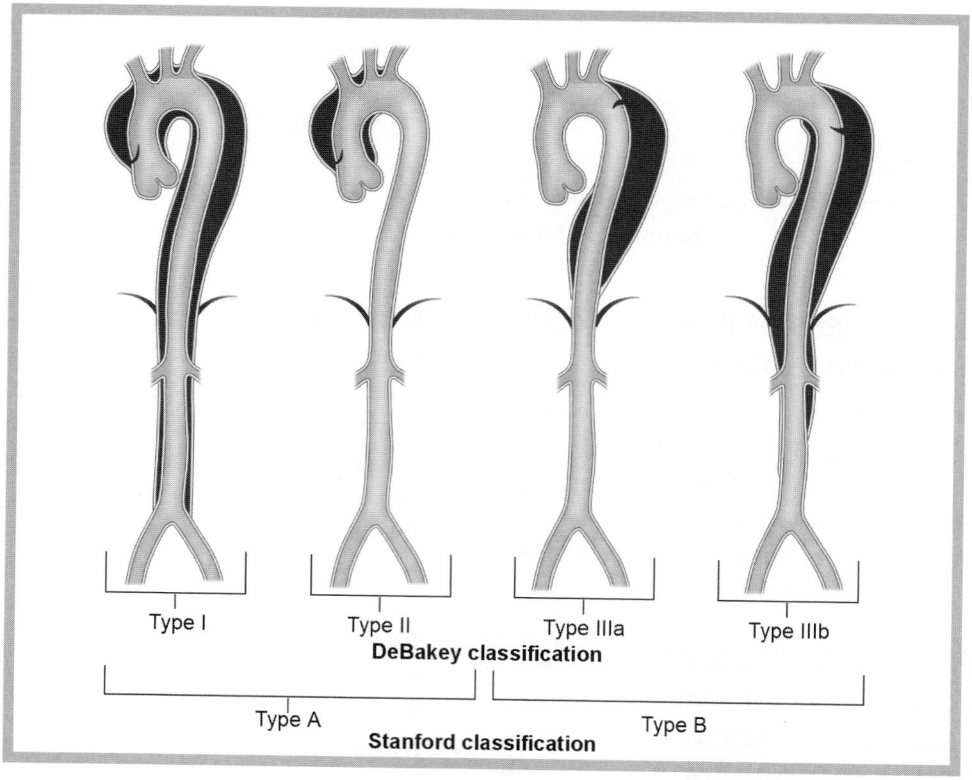

## TRANSTHORACIC ECHOCARDIOGRAM IN AORTIC DISSECTION

Reported sensitivity is 77–80%, while specificity is 93–96%. Although we can detect early with TTE, always confirm dissection by using other imaging modalities.

| *Signs* | *Clinical features* |
|---|---|
| Sign of blood extravasation | • Hemopericardium ± tamponade<br>• Left hemothorax |
| Indirect signs of involvement of the ascending aorta | • Dilatation (symmetrical) of the ascending aorta<br>• New-onset aortic insufficiency (color Doppler) |
| Specific findings | • Aortic dissection: Intimal flap (mobile)<br>• New regional wall motion abnormality |

Algorithm for diagnostics in AAS.

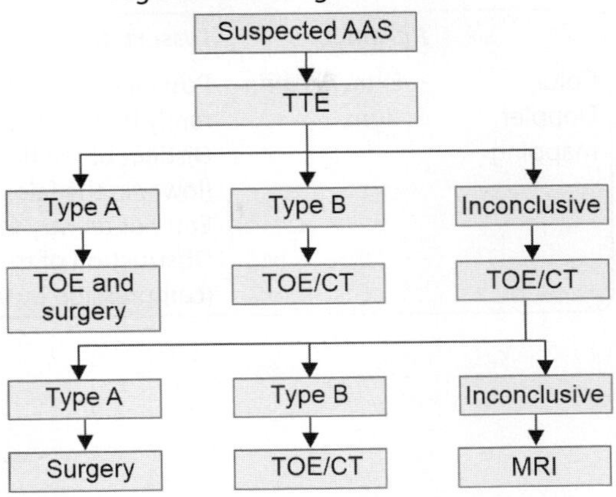


(AAS: acute aortic syndrome; CT: computed tomography; MRI: magnetic resonance imaging; TOE: transesophageal echocardiogram; TTE: transthoracic echocardiogram)

Difference between true and false lumen.

| | *True lumen* | *False lumen* |
|---|---|---|
| Size | True < false | *Most often:* False > true lumen |
| Pulsation | Systolic expansion | Systolic compression |
| Flow direction | Systolic antegrade flow | Systolic antegrade flow reduced or absent or retrograde flow |
| Communication flow | From true to false lumen in systole | |
| Contrast echo flow | Early and fast | Delayed and slow |

ECHO difference between dissection disruption.

| | *Parameters* | *Dissection* | *Disruption* |
|---|---|---|---|
| 2D parameters | • Aortic size<br>• Aortic contour<br>• Aortic flap<br>• Spatial extension<br>• Number of aortic lumens<br>• Thrombus | Increased<br>Symmetrical<br>Thin (intimal), mobile<br>Extended (according to anatomical type), parallel to aortic walls<br>Two<br>Possible in false lumen | Normal or increased<br>Asymmetrical (false aneurysm formation)<br>Thick (medial), less mobile<br>Confined to the aortic isthmus, almost perpendicular to aortic walls<br>One<br>None |

*Contd...*

*Contd...*

| | *Parameters* | *Dissection* | *Disruption* |
|---|---|---|---|
| Color Doppler mapping | • Extravasation signs | Possible (hemopericardium, rarely hemothorax)<br>Distinct blood flow velocities (lower in the false channel)<br>Entry or reentry tear<br>Obstruction of true lumen (compression by false lumen) | Possible (hemomediastinum, hemothorax)<br>Similar blood flow velocities on both sides of the medial flap<br>None<br>Pseudocoarctation (protrusion of disrupted aortic wall in lumen) |

CHAPTER 19

# Arrhythmias and Echocardiography: How can We Integrate Electrical and Imaging Together?

*Puneet Khanna, Gourav Mittal*

## ATRIAL FIBRILLATION AND ECHOCARDIOGRAPHY

### Evaluation of Cardiac Function

- *Left ventricular/right ventricular (LV/RV) systolic function:* Assessment of LV systolic function using two-dimensional (2D) LV volumes and ejection fraction (EF)
- *Diastolic function:* Evaluation of LV diastolic function parameters
- *Left atrial (LA) function:*
    - Measurement of LA maximum, minimum, and pre-A volume
    - Assessment of LA reservoir, conduit, and contractile function
- *Valvular function:* Evaluation of valvular structure and function, especially in cases of hemodynamically significant valve disease such as rheumatic heart disease or prosthetic valves
- *Pericardium:* Detection of pericardial effusion or constrictive pericarditis.

### Diagnosis (Etiology or Structural Heart Disease Associated with Atrial Fibrillation)

- *Valvular atrial fibrillation (AF):* Assessment for hemodynamically significant valve disease (e.g., rheumatic heart disease)
- *Nonvalvular AF:* Evaluation for structural heart diseases such as ischemic cardiomyopathy (ICMP) or non-ICMP, including tachycardia-induced cardiomyopathy
- *Pharmacological stress/stress echocardiography (ECHO):* Utilization of stress ECHO to assess myocardial ischemia or viability.

### Prognosis

- *Thrombogenic risk:* Assessment of thrombotic risk factors such as LV systolic dysfunction (LVEF <40%) and LV longitudinal strain
- *Prediction of successful cardioversion to sinus rhythm:* Evaluation of atrial size (indexed LA volume), LV systolic and diastolic function, severity of valvular diseases, and LV hypertrophy.

### Management Decisions

- *Pharmacological therapy for rhythm/rate control:* Choice of antiarrhythmic agents based on the presence of structural heart disease and LV function
- *Guidance of cardioversion [transesophageal ECHO (TEE) guided]:* Detection of LA appendage (LAA) thrombus and assessment for other abnormalities [e.g., spontaneous ECHO contrast (SEC), sludge, emptying velocity (EFv)]

- *Cardiac ablation procedure:*
  - Preprocedural evaluation to rule out thrombus, assess LA size, and define pulmonary vein (PV) anatomy
  - Intraprocedural guidance including visualization of interatrial septum (IAS) and puncture sites
  - Follow-up to monitor LV function and LA volumes postprocedure

Echocardiography plays a critical role in the comprehensive assessment and management of patients with AF, providing valuable insights into the cardiac structure, function, and potential underlying pathologies influencing the arrhythmia and treatment outcomes.

## Algorithm for Approach

**Flowchart 1** shows the integration of ECHO for management of arrhythmias.

# EVALUATION OF CARDIAC FUNCTION IN VENTRICULAR ARRHYTHMIAS

- *LV/RV systolic function:*
  - *2D and 3D LV volumes and EF:* Assessment of LV volumes and EF to evaluate systolic function
  - *Deformation imaging (longitudinal function):* Evaluation of longitudinal strain to assess regional and global LV function
- *Diastolic function/LV filling pressures (LVFP):* Assessment of LV diastolic function and LVFP using parameters such as E/A ratio, E/e' ratio, and tissue Doppler imaging
- *Valvular function:* Evaluation of valvular structure and function, including detection of regurgitation or stenosis, and

**Flowchart 1:** Integration of ECHO for management of arrhythmias.

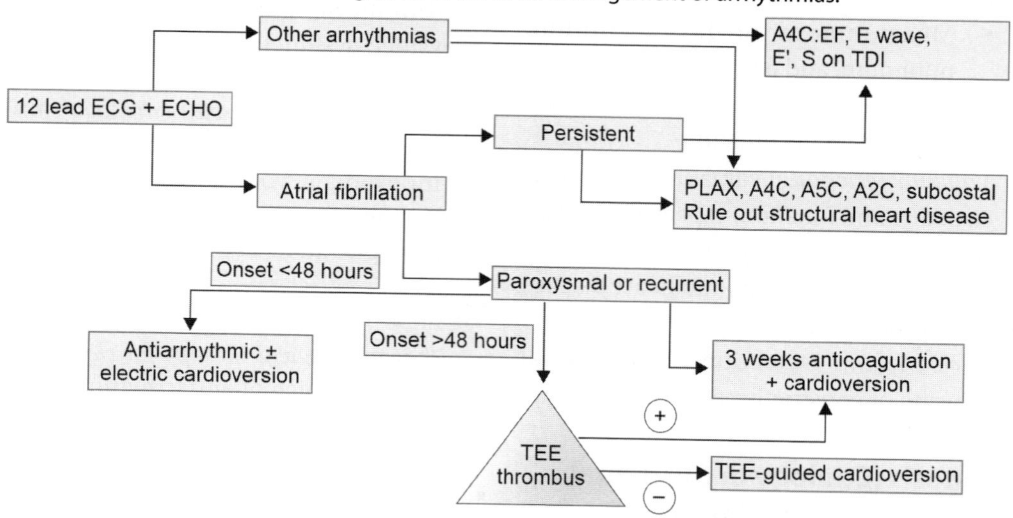


(ECG: electrocardiogram; ECHO: echocardiography; EF: ejection fraction; PLAX: parasternal long axis; TDI: tissue Doppler imaging; TEE: transesophageal echocardiography)

assessment of severity using Doppler techniques

- *Pericardium:* Assessment for the presence of pericardial effusion or constrictive pericarditis

## Diagnosis (Detection of the Potential Organic Substrate)

- *Structural heart disease:* Identification of myocardial abnormalities (e.g., hypertrophy and fibrosis) and valvular pathologies (e.g., congenital defects and endocarditis).
- *Myocardial ischemia:* Utilization of pharmacological stress ECHO with or without contrast to assess myocardial perfusion and function under stress conditions. Evaluation of coronary flow reserve may also be performed.

## Prognosis (Evaluation for Sudden Cardiac Death)

- *ICMP:* Parameters such as LVEF (<35%), wall motion score index (WMSI), and relative wall thickness (RWT) are evaluated.
- *Dilated cardiomyopathy (DCMP):* LVEF (<35%), LV global longitudinal strain (GLS), and mechanical dispersion are assessed to gauge prognosis.
- *Hypertrophic cardiomyopathy (HCM):* Evaluation includes maximum LV wall thickness, LV outflow tract (LVOT) gradient, LA size, LV GLS, and mechanical dispersion.
- *Arrhythmogenic right ventricular cardiomyopathy/dysplasia (ARVC/D):* Assessment involves regional RV wall motion abnormalities (akinesia, dyskinesia, and aneurysm), RV diameter, and RV mechanical dispersion.

These parameters provide essential information for diagnosing underlying cardiac conditions associated with ventricular arrhythmias and predicting the risk of adverse outcomes, including sudden cardiac death. ECHO plays a crucial role in the comprehensive evaluation and management of patients with ventricular arrhythmias, guiding therapeutic decisions and prognostic assessments.

# HOW DOES THE PRESENCE OF ARRHYTHMIAS INFLUENCE/ IMPACT ECHOCARDIOGRAPHY ASSESSMENT?

## Sinus Tachycardia

*Impact on ECHO parameters:*

- *Volumes and EF underestimation:* Rapid heart rate shortens diastole, reducing the filling time and potentially underestimating end-diastolic volume and EF.
- *E and A waves fusion:* Tachycardia can lead to fusion of the E and A waves in the mitral inflow pattern, complicating assessment of diastolic function.
- *Valvular stenosis:*
  - *Maximal valve opening underestimation*: Shortened diastole may underestimate the maximal opening of stenotic valves.
  - *Doppler velocities and mean pressure gradient (MPG) overestimation*: Higher heart rates can lead to overestimation of Doppler velocities and MPG in stenotic valves.
  - *Pressure half-time (PHT) not accurately measured:* PHT for valvular stenosis is not accurately measured at heart rates >100 beats/min.

## Ectopic Beats

*Impact:*

- *Inaccurate evaluation of systolic and diastolic function:* Ectopic beats disrupt normal cardiac cycle timing, affecting the assessment of both systolic and diastolic function.

- *Important information:*
  - *Aortic stenosis (AS) severity and contractile reserve:* Evaluation post-extrasystole can provide information on AS severity and contractile reserve.
  - *Separation of E and A waves:* After an ectopic beat, distinguishing between the E and A waves in the mitral inflow pattern becomes important.

## Atrial Fibrillation/Flutter

*Impact:*

- *Limited accuracy of LV systolic and diastolic function:* Irregular ventricular response in AF/flutter makes accurate assessment of LV systolic and diastolic function challenging.
- *Parameters for left ventricle filling pressure evaluation:*
  - *Isovolumic relaxation time (IVRT) <65 ms, deceleration time (DT) <150 ms, E/E′ septal >11:* These parameters are less reliable in AF/flutter.
  - *Average of ≥10 consecutive cycles*: Averaging data over multiple cycles or selecting cycles corresponding to an optimal heart rate (60–80 beats/min) improves accuracy.

## Bradycardia

*Impact:*

- *Ventricular size and stroke volume increase:* Prolonged diastole in bradycardia increases filling time, potentially leading to increased ventricular size and stroke volume.
- *Overestimation of valvular regurgitations:* Color Doppler may exaggerate the extent of valvular regurgitations due to prolonged diastole.
- *Underestimation of AV valve stenosis:* MPG-based assessment of AV valve stenosis may underestimate the severity due to prolonged diastole.

## Atrioventricular Block

*Impact:*

- *Atrioventricular (AV), ventriculoventricular (VV), and LV asynchrony:* AV block disrupts the coordinated atrial and ventricular contraction, leading to asynchrony.
- *First-degree AV block:*
  - *PR >280 ms:* Usually results in fusion of E and A waves.
  - *PR values > 320 ms:* Marked fusion of E and A waves, with filling occurring predominantly during atrial contraction, potentially leading to diastolic mitral regurgitation
- *Second- or third-degree AV block:* Results in highly variable patterns of mitral inflow due to irregular and asynchronous atrial and ventricular contraction.

Understanding these effects is crucial for accurate interpretation of ECHO findings in patients with various arrhythmias, allowing for appropriate adjustments in imaging protocols and interpretation criteria to ensure reliable diagnostic information.

CHAPTER 20

# Emergency Intraoperative and Postoperative Echocardiography

Richa Saroa, Sanjeev Palta, Avneet Singh

## INTRODUCTION

In 1972, Johnson et al. described for the first time the intraoperative use of echocardiography for mitral valve surgery using M-mode.[1] Gradually, over the years, intraoperative echocardiography has evolved from comprehensive assessment to a simple, focused approach, providing a simple "yes" or "no" answer for modification of patient management.[2] The perioperative echocardiography can be easily performed and interpreted by noncardiologists and can alter management in 52–77% of patients with preexisting or new hemodynamic instability.[3]

## TRANSTHORACIC ECHOCARDIOGRAPHY

There are several terminologies to describe intraoperative echocardiography, namely focused cardiac ultrasound (FOCUS), point-of-care ultrasound (POCUS), focused-assessed transthoracic echocardiography (FATE), or rapid on-site evaluation (ROSE).[3-5] The primary objective is to obtain limited "focused" views in a short time to make a rapid diagnosis.[6]

### Views

There are three transthoracic echocardiography (TTE) windows—parasternal, apical, and subcostal—used for focused imaging.

The images are acquired with the following views **(Table 1)**.

**TABLE 1:** Focused echo view and their application in elective intraoperative conditions.

| *Focused TTE view* | *Application* |
|---|---|
| Parasternal long axis | • LV/RV size and function<br>• Regional wall motion abnormality<br>• Intracardiac thrombus<br>• Pericardial effusion |
| Parasternal short axis | • LV/RV size and function<br>• Regional wall motion abnormality corresponding to segments perfused by all coronary arteries<br>• Hypovolemia |
| Apical four chamber | • LV/RV size and function<br>• Regional wall motion abnormality<br>• Pericardial effusion<br>• Placement of transvenous pacing wires |
| Subcostal four chamber | • Pericardial effusion<br>• Guiding pericardiocentesis<br>• Cardiac pulsatility during cardiac compressions |
| Subcostal inferior vena cava | Intravascular volume status |

(LV: left ventricle; RV: right ventricle; TTE: transthoracic echocardiography)

## Indications

The "Five-F approach" for pericardial and pleural fluid, chamber form, function, flow, and filling of inferior vena cava (IVC) is utilized.[7] There are numerous clinical scenarios where a timely focused assessment yields improved patient management.

- Identification of hypoechoic fluid around the heart, suggesting pericardial effusion **(Fig. 1A)** or pericardial tamponade with diastolic collapse of atria and ventricles **(Fig. 1B)**.
- To identify hematoma and cardiac contusions in cardiac trauma
- The parasternal short axis view with kissing papillary muscles and subcostal view showing >50% collapsibility of IVC is suggestive of hypovolemia **(Figs. 2A and B)**. The vasodilatory shock has a similar echocardiographic picture; however, it can be differentiated on the basis of a hyperdynamic left ventricle and a normal to supranormal cardiac output.
- To assess venous excess grade (VExUS), by measuring the IVC diameter, hepatic, portal, and renal vein Doppler pattern and ascertain the need for diuretics or inotropes.

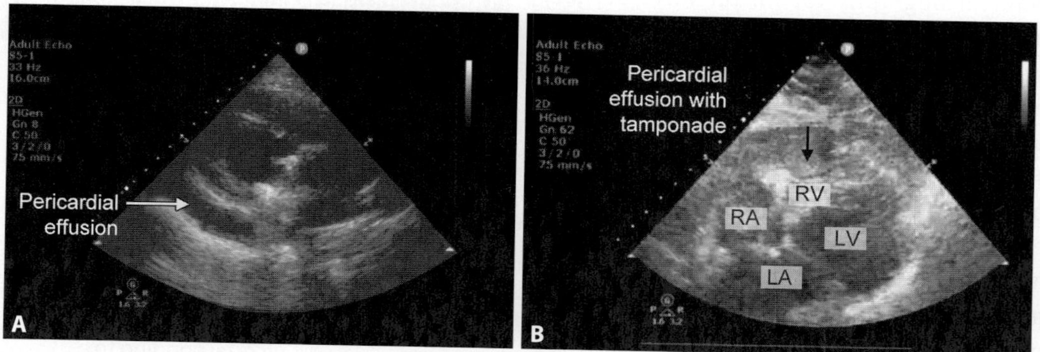


**Figs. 1A and B:** (A) Transthoracic parasternal long axis view showing pericardial effusion (arrow) behind left ventricle; (B) Transthoracic subcostal four-chamber view showing pericardial effusion with tamponade causing right ventricle collapse (arrow). (LA: left atria; LV: left ventricle; RA: right atria; RV: right ventricle)

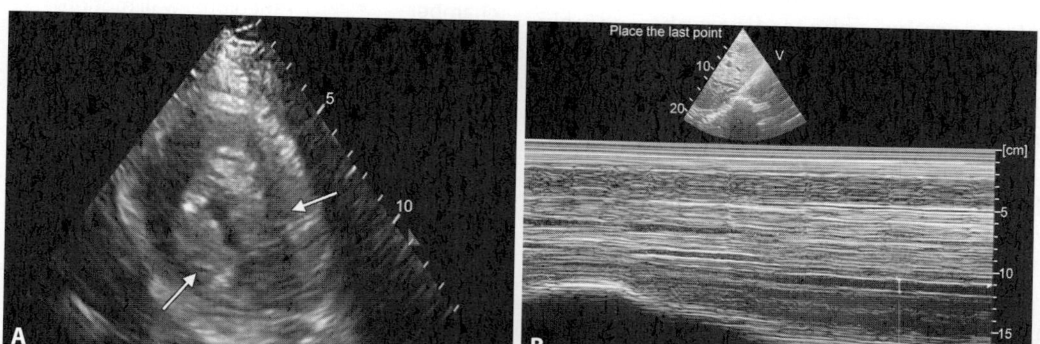


**Figs. 2A and B:** (A) Transthoracic parasternal short axis view showing "kissing" papillary muscles (arrow) suggesting hypovolemia; (B) Transthoracic subcostal inferior vena cava view showing more than 50% collapsibility suggesting hypovolemia.

- A new-onset dyspnea can be due to a worsening valvopathy or pulmonary thromboembolism—right ventricle dilatation, right ventricle free wall akinesia (McConnell's sign), pulmonary artery acceleration time <60 milliseconds, and tricuspid regurgitation jet gradient <60 mm Hg (the 60/60 sign) **(Fig. 3)**.
- In evaluating chest pain, with or without electrocardiogram abnormalities, the parasternal long and short axis and apical four-chamber view identify new regional wall motion abnormality **(Fig. 4)** or aortic dissection.
- During cardiac arrest, the subcostal view can be used to identify the cause of cardiac arrest, identify organized cardiac contractility, and guide insertion of transvenous pacing wires or extracorporeal life support cannulas.

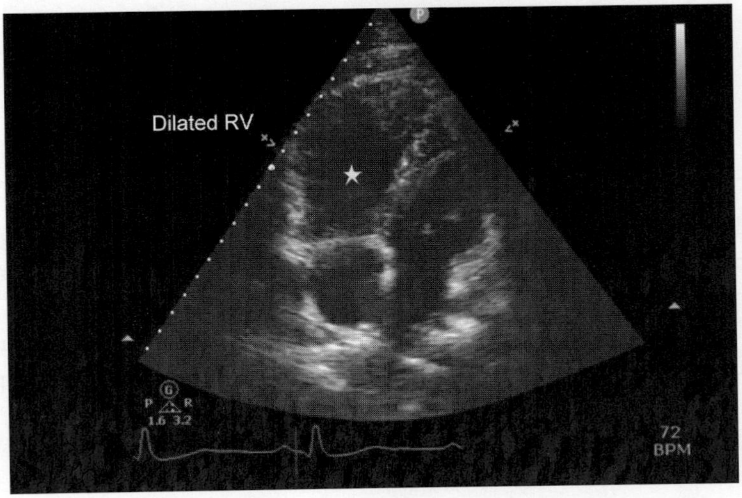


**Fig. 3:** Transthoracic four-chamber view dilated right ventricle (star) in pulmonary embolism. (RA: right atria)

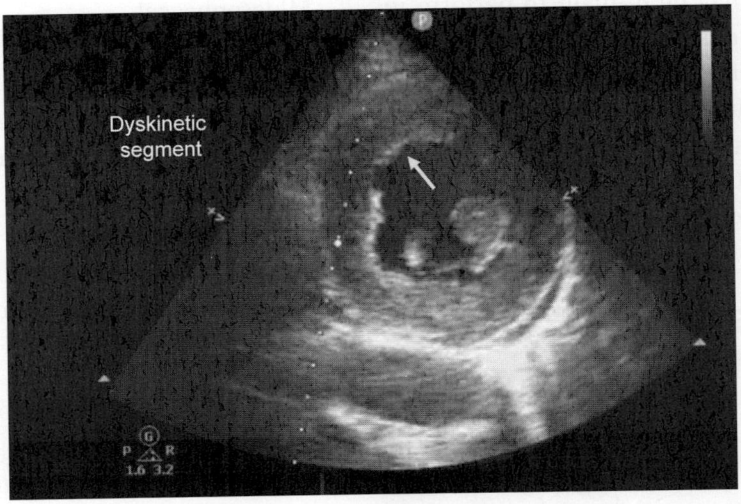


**Fig. 4:** Parasternal midpapillary short axis view showing segmental dyskinesia (arrow).

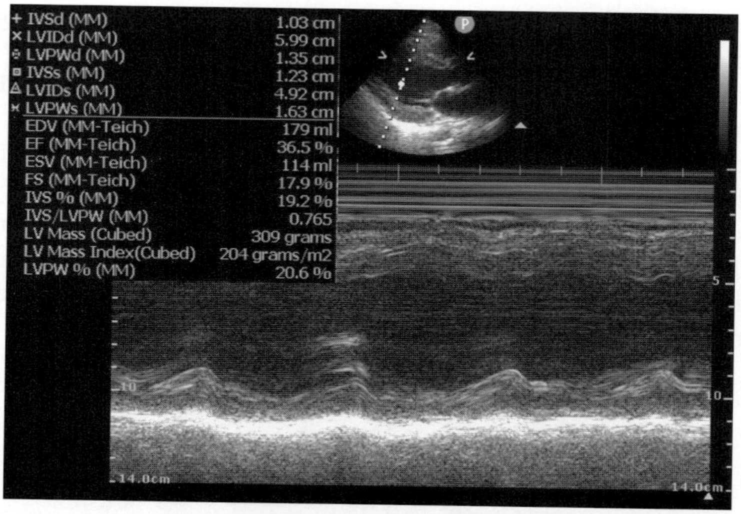


**Fig. 5:** M-mode at the parasternal long axis showing enlarged left ventricle with reduced ejection fraction.

- The rapid obstetrics screening echocardiography (ROSE) identifies obstetric emergencies such as hemorrhage-induced hypovolemia, peripartum cardiomyopathy **(Fig. 5)**, myocardial infarction, pulmonary embolism, and gross estimation of fetal heart rate.

## Contraindications

The TTE has no absolute contraindications. However, it may be difficult to perform in persons with obstructive pulmonary disease or extremes of body habitus. Truncal obesity with thick anterior chest wall may impede passage of ultrasonic waves.[8] Narrow inter-rib space in a thin person may cause difficulty in probe placement, and a smaller footprint may be useful for such situations.

# TRANSESOPHAGEAL ECHOCARDIOGRAPHY

The perioperative use of transesophageal echocardiography (TEE) has evolved to include patients undergoing high-risk noncardiac procedures and patients with cardiac disease undergoing noncardiac surgery.[9-11] The TEE provides superior images compared to TTE because of its proximity to heart and avoidance of lungs and ribs or sterile surgical area as impediments to imaging.[12,13]

## Views

*There are four windows for the examination:*[11]

1. Upper esophageal
2. Midesophageal
3. Transgastric
4. Deep transgastric

The 11 basic and 28 comprehensive views are recommended for intraoperative TEE.

## Indications

The American Society of Anesthesiology Practice guidelines[10] recommend the use of TEE based on patient risk factors, type of surgery, and in cases of unexplained hemodynamic instability. The following are the indications for perioperative uses of TEE:

- Patients undergoing cardiac or aortic procedures

- Catheter-based intracardiac procedures, for example, occluder device placement, percutaneous valvular procedures, and intracardiac ablation procedures
- The nature of the planned surgery (e.g., liver transplantation and neurosurgery in sitting position) **(Fig. 6)** or the patient's known or suspected cardiovascular pathology might result in severe hemodynamic, pulmonary, or neurologic compromise.
- Persistent unexplained life-threatening circulatory instability and hypoxemia **(Fig. 7)**
- In critical care conditions, where the hypotension might be the result of

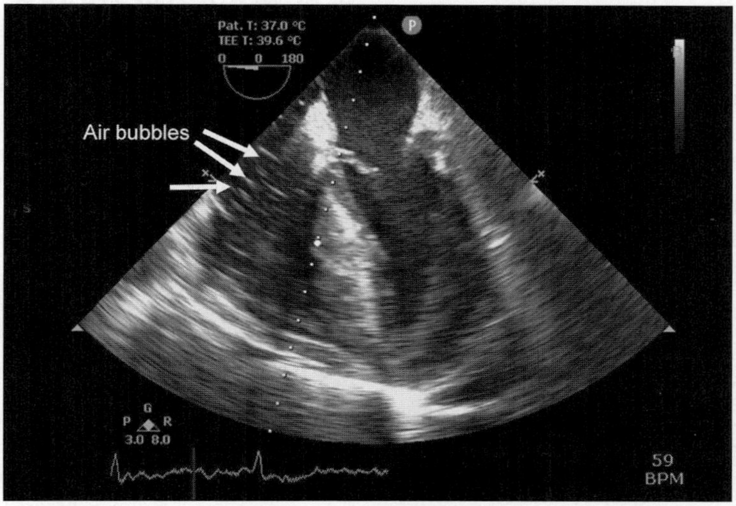


**Fig. 6:** Transesophageal midesophageal four-chamber view showing multiple air bubbles.

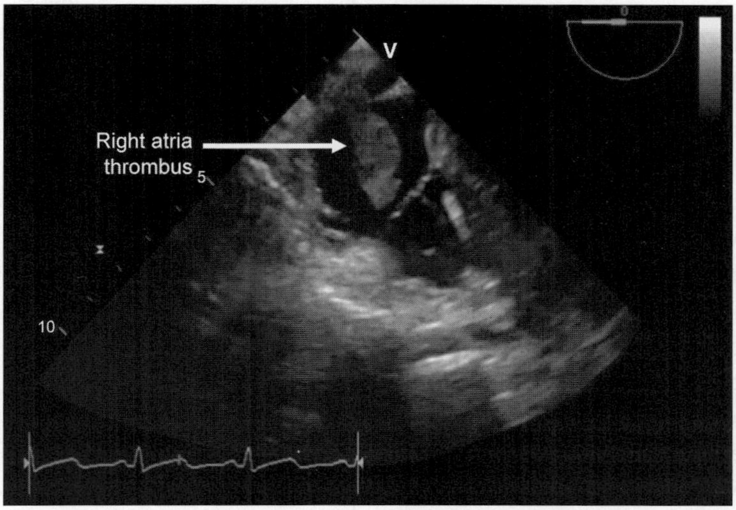


**Fig. 7:** Transesophageal midesophageal four-chamber right ventricle focused view showing thrombus in right atrium causing hypoxemia.

previously undetected valvular lesions, wall motion abnormalities, aortic dissection, or pericardial tamponade
- Patients in whom TTE is unable to provide a useful diagnosis

## Contraindications

- *Absolute contraindications:*
    - Esophageal stricture
    - Transesophageal fistula
    - Postesophageal surgery
    - Esophageal trauma
- *Relative contraindications:*
    - Zenker diverticulum
    - Esophageal varices
    - Postradiation therapy
    - Pervious bariatric surgery

In such situations, the services of the most experienced echocardiographer must be utilized, if the expected benefit outweighs the potential risk. The appropriate precautions that can be utilized in such situations can be epicardial echocardiography using a smaller footprint TEE probe and limiting probe manipulations.

## EMERGENCY ECHOCARDIOGRAPHY

The emergency use of TTE, using a focused assessment-focused echocardiographic evaluation in life support and peri-resuscitation of emergency patients "FEEL", helps to diagnose conditions precipitating shock or cardiac arrest.[14,15] The transthoracic subcostal view identifies tamponade or cardiac motion with minimal interference to cardiac compressions.[15] The "rescue TEE"[16] is superior to TTE in such situations and can provide real-time feedback of chest compression quality, identify cardiac arrhythmias, reduce pauses for pulse checks, and deliver defibrillation. The TEE views should be limited to a few focused views during cardiac arrest[16,17] **(Table 2)**.

During the postcardiac arrest setting, echocardiography may be utilized to optimize the cardiac output and identify myocardial ischemia resulting from the cardiac arrest.[14]

## ADVANCED ECHOCARDIOGRAPHY MODALITIES

The three-dimensional echocardiography, speckle tracking, and contrast echocardiography have a limited role in the perioperative period.[18,19]

**TABLE 2:** Focused echo view and their application in emergency conditions.

| *Focused TEE view* | *Applications* |
|---|---|
| Midesophageal four chamber | • Tamponade<br>• Cardiac activity<br>• Intracardiac thrombus<br>• Assess LV/RV size and function<br>• Define fine ventricular fibrillation |
| Midesophageal long axis view | • Aortic dissection<br>• Area of maximum compression during chest compression |
| Transgastric short axis view | • Cardiac filling status<br>• Assess LV/RV size and function<br>• Tamponade |
| Bicaval | ECMO canula insertion guidance |
| Descending thoracic aorta long axis | • Aortic dissection<br>• ECMO canula insertion guidance |

(ECMO: extracorporeal membrane oxygenation device; LV: left ventricle; RV: right ventricle; TEE: transesophageal echocardiography)

## CONCLUSION

An echocardiography during the perioperative period provides important diagnostic value for a critically ill patient. The resuscitative echocardiography improves patient care and outcomes.

## REFERENCES


1. Johnson ML, Holmes JH, Spangler RD, Paton BC. Usefulness of echocardiography in patients undergoing mitral valve surgery. J Thorac Cardiovasc Surg. 1972;64:922-34.
2. Spencer KT, Kimura BJ, Korcarz CE, Pellikka PA, Rahko PS, Siegel RJ. Focused cardiac ultrasound: recommendations from the American Society of Echocardiography. J Am Soc Echocardiogr. 2013;26:567-81.
3. Kratz T, Steinfeldt T, Exner M, Dell Orto MC, Timmesfeld N, Kratz C, et al. Impact of focused intraoperative transthoracic echocardiography by anesthesiologists on management in hemodynamically unstable high-risk noncardiac surgery patients. J Cardiothorac Vasc Anesth. 2017;31:602-9.
4. Labovitz AJ, Noble VE, Bierig M, Goldstein SA, Jones R, Kort S, et al. Focused cardiac ultrasound in the emergent setting: a consensus statement of the American Society of Echocardiography and American College of Emergency Physicians. J Am Soc Echocardiogr. 2010;23:1225-30.
5. Griffiths SE, Waight G, Dennis AT. Focused transthoracic echocardiography in obstetrics. BJA Educ. 2018;18:271-6.
6. Holm JH, Frederiksen CA, Juhl-Olsen P, Sloth E. Perioperative use of focus assessed transthoracic echocardiography (FATE). Anesth Analg. 2012;115:1029-32.
7. Atkinson P, Peach M, Lewis D. Just the Facts: The Five F's of Focused Echocardiography in Shock. CJEM. 2020;22:655-7.
8. Styczynski G, Sinski M, Szmigielski C. Feasibility of transthoracic echocardiography in obese patients and its relation to the distance between the skin surface and the left ventricular apex. J Am Soc Echocardiogr. 2020;33:520.
9. Brandt RR, Oh JK, Abel MD, Click RL, Orszulak TA, Seward JB. Role of emergency intraoperative transesophageal echocardiography. J Am Soc Echocardiogr. 1998;11:972-7.
10. American Society of Anesthesiologists and Society of Cardiovascular Anesthesiologists Task Force on Transesophageal Echocardiography. Practice guidelines for perioperative transesophageal echocardiography. An updated report by the American Society of Anesthesiologists and the Society of Cardiovascular Anesthesiologists Task Force on Transesophageal Echocardiography. Anesthesiology. 2010;112:1084-96.
11. Reeves ST, Finley AC, Skubas NJ, Swaminathan M, Whitley WS, Glas KE, et al. Basic perioperative transesophageal echocardiography examination: a consensus statement of the American Society of Echocardiography and the Society of Cardiovascular Anesthesiologists. J Am Soc Echocardiogr. 2013;26:443-56.
12. Kronzon I, Tunick PA, Freedberg RS, Trehan N, Rosenzweig BP, Schwinger ME. Transesophageal echocardiography is superior to transthoracic echocardiography in the diagnosis of sinus venosus atrial septal defect. J Am Coll Cardiol. 1991;17:537-42.
13. de Bruijn SF, Agema WR, Lammers GJ, van der Wall EE, Wolterbeek R, Holman ER, et al. Transesophageal echocardiography is superior to transthoracic echocardiography in management of patients of any age with transient ischemic attack or stroke. Stroke. 2006;37:2531-4.
14. Price S, Uddin S, Quinn T. Echocardiography in cardiac arrest. Curr Opin Crit Care. 2010;16:211-5.
15. Breitkreutz R, Price S, Steiger HV, Seeger FH, Ilper H, Ackermann H, et al. Focused echocardiographic evaluation in life support and peri-resuscitation of emergency patients: a prospective trial. Resuscitation. 2010;81:1527-33.
16. Kegel F, Chenkin J. Resuscitative transesophageal echocardiography in the emergency

department: a single-centre case series. Scand J Trauma Resusc Emerg Med. 2023; 31:24.

17. Teran F, Prats MI, Nelson BP, Kessler R, Blaivas M, Peberdy MA, et al. Focused Transesophageal Echocardiography During Cardiac Arrest Resuscitation: JACC Review Topic of the Week. J Am Coll Cardiol. 2020;76: 745-54.
18. Neskovic AN, Hagendorff A, Lancellotti P, Guarracino F, Varga A, Cosyns B, et al. Emergency echocardiography: the European Association of Cardiovascular Imaging recommendations. Eur Heart J Cardiovasc Imaging. 2013;14:1-11.
19. Matthews S, Levy PD. Emergency department-based 3D echocardiogram use: a case series. Ultrasound J. 2020;12:44.

CHAPTER

# 21 Echocardiography in Complications of Percutaneous Interventions

*Kandaswamy N*

## INTRODUCTION

Percutaneous interventions are performed widely in critically ill patients and also patients post percutaneous coronary interventions (PCI) get admitted to the intensive care unit (ICU) for further care. It is imperative for the intensivist to be aware of the complications involved with the percutaneous procedures so that they can be recognized early and managed aptly. Echocardiography in this setting is a useful tool as it helps in recognizing the complications bedside, obviating the risk and delay associated with transfer to imaging suite. Both transthoracic echocardiography (TTE) and transesophageal echocardiography (TEE) have their own place in the ICU echocardiography.

*The complications associated with percutaneous interventions can be grouped into two categories:*

1. Percutaneous interventions performed in the ICU
2. Percutaneous interventions in the cardiac catheterization laboratory

## PERCUTANEOUS INTERVENTIONS PERFORMED IN THE INTENSIVE CARE UNIT

- Central venous catheter and hemodialysis catheter insertion
- Pulmonary artery catheter insertion
- Temporary transvenous pacemaker (TTP) insertion
- Pericardiocentesis
- Intra-aortic balloon pump (IABP) insertion
- Extracorporeal membrane oxygenation (ECMO) cannula insertion

### Central Venous Catheter and Hemodialysis Catheter

Most common complications are related to the guidewire placement. Advancement of the guidewire too much inside might irritate the right heart which can lead to arrhythmias. It can be prevented by continuous subcostal view monitoring of the heart. Guidewire getting lost during railroading of the catheter over the guidewire is a rare but potential problem in the hands of less experienced clinicians. TTE can determine the location of the guidewire and appropriate help can be sought from interventional cardiology. Direct tricuspid valve injuries can be assessed by evaluating the tricuspid regurgitation (TR) jet and comparing it with the baseline.[1]

### Pulmonary Artery Catheter

Though the practice of using pulmonary artery catheters (PAC) has dwindled with time in general ICUs, cardiac ICUs still use them in postcardiac surgery patients frequently.

The guidewire of PACs is longer and can cause atrial or ventricular arrhythmias due to irritation or contact of the catheter with the cardiac walls. Valve rupture or cardiac wall perforation are rare but serious complications. Vessel rupture can happen at the moment of balloon inflation into the pulmonary artery, which can lead to pulmonary artery perforation, pseudoaneurysm formation, and rupture. The pulmonary artery can be visualized with the parasternal short-axis view at aortic valve level, which is obtained by anterior angulation of the probe from a standard parasternal short-axis view at midpapillary level. Myocardial perforation leading to pericardial effusion and cardiac tamponade may happen in patients with dilated right atrium (RA) and right ventricle (RV). Thrombosis due to the indwelling catheter acting as a nidus for thrombus is possible and both TTE and TEE with right ventricular outflow tract view can identify the same.

## Temporary Transvenous Pacemaker Insertion

Temporary transvenous pacemaker insertion is done to treat patients with severe heart block and life-threatening arrhythmias. Myocardial perforation and pericardial tamponade complicating TTP insertion occur in about 0.6% of patients[2] undergoing the procedure and is associated with a fivefold increase in risk for inhospital mortality. TTE might help in rapid identification of the cardiac tamponade and aid in urgent pericardiocentesis.

## Pericardiocentesis

In the ICU, pericardiocentesis is usually performed as an emergency procedure and has high risk of complications such as injury to the myocardium with hemorrhage into the pericardium, leading to iatrogenic cardiac tamponade. TTE can be both a diagnostic tool in the identification of cardiac tamponade and grading pericardial effusion and also a guide for pericardiocentesis. Complication rates with pericardiocentesis are relatively lower with the parasternal or apical approach compared to the subxiphoid approach as the distance from the skin-to-fluid collection is the least in the former views and posteriorly placed effusions are not accessed via the subxiphoid approach.[3] Echocardiographic features of cardiac tamponade are given in **Box 1**.

## Intra-aortic Balloon Pump Insertion

Transthoracic echocardiography and TEE can both be used to position IABP catheter

**BOX 1:** Echocardiographic features of cardiac tamponade.

- *2D and M-Mode:*
  - Pericardial effusion
  - Underfilled heart
  - Late systolic RA free wall inversion
  - Early diastolic RV free wall inversion (may precede actual clinical hemodynamic compromise)
  - IVC plethora with decreased respiratory variation
- *Doppler:*
  - Increased MV flow variation (PW Doppler) >25% decrease with inspiration
  - Increased TV flow velocity variation (PW Doppler) >50% increase during inspiration
  - Increased LVOT VTI variation with PW Doppler >10% decrease with inspiration
  - Low LVOT VTI and corresponding stroke volume consistent with hemodynamic impairment
  - Absence of diastolic inflow (PW Doppler) of HV
  - Increased IVRT

(2D: two dimensional; HV: hepatic veins; IVC: inferior vena cava; IVRT: isovolumic relaxation time; LVOT VTI: left ventricular outflow tract velocity time integral; MV: mitral valve; PW: pulse wave; RA: right atrium; RV: right ventricle; TV: tricuspid valve) insertion. In TTE, an off-axis apical two-chamber view of the descending aorta and a suprasternal view of the aortic arch are performed. In TEE, a midesophageal 0° short-axis view and a 90° long-axis view of the descending aorta, and an upper esophageal 0–10° view of the aortic arch is performed.[4] The tip of the balloon catheter must be located just distal to the origin of the left subclavian artery. Complications such as catheter tip misplacement leading to occlusion of the left subclavian artery origin can be identified with the aortic arch views. Moreover, screening of aortic valvular insufficiency with an echocardiogram is a basic prerequisite for IABP insertion.

### Extracorporeal Membrane Oxygenation

Echocardiography is critical in the detection and management of specific complications that may arise during ECMO support. TEE is usually used to detect these complications as TTE has limited spatial resolution. TEE helps with rapid assessment of cannula malpositioning, overloading or excessive cardiac offloading, cardiac function, and evidence of cardiac tamponade.[5] In venovenous ECMO, the position of the access cannula tip is in the proximal inferior vena cava (IVC), just before the entry into the RA and the optimal position for the return cannula is in the mid-RA and away from the interatrial septum and the tricuspid valve. In the absence of TEE probe, even TTE can be used for cannula position determination with the subcostal bicaval view. It can be obtained by tilting the probe more cephalad from the traditional sagittal IVC view. **Figure 1** shows a pericardial effusion with cardiac tamponade after ECMO cannula insertion.

## COMPLICATIONS AFTER PRIMARY PERCUTANEOUS CORONARY INTERVENTION

Transthoracic echocardiography after PCI is routinely practiced to assess left ventricle (LV) and RV systolic function.[6] In case of suspected reperfusion injury and sudden hemodynamic deterioration, TTE can diagnose new regional wall motion abnormality and mechanical complications such as ventricular septal

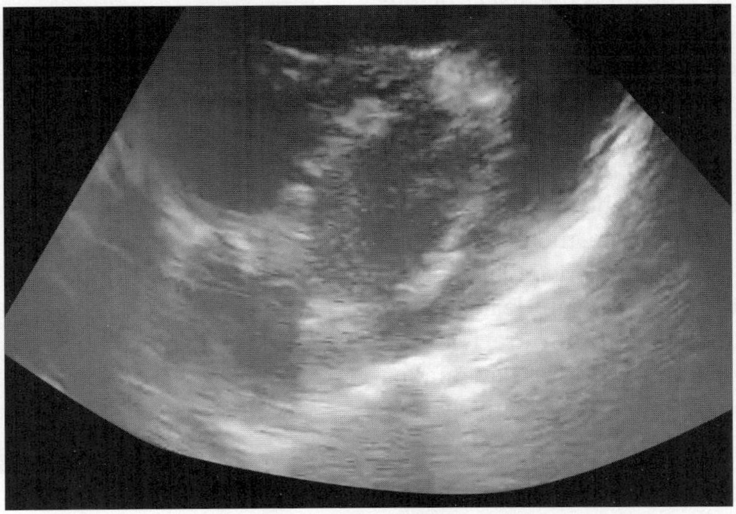

**Fig. 1:** Pericardial effusion with tamponade indicated by early diastolic right ventricular free wall collapse.

defect, papillary muscle rupture, valve dysfunction, pericardial effusion, or tamponade. The overall complication risk associated with PCI is ~3% but varies widely between studies and increases with higher lesion complexity. A stent abscess is an extremely rare and late complication which might be seen as an echodense myocardial mass in TTE.

## COMPLICATIONS AFTER ELECTROPHYSIOLOGICAL PROCEDURES

Electrophysiological procedure (EP) includes implantation of pacemaker and implantable cardioverter defibrillator (ICD) and ablation procedures for atrial fibrillation. They are usually low-risk procedures. However, complications can arise at different stages of the procedure. In procedures for atrial fibrillation, a prior TEE examination of the left atrial (LA) appendage and anatomy of the interatrial septum must be noted.

*Acute complications:* Pericardial effusion during an EP procedure can be associated with sudden hemodynamic instability. The easiest and best approach is to opt for the subcostal view of the heart. The RA is the first structure to be affected. Urgent pericardiocentesis might be needed and in some cases, might have to place a pericardial catheter.

Perforation of the myocardium by the pacemaker lead can be observed in the TTE focused on the RV. The beam width should be narrowed in order to increase spatial and temporal resolution. Pericardial effusion and visualization of the tip of the lead floating outside the RV myocardium are features consistent with perforation. Pacemaker lead detachment, which is a relatively rare complication, can also be seen by TTE.

*Long-term complications:* These include infection of the pacemaker and endocarditis of the pacemaker leads. TEE is superior and mandatory in suspected pacemaker lead endocarditis. The entire lead should be followed, beginning from the superior vena cava to the tip of the lead. Biplanar imaging is recommended to ensure proper visualization, especially in case of multiple leads. Clinical correlation such as inflammatory parameters, blood cultures, and fever should be made to differentiate between vegetation and thrombus as both are seen as echogenic structures in TTE/TEE. **Figure 2** shows a mitral valve vegetation/thrombus after removal of a long-standing pacemaker lead.

Cardiac resynchronization therapy (CRT) lead endocarditis is a delayed complication. It requires the visualization of the coronary sinus which can be obtained by posterior angulation of the transducer from an apical four-chamber view.

## COMPLICATIONS FOLLOWING PERCUTANEOUS VALVULAR PROCEDURES

Percutaneous valvular procedures are becoming frequent in developing nations,

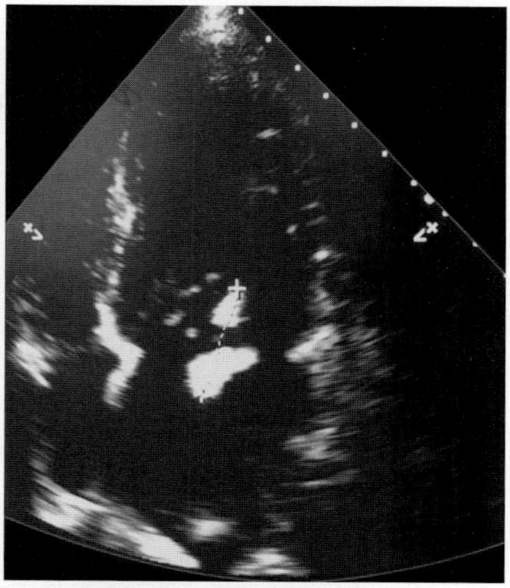

**Fig. 2:** Mitral valve vegetation/thrombus seen as hyperechogenic shadow.

**TABLE 1:** Complications detected by echocardiography after percutaneous valvular procedures.

| *Procedure* | *Complications detected by ECHO* |
|---|---|
| TAVI | • Incomplete expansion during deployment<br>• Transcatheter heart valves migrating into the aorta or left ventricle<br>• Aortic embolization during implantation |
| Indirect mitral valve annuloplasty | • Coronary sinus dissection or perforation<br>• Extrinsic left coronary artery compression causing RWMA<br>• Partial device dislodgment or fracture |
| Mitral valve edge-to-edge | • Iatrogenic ASD seen as turbulent flow across the interatrial septum<br>• Acute RV failure is seen as reduced TAPSE |
| Tricuspid valve direct annuloplasty | • RCA extrinsic compression causing RWMA<br>• Partial device dislodgment or fracture<br>• Tricuspid regurgitation |

(ASD: atrial septal defect; ECHO: echocardiography; RCA: right coronary artery; RV: right ventricle; RWMA: regional wall motion abnormality; TAPSE: tricuspid annular plane systolic excursion; TAVI: transcatheter aortic valve implantation)

such as India, with an increased incidence of rheumatic heart disease. It can involve either aortic, tricuspid, or mitral valves. Myocardial perforation followed by pericardial effusion and tamponade can be seen in procedures involving all valves. Other valve-specific complications are listed in **Table 1**.

## CONCLUSION

The critical care physician should be well versed with all the basic views of TTE and TEE to detect the complications associated with percutaneous interventions, be it ICU procedures or cardiac catheterization laboratory procedures. Sometimes, special views such as the suprasternal aortic arch view, coronary sinus view, LA appendage view, and bicaval view might be useful to detect specific complications. Of all, cardiac tamponade is the most life-threatening complication and bedside echocardiography is a vital tool in both diagnosis and intervention for treatment by pericardiocentesis.

## REFERENCES

1. Kornbau C, Lee KC, Hughes GD, Firstenberg MS. Central line complications. Int J Crit Illn Inj Sci. 2015;5(3):170-8.
2. Metkus TS, Schulman SP, Marine JE, Eid SM. Complications and outcomes of temporary transvenous pacing: an analysis of >360,000 patients from the national inpatient sample. Chest. 2019;155(4):749-57.
3. Stolz L, Situ-LaCasse E, Acuña J, Thompson M, Hawbaker N, Valenzuela J, et al. What is the ideal approach for emergent pericardiocentesis using point-of-care ultrasound guidance? World J Emerg Med. 2021;12(3):169-73.
4. Baldetti L, Beneduce A, Boccellino A, Pagnesi M, Barone G, Gallone G, et al. Bedside intra-aortic balloon pump insertion in cardiac intensive care unit: a single-center experience. Catheter Cardiovasc Interv. 2022;99(7):1976-83.
5. Platts DG, Sedgwick JF, Burstow DJ, Mullany DV, Fraser JF. The role of echocardiography in the management of patients supported by extracorporeal membrane oxygenation. J Am Soc Echocardiogr. 2012;25(2):131-41.
6. Parasuraman SK, Srinivasan J, Broadhurst P. Is follow-up echocardiogram mandatory after a STEMI? Echo Res Pract. 2020;7(3):K27-30.

CHAPTER 22

# Fluid for Critically Ill Responsiveness, Tolerance and Removal: Echocardiography Integrated Approach

*Gourav Mittal, Puneet Khanna*

## INTRODUCTION

Critically ill patients have complex physiology with intricate interactions between physiological, pathological, and compensatory mechanisms. Deciding whether to administer fluids remains a gray area, even with advanced hemodynamic monitoring in place. As the literature and evidence continue to evolve, we now recognize that fluids can be considered a form of medicine, carrying potential side effects. Incorrect fluid administration can lead to increased organ dysfunction and higher mortality rates.

When a critically ill patient's hemodynamics are crashing, intensivists often face the dilemma of whether to administer fluids. From a physiological perspective, this situation brings to mind two key states:

1. *Fluid responsiveness:* This is the scenario where administering fluid leads to an increase in cardiac output and subsequently improves hemodynamics.
2. *Fluid tolerance:* This refers to whether the patient can tolerate the administered fluid, regardless of responsiveness, without causing further organ dysfunction.

These considerations are crucial in making informed decisions about fluid administration in critical care.

The interplay between fluid tolerance and fluid responsiveness can lead to four distinct hemodynamic profiles (proposed), each requiring different management strategies.

1. *Fluid tolerant, fluid responsive (D-dry):* These patients benefit from fluid administration as it increases cardiac output without causing harm
2. *Fluid tolerant, fluid unresponsive (R-at risk):* These patients can tolerate fluids but do not show improved cardiac output, posing a risk for fluid overload
3. *Fluid intolerant, fluid responsive (L-leaky):* These patients show improved cardiac output with fluids but are at risk of organ dysfunction due to poor fluid tolerance
4. *Fluid intolerant, fluid unresponsive (F-full):* These patients neither benefit from fluid administration nor tolerate it well, often leading to worsened organ function

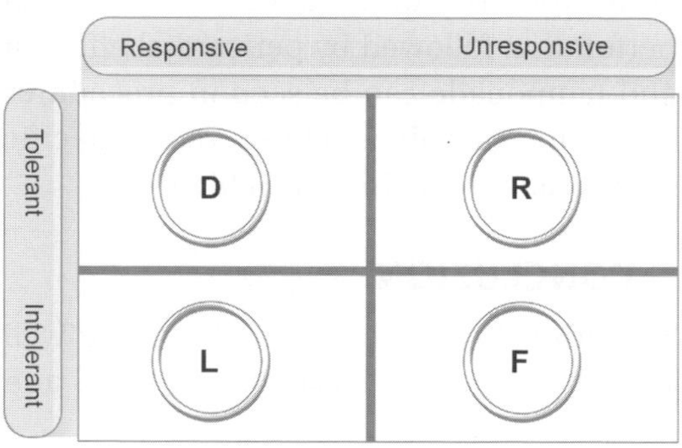

It is important to note that there can be overlap between these profiles and that they can change dynamically in response to pathological states and interventions.

Echocardiography and ultrasonography can help identify which phenotype predominates in a patient at the time of assessment. Consider the following points before proceeding with the examination:

- A single parameter or examination will not provide an accurate assessment; it is the trend over time that should guide treatment.
- Do not check for fluid responsiveness when the patient is hemodynamically stable. Instead, assess for congestion, particularly after resuscitation is complete.
- Prediction of fluid responsiveness and actual fluid responsiveness are two different concepts. Prediction depends on certain loading conditions applied to the cardiovascular system under standardized conditions to determine the probability of the cardiac axis lying on the steep portion of the Frank–Starling relationship. Actual fluid responsiveness is assessed by administering fluids and observing whether cardiac output and organ perfusion improve.
- Some parameters are static, while others are dynamic concerning fluid responsiveness. Static parameters are measured without applying any stress or challenge to the cardiovascular system, capturing a snapshot of the values. Dynamic variables are measured after adding stress to the cardiovascular system, such as thorough mechanical ventilation or fluid loading (active or passive).
- Static parameters are easier to obtain but are meaningful only in extreme conditions, such as profound hypovolemia or congestion. They have limited value in determining intermediate conditions, which are often encountered by intensivists.

## PARAMETERS USEFUL IN ASSESSING FLUID RESPONSIVENESS

*Static:*
- CVP assessment with IVC diameter
- *ECHO:*
  - A4C view—mitral inflow—E/A, E/E', interatrial septal ballooning
  - PSAX—LV end-diastolic area, LV cavity visual assessment

*Dynamic:*
- On MV
  - *TEE:* SVC shape change with respiratory variations
  - *TTE:* Subcostal view; IVC size and size variations with respiration
  - *TTE:* A5C—LVOT VTI variations with respiration
- Spontaneously breathing
  - *TTE:* Subcostal view; IVC size and size variations with respiration
- Either on MV or spontaneous breathing
  - PLR (or mini fluid challenge)
  - *A5C view:* LVOT VTI change before and after

(CVP: central venous pressure; ECHO: echocardiography; IVC: inferior vena cava; LV: left ventricular; LVOT: left ventricular outflow tract; MV: mechanical ventilation; PLR: passive leg raising; SVC: superior vena cava; TEE: transesophageal echocardiography; TTE: transthoracic echocardiography; VTI: velocity time integral)

## PARAMETERS USEFUL IN ASSESSING FLUID INTOLERANCE

*Right-side intolerance:*
- *TTE:* Subcostal—IVC ≥2 cm, full cardiac chambers
- Venous Doppler (IVC, hepatic vein, portal vein, intrarenal veins)
  - VEXUS ≥2
  - Pulsating femoral vein Doppler

*Left-side intolerance:*
- Lung ultrasound
  - EVLW ≥10 mL/kg (with the help of LUS score)
  - B/B profile involving nondependent chest area also
- *TTE:* A4C
  - E/e' ≥14 or E/A >2

(EVLW: extravascular lung water; IVC: inferior vena cava; LUS: lung ultrasound; TTE: transthoracic echocardiography)

## Patient on Mechanical Ventilation

| *Echo indices* | *Hypovolemia* | *Fluid responsive* | *Normovolemia* | *Hypervolemia* |
|---|---|---|---|---|
| Shape, size, and respiratory variation in SVC | Triangular vessel with significant respiratory variations | Triangular vessel with significant respiratory variations[1] | Triangular vessel with minimal respiratory variations | Round-shaped, dilated vessel with minimal respiratory variations |
| Shape, size, respiratory variation in IVC | Ellipsoid vessel with AP diameter <10 mm with minimal respiratory variations | Significant respiratory variations[2] | Minimal respiratory variations | Round-shaped, dilated vessel (diameter >23 mm) with minimal respiratory variations |
| Respiratory variations in LVOT VTI | Significant respiratory variations | Significant respiratory variations | Minimal variations | No variations |

(AP: anteroposterior; IVC: inferior vena cava; LVOT: left ventricular outflow tract; PLR: passive leg raising; SVC: superior vena cava; VTI: velocity time integral)

[1]ΔSVC ≥21%; sensitivity 65%, specificity 84% to predict change of 10% in LVOT VTI in response to PLR

[2]ΔIVC ≥10%; sensitivity 79%, specificity 64% to predict change of 10% in LVOT VTI in response to PLR

## Spontaneously Breathing Patients

| *Echo indices* | *Hypovolemia* | *Fluid responsive* | *Normovolemia* | *Hypervolemia* |
|---|---|---|---|---|
| Shape, size, respiratory variation in inferior vena cava (IVC) | Total inspiratory collapse or end-expiratory diameter <13 mm | ΔIVC >50% | End-expiratory diameter > 13 mm, <20 mm with inspiratory collapse <50% | Round-shaped, dilated vessel (diameter >23 mm) with minimal respiratory variations |

## All Patients

| *Echo indices* | *Hypovolemia* | *Fluid responsive* | *Normovolemia* | *Hypervolemia* |
|---|---|---|---|---|
| LV visual assessment | Kissing papillary muscles | | | Dilated/ballooned LV |
| LV end-diastolic area | <10 $cm^2$ | | | >20 $cm^2$ |
| LV filling pressures qualitative | | | | Continuous bulging of interatrial septum |
| MV inflow in reduced LVEF | | | Normal pattern for age | E/A >2/DTE <150 ms |
| MV inflow in normal LV | | | Mean E/E' <8 | Mean E/E' >14 |
| LVOT VTI change in PLR | Marked increase >>12% | Increased ≥12% | Minimal increase | No change |

(DTE: deceleration time; LV: left ventricular; LVEF: LV ejection fraction; LVOT: LV outflow tract; MV: mechanical ventilation; PLR: passive leg raising; VTI: velocity time integral)

## WHICH TEST ONE SHOULD USE FOR FLUID ASSESSMENT

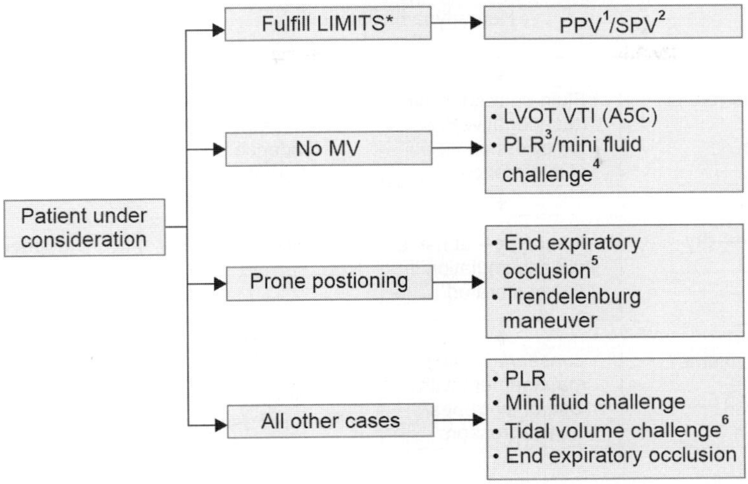


(HR: heart rate; LVOT: left ventricular outflow tract; MV: mechanical ventilation; PLR: passive leg raising; PPV: pulse pressure variation; RR: respiratory rate; SPV: systolic pressure variation; VTI: velocity time integral)
*L: Low HR/RR <3.6, I: Irregular heart rhythm, M: MV tidal volume <8 mL/kg, I: Increased abdominal pressure, T: Thorax open, S: Spontaneous breathing
[1,2]>12% variation; [3]>10% VTI variation; [4]>6% prefer continuous CO monitoring (after 100 mL); [5]5% change in LVOT VTI on 15-second end-expiratory hold; [6]from 6 to 8 mL/kg for 1 minute—ΔPPV >3.5%, ΔSPV >2.5%

## INFERIOR VENA CAVA ASSESSMENT LIMITATIONS IN FLUID RESPONSIVENESS

| | |
|---|---|
| MV with high PEEP and/or low TV | • False negative fluid resposiveness |
| Assisted ventilation modalities, NIV, CPAP | • Both false negative or false positive fluid resposiveness |
| Varrying respiraory pattern | • Significant efforts—false positive<br>• Shallow efforts—false negative |
| Asthma/COPD exacerbation | • Hyperinflation—false negative<br>• Active expiration—false positive |
| Chronic RV dysfuntion/SEV TR | • False negative |
| RV MI | • False negative |
| Cardiac temponade | • False negative |
| Intraabdominal hypertension | • Either of two possible false positive/false negative |
| Local mechanical factors | • Venous return hindrance, IVC dilatation (stenosis, thrombosis)—False negative<br>• IVC compression (masses)—False negative<br>• Hindrance to IVC size change (ECMO cannulae, cava filters)—False negative |
| Pronounced lateral IVC deviation | • False positive |

(COPD: chronic obstructive pulmonary disease; CPAP: continuous positive airway pressure; ECMO: extracorporeal membrane oxygenation; IVC: inferior vena cava; MI: myocardial infarction; MV: mechanical ventilation; NIV: noninvasive ventilation; PEEP: positive end-expiratory pressure; RV: right ventricular; TR: tricuspid regurgitation; TV: tricuspid valve)

## COMBINING ALL TOGETHER WITH PHENOTYPES AND MANAGEMENT

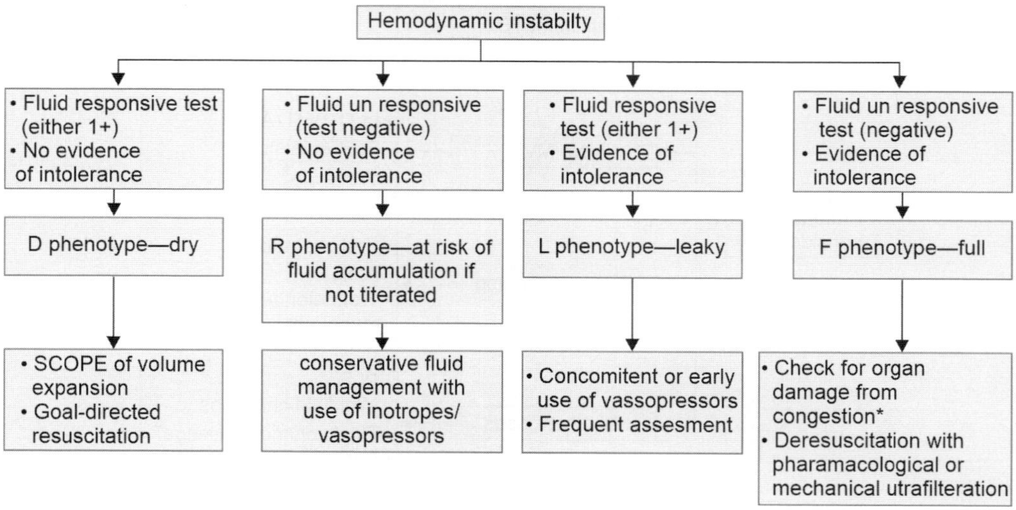


*Organ dysfunction induced by fluid congestion

- Lungs
  - Alteration in gas exchange
  - Reduction in complacency
  - Increased work on breathing
- Heart
  - Conduction disorders
  - Change in contractility
  - Diastolic dysfunction
- Brain
  - Cognitive dysfunction
  - Delirium
- Kidney
  - Increased interstitial pressure
  - Reduction in renal blood flow
  - Decreased glomerular filtration rate
  - Uremia
  - Retention of salt and water
- Liver
  - Cholestasis
  - Dysfunction of hepatic synthesis
- Intestine
  - Ileum
  - Malabsorption
- Skin
  - Reduction in the healing process
  - Pressure ulcer
- Wound infection

## BASIC POINTS

### Subcostal Inferior Vena Cava

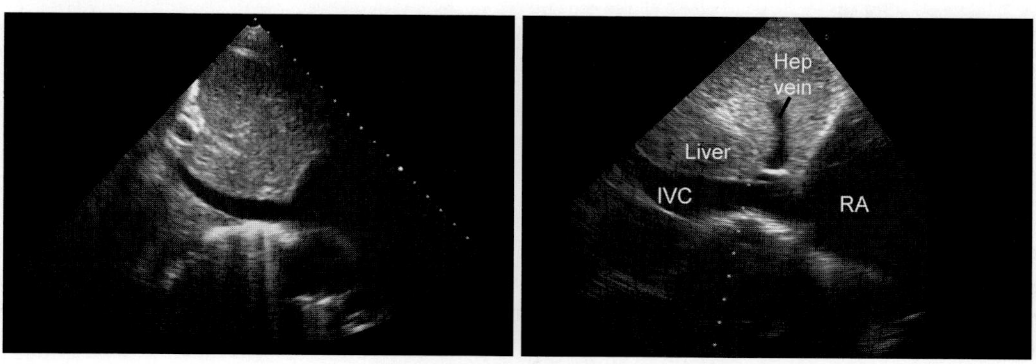


**Inferior vena cava for Volume Status: Where to measure?**

***Volume status:* Based on IVC diameter**

- Normal IVC diameter = 1.5–2.5 cm
    - IVC <1 cm: Sever volume depletion
    - IVC <1.5 cm: Volume depletion
    - IVC >2.5 cm: Volume overload

**Volume status: IVC diameter—respiratory variations**

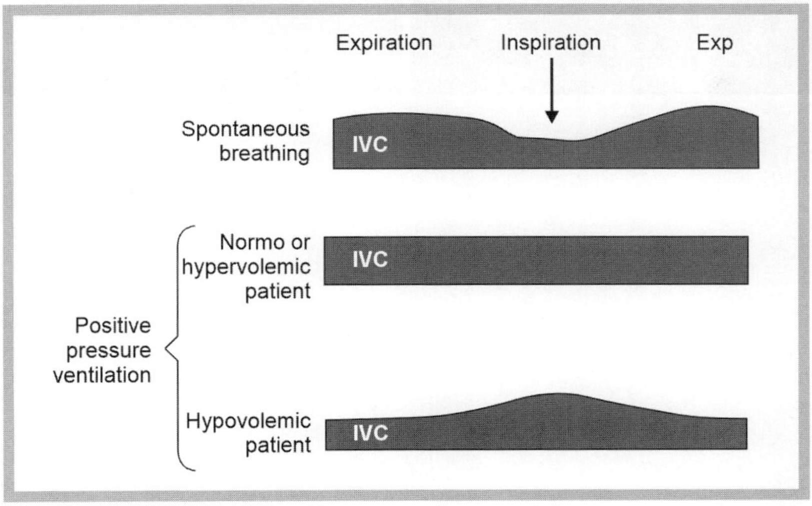


**Volume status: Based on IVC Collapsibility—collapsibility or caval index**

*Spontaneously breathing patient:* IVC normally collapses >50% with inspiration or sniffing.

*Collapse <50%:* Volume overload
*Collapse >50%:* Volume responsive
Caval index (CI)

$$CI = \frac{\text{Maximum (expiratory) diameter} - \text{minimal (inspiratory) diameter}}{\text{Maximum (expiratory) diameter}}$$

- In adults, the following correlation is present between central venous pressure, IVC diameter, and respiration
    - Size ≤2.1 cm; collapse >50% during sniff = Right atrial pressure (RAP) 0–5 mm Hg
    - Size >2.1 cm; collapse >50% during sniff = RAP 5–10 mm Hg
    - Size >2.1 cm; collapse <50% during sniff = RAP 10–20 mm Hg

## Volume Status: Distensibility and Variability Index

- In fully supported, mechanically ventilated patients (no respiratory effort, TV >8 mL/kg)
- *Distensibility index (DI) <18%:* Not volume responsive
- ΔIVC = (Maximum diameter – minimum diameter)/(mean diameter) × 100 ΔIVC >12%: Fluid responsive

## Passive Leg Raising Test

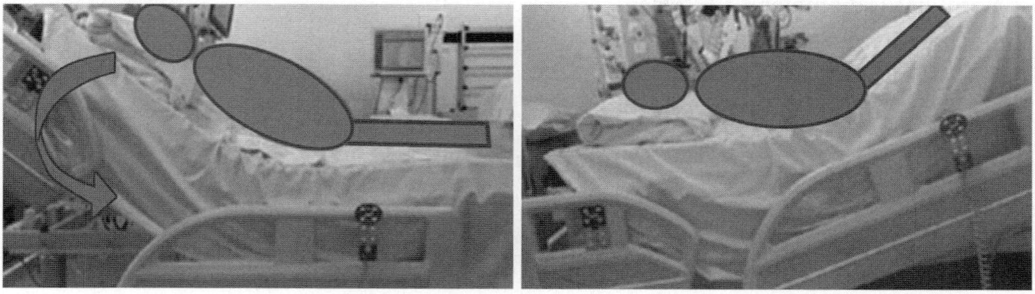

CHAPTER 23

# Echocardiography in Critically Ill Children

*Aravindhan Manoharan, Rakesh Lodha*

## INTRODUCTION

Cardiac point-of-care ultrasound (POCUS) is a specialized, physiology-based imaging tool used by noncardiology clinicians to enhance clinical assessments and improve patient management. It has evolved widely and has become a common practice in most Intensive care units. However, its application in children requires careful consideration based on the anatomical and physiological differences.

## INDICATIONS

According to the 2023 guidelines from the American Society of Echocardiography for children,[1] Cardiac POCUS is indicated for:

- Qualitative and semiquantitative assessment of systolic function.
- Evaluation of preload and volume responsiveness.
- Evaluation and guidance for pericardiocentesis in pericardial effusion.
- Evaluation of pulmonary systolic pressure and pulmonary hypertension (semiquantitative).

These guidelines also specify certain limitations:[1]

- Any child with clinical features suggestive of congenital heart disease (CHD), such as cyanosis and murmurs, cardiac POCUS is considered not appropriate for evaluation.
- Cardiac POCUS is not appropriate for diagnosing/excluding CHD.
- In children with known CHD, Cardiac POCUS is not advised.
- Routine use of cardiac POCUS in a non-emergent setting is not yet established.

## TECHNICAL CONSIDERATIONS

Both low-frequency (2–2.5 MHz) and high-frequency (≥7.5 MHz) probes/transducers are available for performing cardiac POCUS in children due to variations in imaging depths. Also, the low-frequency adult probe, due to its large footprint, would be difficult to negotiate in between the narrow rib spaces in children making it difficult to get a proper view. So, it is advisable to have both low and high-frequency probes with smaller footprints when performing pediatric echocardiography.[2]

## VIEWS

The most challenging part of pediatric echocardiography is obtaining the proper images. The five important views in pediatric cardiac POCUS are:

1. Parasternal long-axis view
2. Parasternal short-axis view
3. Apical four-chamber view

4. Subcostal view
5. Subcostal inferior vena cava (IVC) view.

The views, transducer position, and possible assessment goals are summarized in **Table 1**.

# EVALUATION OF LEFT VENTRICULAR SYSTOLIC FUNCTION

## Qualitative Assessment

Clinicians can qualitatively assess the LV function (eyeballing technique) by looking at the global and focal contractility of the left ventricle in various views. A poor function may be indicated when the left ventricular walls appear to contract less vigorously than normal, the walls of the left ventricle do not thicken appreciably during systole, the anterior leaflet of the mitral valve does not move close to the interventricular septum during systole, and/or the overall contraction of the left ventricle appears weak or sluggish, with less inward movement of the walls.[3]

## Quantitative Assessment

### *Fractional Shortening Method*

The fractional shortening (FS) method quantifies contractility by measuring the left ventricular end-diastolic diameter (LVEDD) and the left ventricular end-systolic diameter (LVESD) in either the parasternal long axis or short axis view at the level of the papillary muscle **(Fig. 6)**. Fractional shortening is calculated as:[4]

$$FS(\%) = \frac{(LVEDD - LVESD) \times 100}{LVEDD}$$

**TABLE 1:** Imaging views for pediatric cardiac POCUS **(Figs. 1 to 5)**.[1]

| *View* | *Transducer placement** | *Potential goals* |
|---|---|---|
| 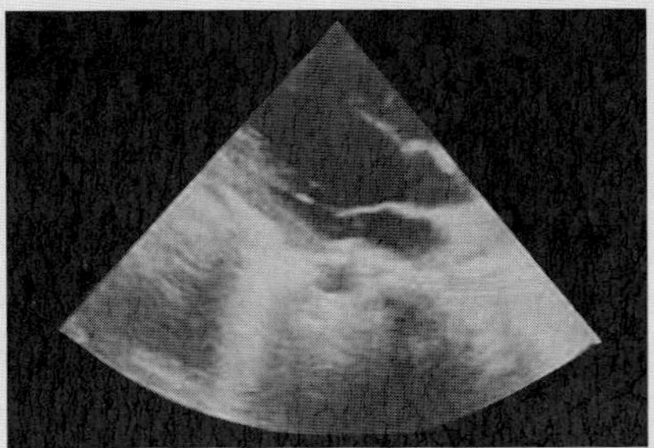 **Fig. 1:** Parasternal long-axis view. | • *Position:* Left of the sternum<br>• *Indicator:* 10–11 o'clock (toward the right shoulder)* | • Assessment of LV systolic function<br>• Differentiating pericardial from pleural effusion |
| 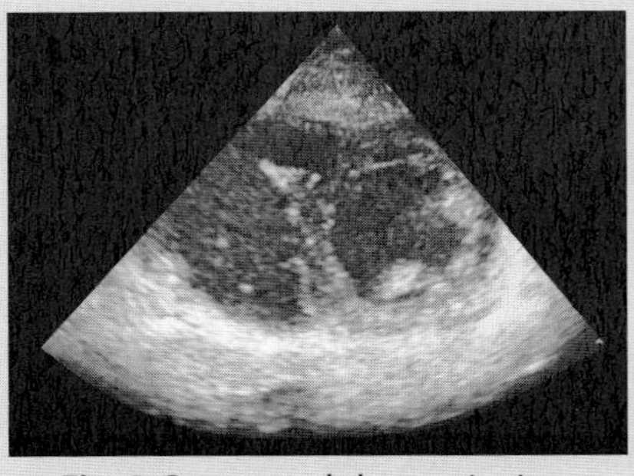 **Fig. 2:** Parasternal short-axis view. | • *Position:* Left of the sternum<br>• *Indicator:* 1–2 o'clock (toward the left shoulder)* | • Evaluation of LV size and systolic function<br>• Evaluation of RV size and systolic function<br>• Evaluation of interventricular septal position<br>• Evaluation of pericardial effusion |

*Contd...*

*Contd...*

| ***View*** | ***Transducer placement**** | ***Potential goals*** |
|---|---|---|
| 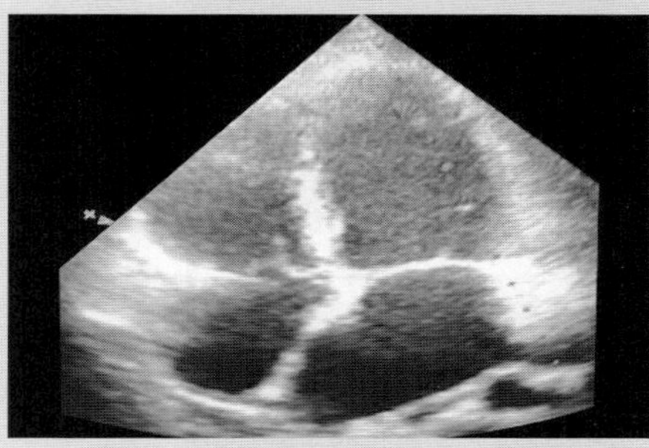 **Fig. 3:** Apical 4 chamber view. | • *Position:* Point of maximal impulse<br>• *Indicator:* 3 o'clock (toward the left axilla)* | • LV systolic function<br>• Evaluation of pericardial effusion<br>• Evaluation of mitral and tricuspid regurgitation |
| 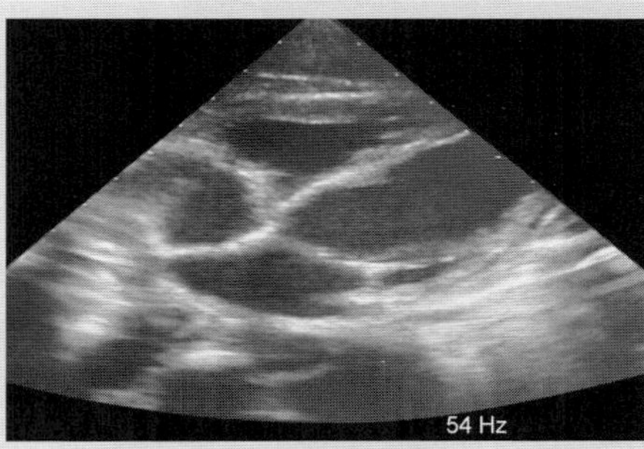  **Fig. 4:** Subcostal view. | • *Position:* Subxiphoid<br>• *Indicator:* 3 o'clock (toward left flank) | • Evaluation of pericardial and pleural effusion<br>• Evaluation of biventricular function |
| 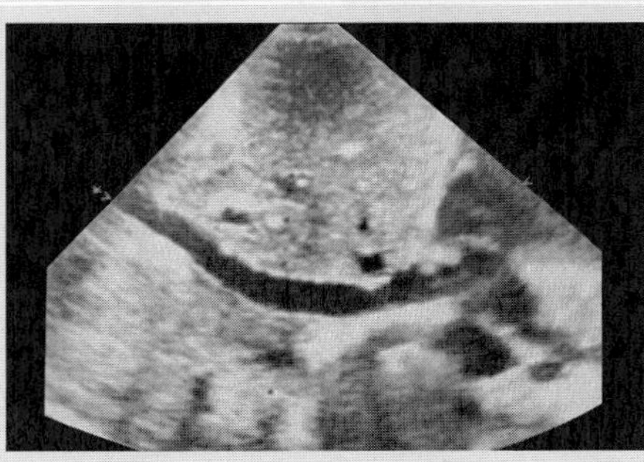 **Fig. 5:** Subcostal IVC view. | Subxiphoid, indicator at 12 o'clock (toward the head) | Evaluation of fluid status |

*Better visualized with a child in the lateral decubitus position.
(IVC: inferior vena cava; LV: left ventricle; RV: right ventricle)

Doubling the FS value provides the ejection fraction. It is important to note that in conditions with the altered shape of the ventricle, the fractional shortening method is not reliable. It can happen in children with CHD, preload, and afterload changes, and those with ventricular interactions.[5]

### *Simpson Biplanar Technique*

It is considered one of the most reliable methods for estimating EF. However, it requires proper image acquisition and is time-consuming. This technique is performed in the apical four-chamber view, by tracing

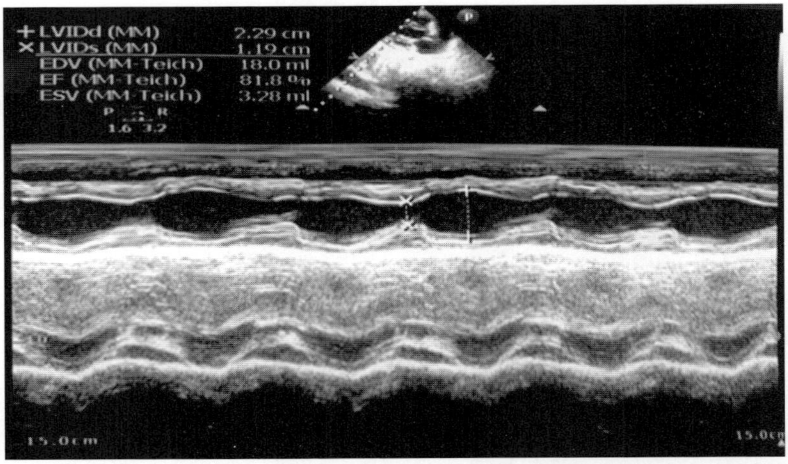


**Fig. 6:** M-mode in parasternal long-axis view for calculating fractional shortening and ejection fraction (EF).
*Source:* Pediatric Intensive Care Unit, AIIMS New Delhi.

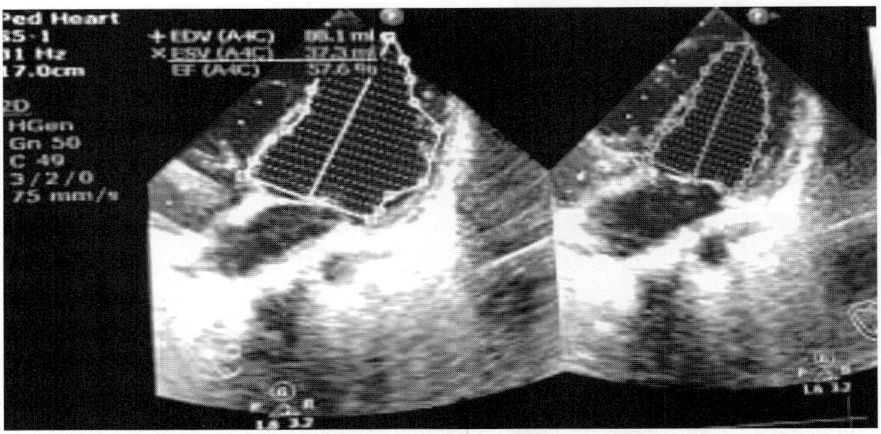


**Fig. 7:** Apical four-chamber view with both systolic and diastolic volumes traced (biplanar technique).
*Source:* Pediatric Intensive Care Unit, AIIMS New Delhi.

**TABLE 2:** Condition of the heart according to EF.

| | ***Hyperdynamic*** | ***Normal*** | ***Mildly reduced*** | ***Moderately reduced*** | ***Severely reduced*** |
|---|---|---|---|---|---|
| Ejection fraction (EF) | ≥70% | 55–69% | 45–54% | 30–44% | <30% |

the endocardial borders at the end systole and diastole **(Fig. 7)**.[6] Normal EF is above 55%. Various ranges of Ef and conditions are labeled **(Table 2)**.

## EVALUATION OF CARDIAC OUTPUT

For measuring the cardiac output (CO), we have to measure the stroke volume first. The

LVOT area is multiplied by the velocity time integral (VTI) at the LVOT to give the stroke volume. The LVOT diameter is measured in the parasternal long-axis view, just below the hinge point of the aortic leaflets **(Fig. 8)**. The LVOT area is then calculated as:[7]

$$\text{LVOT area} = \pi \times (\text{LVOT diameter}/2)^2$$

The VTI is measured in the apical five-chamber view using pulse wave Doppler at the LVOT, tracing the ejection wave **(Fig. 9)**. Different sizes of ejection wave may be obtained which is due to the stroke volume variation as part of cardiorespiratory interaction due to respiration.

$$\text{Stroke volume} = \text{LVOT area} \times \text{Velocity time integral}$$

$$\text{CO} = \text{SV} \times \text{Heart rate}$$

$$\text{Cardiac index} = \text{CO} \times \text{Body surface area}$$

A recent study[7] comparing cardiac output measured by POCUS with invasive cardiac output monitoring (pulse index continuous cardiac output monitoring) found that cardiac output measured by both strongly correlated ($p < 0.001$, $r = 0.985$).

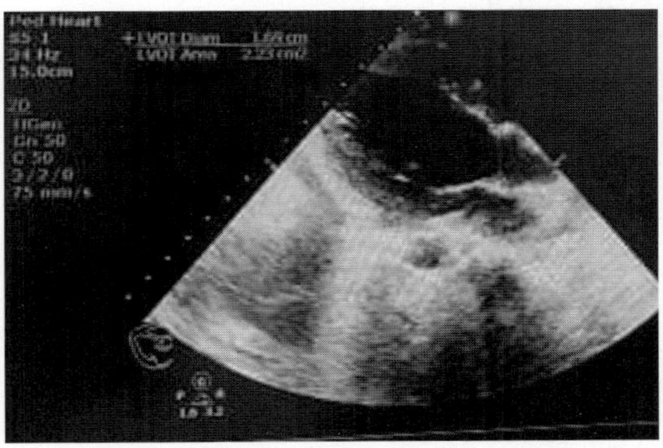

**Fig. 8:** LVOT diameter is calculated in the PLAX view. (LVOT: left ventricular outflow tract; PLAX: parasternal long axis view)
*Source:* Pediatric Intensive Care, AIIMS New Delhi.

## PRELOAD AND VOLUME RESPONSIVENESS

Fluid therapy remains the cornerstone in the management of any child who presents with unstable PICU. However, whether the child requires, and will clinically respond to fluids remains a challenge to the treating physician.[8] If the cardiac output increases by 10–15% after giving a fluid challenge, then it is said to be fluid-responsive.[9-11] Early fluid administration improves survival, but overzealous fluid administration results in

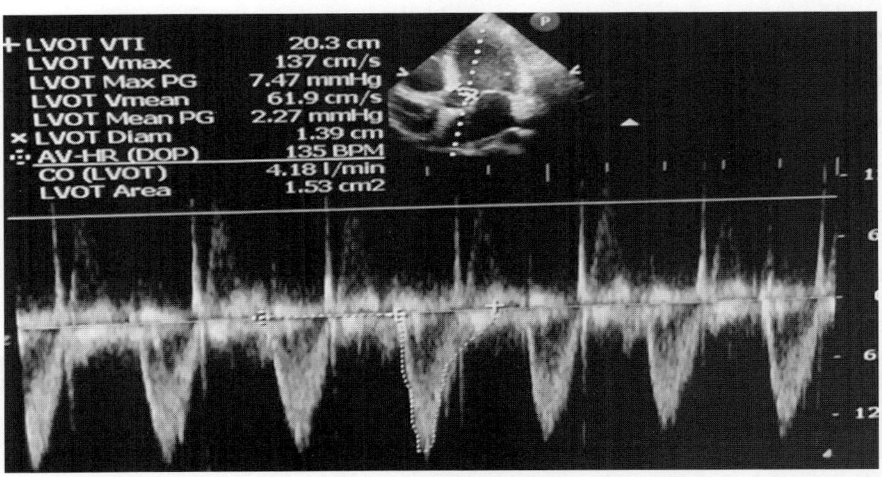


**Fig. 9:** Pulse wave doppler at the LVOT tracing the VTI. (LVOT: left ventricular outflow tract; VTI: velocity time integral)
*Source:* Pediatric Intensive Care Unit, AIIMS New Delhi.

fluid overload, prolonged ventilation, and mortality.[12-14]

Point-of-care ultrasonography can predict fluid responsiveness by measuring static and dynamic parameters **(Table 3)**. Dynamic parameters, which are more physiology-based and dependent on cardiopulmonary interactions, are considered more accurate than static parameters for predicting fluid responsiveness.[15-16,8]

## Respiratory Variation in Aortic Blood Flow Peak Velocity (ΔVpeak)/Velocity Time Integral (Delta Vti)

In the apical five-chamber view, ΔVpeak is measured at the aortic annulus or the left ventricular outflow tract by using pulsed wave Doppler.

$\Delta$Vpeak (%) = 100 × (Vpeak max – Vpeak min)/[(Vpeak max + Vpeak min)/2]

A value of >12% is predictive of fluid responsiveness.[8] ΔVpeak is the most consistent predictor of fluid responsiveness in pediatric patients.[16] Instead of ΔVpeak, ΔVti can be used, and >15% is taken as a predictor of fluid responsiveness.[17]

## Respiratory Variation in the Inferior Vena Cava Diameter

### *Collapsibility Index*

In a spontaneously breathing child, the IVC collapses during inspiration (due to decreased intrathoracic pressure causing forward flow of blood into the right atrium). Though this is physiological, an exaggerated collapsibility of >50% has been taken to be a marker of volume responsiveness.[18] This value has been extrapolated from an adult population as there a still limited data available in the child population. The measurement of IVC diameter is made about 1–2 cm distal to the hepatic vein inlet **(Fig. 10)**.

*Inferior vena cava collapsibility index:* 100 × (IVC diameter at end-expiration—IVC diameter at inspiration)/IVC diameter at end-expiration.

### *Distensibility Index*

On positive pressure ventilation, during inspiration the positive pressure given by the ventilator increases the intra thoracic pressure causing a decrease in the venous return; this causes the IVC to dilate during inspiration, and during expiration, the intra thoracic pressure falls causing venous drainage from the IVC into the right atrium causing IVC to collapse. Therefore, the IVC distensibility index be used in children on mechanical ventilation.

*Inferior vena cava distensibility index:* 100 × (IVC diameter at end inspiration – IVC diameter at end-expiration)/IVC diameter at end inspiration.

Inferior vena cava distensibility index values of >18% were in favor of fluid deficit.[18] The cutoffs are again taken from the adult population. Pediatric studies are scarce and more studies are required to get optimal cutoff in children. It is important to remember that the distensibility index may not be reliable

**TABLE 3:** Static and dynamic parameters for predicting fluid responsiveness by echocardiography.

| *Static parameters* | *Dynamic parameters* |
|---|---|
| • Left ventricular end-diastolic area<br>• Stroke volume index<br>• Corrected flow time | • Respiratory variation in aortic blood flow peak velocity<br>• Respiratory variation in the inferior vena cava diameter<br>• Stroke volume variation<br>• Velocity–time integral |

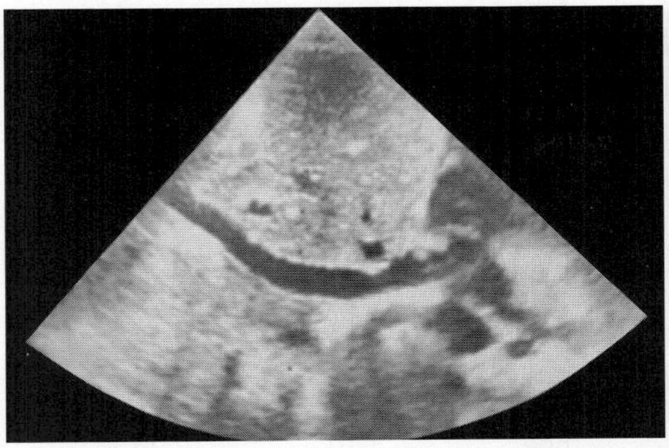

**Fig. 10:** Subcostal view showing the IVC draining in the right atrium.
*Source:* Pediatric Intensive care unit, AIIMS NEW DELHI.

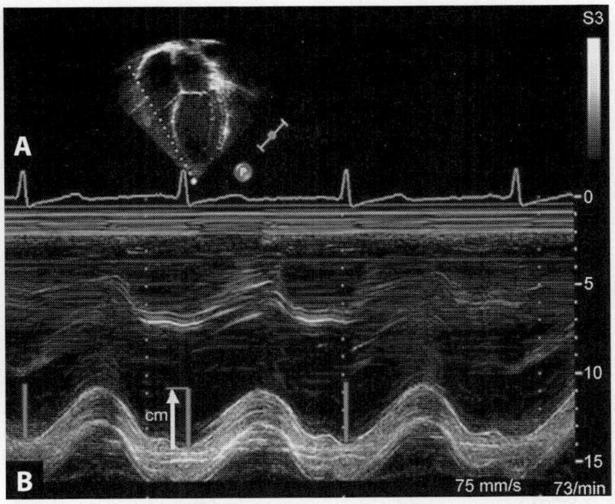

**Figs. 11A and B:** The white broken arrow indicates M mode placement at the lateral annulus with the absolute longitudinal displacement indicated by the red line.[19]

in spontaneously breathing children on mechanical ventilation and a minimum tidal volume of 8 mL/kg is required for its correct assessment.

## EVALUATION OF RIGHT VENTRICULAR FUNCTION AND PULMONARY HYPERTENSION

Evaluation of pulmonary hypertension is another important parameter in managing critically ill children. The main parameters assessed are:

- Right ventricular size and movement
- Tricuspid annular plane systolic excursion (TAPSE)
- Tricuspid regurgitation jet velocity

### Right Ventricular Size and Movement

Right ventricle (RV) size is two-thirds of the LV size normally, so any abnormal dilation may be indicative of right ventricular dysfunction. Bulging of the interventricular septum towards the left side also indicates right ventricular dysfunction.

### Tricuspid Annular Plane Systolic Excursion

Tricuspid annular plane systolic excursion measures RV function by assessing the longitudinal movement of RV fibers. M-mode is applied at the lateral annulus of the tricuspid valve with a line as parallel to the lateral wall in the apical four-chamber view **(Figs. 11A and B)**. Absolute longitudinal displacement indicates TAPSE.

TAPSE is the most utilized index to report RV function. Decreased TAPSE indicates right ventricular systolic dysfunction. TAPSE can help in monitoring the progression of pediatric pulmonary hypertension and assessing the effectiveness of interventions over time.

Unlike adults, children do not have a definite threshold. A study[19] collected reference values from 640 healthy children and calculated Z scores. TAPSE measured 0.91 cm (0.56–1.26 cm) in neonates to 2.47 cm (1.84–3.10 cm) in 18-year-olds. TAPSE readings correlated positively with age and body surface area. There was no significant gender variation in TAPSE. **Table 4** enlisting the various values according to age.

### Tricuspid Regurgitant Jet Velocity

In the apical four-chamber view, focus on the tricuspid valve, then add color to guide the

**TABLE 4:** Tricuspid annular plane systolic excursion (TAPSE) scores for different age groups.[19]

| TAPSE (cm) | | | | | | |
|---|---|---|---|---|---|---|
| Bounds for z-score ranges | | | | | | |
| ***Age*** | ***n*** | ***Mean*** | ***±2SD (95%)*** | | ***±3SD (99%)*** | |
| 0–30 days | 41 | 0.91 | 0.68 | 1.15 | 0.56 | 1.26 |
| 1–3 months | 45 | 1.14 | 0.85 | 1.42 | 0.71 | 1.56 |
| 4–6 months | 20 | 1.31 | 1.01 | 1.65 | 0.86 | 1.77 |
| 7–12 months | 22 | 1.44 | 1.13 | 1.77 | 0.97 | 1.91 |
| 1 year | 25 | 1.55 | 1.25 | 1.88 | 1.10 | 2.00 |
| 2 years | 39 | 1.65 | 1.36 | 1.94 | 1.22 | 2.09 |
| 3 years | 27 | 1.74 | 1.48 | 2.02 | 1.35 | 2.14 |
| 4 years | 47 | 1.82 | 1.56 | 2.07 | 1.43 | 2.20 |
| 5 years | 29 | 1.87 | 1.60 | 2.13 | 1.47 | 2.26 |
| 6 years | 41 | 1.90 | 1.62 | 2.18 | 1.48 | 2.33 |
| 7 years | 32 | 1.94 | 1.64 | 2.25 | 1.49 | 2.39 |
| 8 years | 23 | 1.97 | 1.67 | 2.28 | 1.52 | 2.43 |
| 9 years | 20 | 2.01 | 1.73 | 2.30 | 1.58 | 2.44 |
| 10 years | 27 | 2.05 | 1.79 | 2.31 | 1.65 | 2.46 |
| 11 years | 25 | 2.10 | 1.83 | 2.36 | 1.69 | 2.50 |
| 12 years | 18 | 2.14 | 1.84 | 2.43 | 1.68 | 2.60 |
| 13 years | 20 | 2.20 | 1.85 | 2.54 | 1.68 | 2.71 |
| 14 years | 35 | 2.26 | 1.87 | 2.65 | 1.68 | 2.84 |
| 15 years | 25 | 2.33 | 1.93 | 2.75 | 1.74 | 2.92 |
| 16 years | 34 | 2.39 | 1.98 | 2.78 | 1.78 | 3.01 |
| 17 years | 27 | 2.45 | 2.04 | 2.88 | 1.83 | 3.06 |
| 18 years | 21 | 2.47 | 2.05 | 2.91 | 1.84 | 3.10 |

continuous wave (CW) Doppler. TR jet will appear blue (away from the probe). The line should be drawn through the origin of the jet. The CW line should be aligned parallel to the direction of the TR flow.

A value of ≤2.8 m/s suggests low probability, 2.9–3.4 m/s indicates intermediate probability, and >3.4 m/s suggests a high probability for pulmonary hypertension.

To derive pulmonary pressure from the TR signal one has to use the modified Bernoulli equation:

$$RVSP = 4 \times TRvel^2$$

## ASSESSMENT OF PERICARDIAL EFFUSION AND CARDIAC TAMPONADE

The rate at which fluid accumulates is more important than the actual size, as in a chronic long-standing large effusion may be well tolerated but a rapidly accumulated fluid might result in features of tamponade The position of the fluid in relation to the descending aorta can help in differentiating between pericardial and pleural effusion. The descending aorta will appear posterior

**TABLE 5:** Interpretation of diastolic dysfunction.[21]

| Diastolic dysfunction | Normal | Impaired relaxation or grade 1 diastolic dysfunction | Pseudonormal or grade 2 diastolic dysfunction | Restrictive or grade 3 diastolic dysfunction |
|---|---|---|---|---|
| Finding | • E/A ≥0.8<br>• e′ ≥8 cm/s<br>• E/e′ ≤8 | • E/A <0.8<br>• e′ <8 cm/s<br>• E/e′ <8 | • E/A ≥0.8<br>• e′ <8 cm/s<br>• E/e′ 8–15 | • E/A >2<br>• e′ <8 cm/s<br>• E/e′ >15 |
| Pulse wave Doppler at the mitral annulus | | Impaired relaxation | Increased left atrial pressure causes the push of blood into the ventricles during the ventricular relaxation phase causing the pseudonormalization | A severe increase in left atrial pressure causes the E/A ≥2 |
| Tissue doppler at the level of septal annulus | Normal relaxation | Mild decrease in relaxation speed | Moderate decrease in relaxation speed | Severe decrease in relaxation speed |

to the pericardial effusion and anterior to the pleural effusion.

The largest dimension in end-diastole (<10 mm—mild,10–20 mm—moderate, >20 mm—severe). Moderate to severe effusions are usually circumferential.

### Signs of Cardiac Tamponade

- Right atrial systolic collapse (sensitive not specific)
- Enlarged IVC with no respiratory variation (nonspecific sign)
- Right ventricular diastolic collapse (more specific)
- Significant variation in inspiratory and expiratory blood flows (>10%)—pulses paradoxes.

## ASSESSMENT OF DIASTOLIC DYSFUNCTION

The main utility of assessing diastolic dysfunction is to:

- Optimize the fluid status in critically ill children
- Assess the effectiveness of diuretic therapy in children with congestive cardiac failure
- To assess if the worsening of lung condition is due to cardiogenic or non-cardiogenic cause.

To interpret diastolic dysfunction, we must know how the blood flows in the left ventricle during diastole and how the left ventricle muscle relaxes during diastole **(Table 5)**. Firstly, pulse wave Doppler is used to measure the inflow of blood into the left ventricle at the level of mitral leaflet tips in the apical four-chamber view. This will result in two positively deflected waves the E (passive filling during ventricular relaxation) and A waves (ventricular filling during atrial contraction). Secondly, a tissue Doppler is applied at the level of the septal annulus. The left ventricle relaxes to take the blood coming from the left atrium, this movement is away from the direction of the probe creating a negative deflection e′ (early diastolic filling).[20]

## CONCLUSION

To be effectively utilized, Cardiac POCUS applications should adhere to three fundamental criteria:

- The pathophysiology must be suitable for ultrasound evaluation.

- The clinical scenarios should be common or necessitate urgent intervention.
- Comprehensive and effective training must be widely accessible.

## REFERENCES


1. Lu JC, Riley A, Conlon T, Levine JC, Kwan C, Miller-Hance WC, et al. Recommendations for Cardiac Point-of-Care Ultrasound in Children: A Report from the American Society of Echocardiography. J Am Soc Echocardiogr. 2023;36(3):265-77.
2. Lai WW, Geva T, Shirali GS, Frommelt PC, Humes RA, Brook MM, et al. Guidelines and standards for performance of a pediatric echocardiogram: a report from the task force of the pediatric council of the American society of echocardiography. J Am Soc Echocardiogr. 2006;19(12):1413-30.
3. Sievers B, Kirchberg S, Franken U, Puthenveettil BJ, Bakan A, Trappe HJ. Visual estimation versus quantitative assessment of left ventricular ejection fraction: a comparison by cardiovascular magnetic resonance imaging. Am Heart J. 2005;150(4):737-42.
4. Tissot C, Singh Y, Sekarski N. Echocardiographic evaluation of ventricular function-for the neonatologist and pediatric intensivist. Front Pediatr. 2018;6:79.
5. Moore CL, Rose GA, Tayal VS, Sullivan DM, Arrowood JA, Kline JA. Determination of left ventricular function by emergency physician echocardiography of hypotensive patients. Acad Emerg Med. 2002;9(3):186-93.
6. Otterstad JE. Measuring left ventricular volume and ejection fraction with the biplane Simpson's method. Heart. 2002;88(6):559-60.
7. Aslan N, Yildizdas D, Horoz OO, Coban Y, Demir F, Erdem S, et al. Comparison of cardiac output and cardiac index values measured by critical care echocardiography with the values measured by pulse index continuous cardiac output (PiCCO) in the pediatric intensive care unit:a preliminary study. Ital J Pediatr. 2020;46(1):47.
8. Gan H, Cannesson M, Chandler JR, Ansermino JM. Predicting fluid responsiveness in children: a systematic review. Anesth Analg. 2013;117(6):1380-92.
9. Marlik PE, Monnet X, Teboul JL. Hemodynamic parameters to guide fluid therapy. Ann Intensive Care. 2011;1(1):1.
10. Toscani L, Aya HD, Antonakaki D, Bastoni D, Watson X, Arulkumaran N, et al. What is the impact of the fluid challenge technique on diagnosis of fluid responsiveness? A systematic review and meta-analysis. Crit Care. 2017;21(1):207.
11. Sutherland SM, Zappitelli M, Alexander SR, Chua AN, Brophy PD, Bunchman TE, et al. Fluid overload and mortality in children receiving continuous renal replacement therapy: the prospective pediatric continuous renal replacement therapy registry. Am J Kidney Dis. 2010;55(2):316-25.
12. Li Y, Wang J, Bai Z, Chen J, Wang X, Pan J, et al. Early fluid overload is associated with acute kidney injury and PICU mortality in critically ill children. Eur J Pediatr. 2016;175(1):39-48.
13. Raina R, Sethi SK, Wadhwani N, Vemuganti M, Krishnappa V, Bansal SB. Fluid overload in critically ill children. Front Pediatr. 2018;6:306.
14. Yi L, Liu Z, Qiao L, Wan C, Mu D. Does stroke volume variation predict fluid responsiveness in children: a systematic review and meta-analysis. PLoS One. 2017;12(5):e0177590.
15. Desgranges FP, Desebbe O, Pereira de Souza Neto E, Raphael D, Chassard D. Respiratory variation in aortic blood flow peak velocity to predict fluid responsiveness in mechanically ventilated children: a systematic review and meta-analysis. Paediatr Anaesth. 2016;26(1):37-47.
16. Wang X, Jiang L, Liu S, Ge Y, Gao J. Value of respiratory variation of aortic peak velocity in predicting children receiving mechanical ventilation: a systematic review and meta-analysis. Crit Care. 2019;23(1):372.
17. Sethasathien S, Jariyasakoolroj T, Silvilairat S, Srisurapanont M. Aortic peak flow velocity as a predictor of fluid responsiveness in mechanically ventilated children: a

systematic review and meta-analysis. Pediatr Crit Care Med. 2023;24(7):e352-e361.
18. Yildizdas D, Aslan N. Ultrasonographic inferior vena cava collapsibility and distensibility indices for detecting the volume status of critically ill pediatric patients. J Ultrason. 2020;20(82):e205-9.
19. Koestenberger M, Ravekes W, Everett AD, Stueger HP, Heinzl B, Gamillscheg A, et al. Right ventricular function in infants, children and adolescents: reference values of the tricuspid annular plane systolic excursion (TAPSE) in 640 healthy patients and calculation of z score values. J Am Soc Echocardiogr. 2009;22(6):715-9.
20. Nagueh S, Middleton K, Kopelen H, Zoghbi W, Quiñones M. Doppler tissue imaging: a noninvasive technique for evaluation of left ventricular relaxation and estimation of filling pressures. J Am College of Cardiol. 1997;30(6):1527-33.
21. Nagueh SF, Smiseth OA, Appleton CP, Byrd BF 3rd, Dokainish H, Edvardsen T, et al. Recommendations for the Evaluation of Left Ventricular Diastolic Function by Echocardiography: An Update from the American Society of Echocardiography and the European Association of Cardiovascular Imaging. J Am Soc Echocardiogr. 2016;29(4): 277-314.

CHAPTER 24

# Recent Advances: Role of Artificial Intelligence in Critical Care Echocardiography

*Balaji Rajaram*

*Artificial Intelligence is a tool, not a threat*

**—Rodney Brooks**

## INTRODUCTION

Beginning of artificial intelligence (AI) in medicine had started as early as 1956. During its early inception days, AI has been referred by various names such as "thinking machines" and "cybernetics". The term artificial intelligence was coined by John McCarthy. Since then, AI has made its way across various fields such as communication, robotics, automobiles, education, healthcare, and transportation.

Artificial intelligence refers to the ability of computer systems to perform tasks that requires human intelligence. Machine learning refers to algorithms that can be used to teach a computer to analyze a vast number of data points in a rapid and accurate manner. Machine learning models assess the presence of associations in the datasets and calculate their predictive power. Thereby, these algorithms then apply these predictions acquired from known data sets to the new datasets.[1,2]

Machine learning can be categorized based on the type of feedback received. Machine learning can be supervised, unsupervised, semisupervised, and reinforcement learning.[3] Deep learning involves multiple layers of artificial neural networks to simulate human brain. It helps in analyzing raw and unprocessed data. Complex neural networks (CNN) are mainly used in processing medical image data sets.

The role of AI in healthcare system had started gaining increased recognition in recent times, especially in medical imaging. The ability of AI in interpretation of medical images has been used in other modalities such as chest radiography and mammography.[4,5]

The evolution of technological resources had led on to widespread availability of ultrasound machines outside echocardiography laboratory. Hence, clinicians from various backgrounds use ultrasonography along with the physical examination to improve diagnostic accuracy [FoCUS (focused cardiac ultrasound)].[6,7] Utility of AI is not limited to image interpretation alone. It also plays a role in image acquisition as well. This feature is especially useful in point-of-care ultrasound (POCUS) in the intensive care unit (ICU) settings, where positive pressure ventilation, patient positioning, and presence of surgical drains may interfere with the acquisition of good quality images. **Box 1** summarizes the challenges in implementing AI in echocardiography.

**BOX 1:** Challenge of using artificial intelligence (AI) in echocardiography.

- Echocardiography requires interpretation of moving dynamic images. Moving data sets corresponds to thousands of pixels. Complex algorithms may be required to delineate association with the same.
- Availability
- Cost
- Nonavailability of appropriate echocardiographic database to facilitate deep learning. Even if images are available, it had to be curated, annotated, and correlated with diagnosis/other investigations.
- Need for standardization across various service providers

**BOX 2:** Need for artificial intelligence (AI) in echocardiography.

- Scheduling and triaging of patients who need immediate medical attention
- Appropriate identification of pathologies such as regional wall motion abnormality (RWMA) in resource-limited settings
- Guidance in acquisition of appropriate images
- Focus on identifying pathology rather than quality of image acquisition
- To eliminate subjectivity in the interpretation of imaging
- Improve efficiency (as complex quantification can be done in short period of time)
- Early identification of diastolic dysfunction
- To assess response to therapies such as goal-directed medical therapies
- Detection and differentiation of close mimicking pathologies such as hypertrophic cardiomyopathy and athlete's heart
- Reduction in need for cardiac magnetic resonance imaging (MRI) and 3D echocardiography
- Precise quantification for cardiac tumors

## EVOLUTION OF ARTIFICIAL INTELLIGENCE IN ECHOCARDIOGRAPHY

The application AI to FoCUS involves following steps.[8] It includes acquisition of good quality images, identification and segmentation of various cardiovascular structures, quantification of data sets (such as calculation of ejection fraction and chamber size), and detection of pathologies (such as identification of wall motion abnormalities). AI assists acute care physicians in each of the above-mentioned steps. **Box 2** summarizes the utility of AI in point-of-care echocardiography.

First step in the application of AI in the field of point-of-care ultrasonography is obtaining good-quality images. Image quality will directly affect the diagnostic accuracy. This is especially important in acute care medicine as trainees from various fields will be working in acute care settings. Their level of expertise in getting appropriate good-quality images also varies, leading on to significant inter observer variability. FDA had authorized ultrasound software that uses AI to assist clinicians to obtain good diagnostic quality images.[9] Caption Guidance (Caption Health, Inc.) is based on convolutional neural networks that were created with a database of more than 5 million hand movements of sonographers. It provides a real-time guidance to obtain good-quality images, and it was validated in a trial of over 200 patients.[10]

Identification of appropriate views to get maximum information and identification of appropriate structures is crucial in critical care echocardiography. Feasibility study was conducted by Jeffrey et al. to evaluate the ability of convolutional neural network models to identify the appropriate echocardiographic view and quantify the structural details.[11] More than

14,000 echocardiographic images were used to identify 23 viewpoints and quantification of chamber dimensions (left ventricle volume/mass). It was compared with manual segmentation and measurements. In this study, automated measurements were found to be comparable to manual measurements.

Left ventricular ejection fraction (LVEF) plays an important role in assessing the severity of compromise in cardiac function. LVEF plays an important role in clinical decision making in ICU such as choice of vasoactive agent and judicious usage of fluid resuscitation. LVEF can be determined by various methods including visual gestalt. However, other methodologies carry significant interobserver variability and based on numerous geometric assumptions. Accurate determination of LVEF involves manual tracing of endocardial borders. Manual tracing is time consuming and carries significant interobserver variability, especially with nonexperts. Multicentered study of around 250 patients has revealed that fully automated machine learning-enabled image analysis (AutoLV) **(Figs. 1A and B)** was

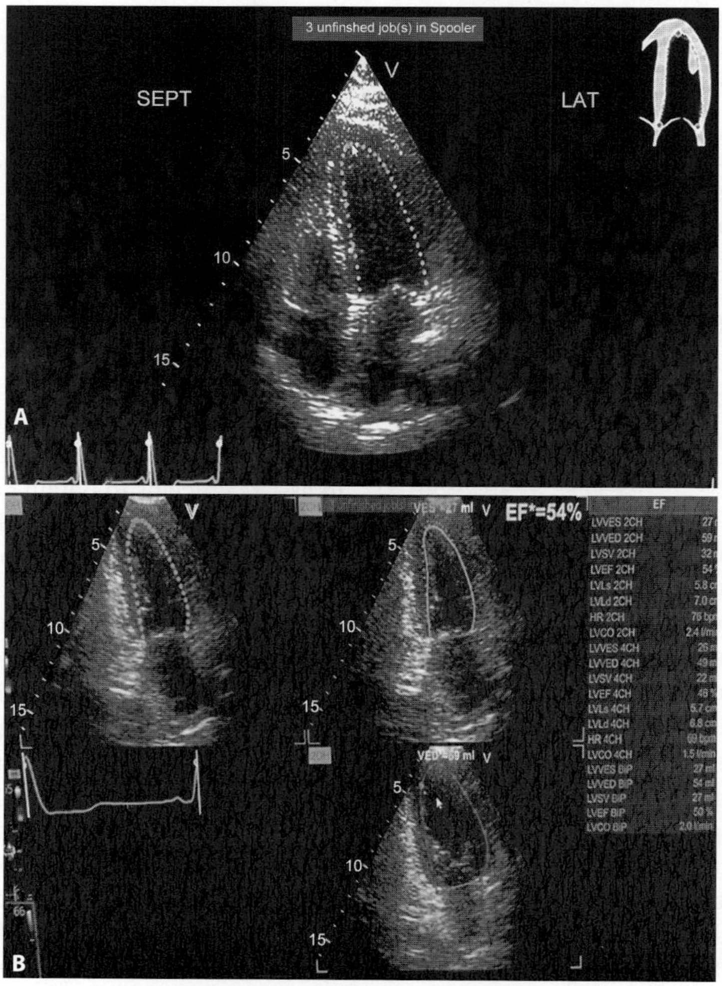


**Figs. 1A and B:** Calculation of ejection fraction (EF) using artificial intelligent (AI). Note the automated tracing of endocardial borders.

feasible in 98% patients. The time consumed was around 8 seconds per patient. Interclass correlation coefficients and Bland-Altman analysis revealed good agreements among automated ejection fraction (EF) measurements. AutoLv measurements were accurate, reproducible with less variability.[12] A blinded, randomized noninferiority clinical trial of over 3,400 studies had demonstrated that initial assessment of LVEF by AI was noninferior to assessment by sonographers. AI-based assessment was less time consuming compared to sonographer-based assessment.[13]

Cardiac output (CO) is an important determinant of the oxygen delivery and perfusion status of the patient. Measurement of CO requires invasive devices such as pulmonary artery catheter (PAC). CO can be measured noninvasively using echocardiography. Echocardiography-derived CO measurements have shown excellent correlation with pulmonary artery (PA) catheter and thermodilution-based derivations.[14-16] Left ventricular outflow tract–velocity time integral (LVOT-VTI) enables the calculation of stroke volume using pulsed wave Doppler (PWD) principle. AI enables automatized measurements of VTI **(Fig. 2)**. SmartVTI (Mindray) or Auto VTI (GE) enables automatic measurements once apical 5-chamber views are obtained. A trend graph depicting VTI, stroke, and CO will be displayed, enabling acute care physician to assess the therapeutic responses.[17]

Epidemiological data suggests that incidence and prognosis of heart failure with preserved ejection fraction (HFpEF) is almost similar to that of heart failure with reduced ejection fraction (HFrEF).[18,19] Left ventricular (LV) relaxation can be impaired by the underlying risk factors (such as old age, hypertension, and coronary artery disease) as well as the current critically ill status of the patient such as sepsis, hypoxia, arrhythmias, acute kidney injury, volume resuscitation therapies, and positive pressure ventilation.[20] The presence of diastolic dysfunction influences critical care interventions such as fluid resuscitation and weaning from mechanical ventilation. Unlike systolic dysfunction, the evaluation of diastology is complex and time consuming. The diagnosis of diastolic dysfunction requires various parameters such as E/A ratio, septal or lateral e′, average E/e′, left atrial volume, and peak

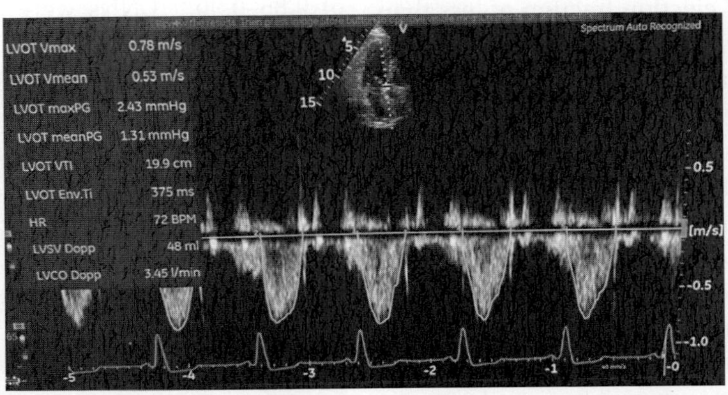


**Fig. 2:** Calculation of left ventricular outflow tract–velocity time integral (LVOT-VTI) using artificial intelligence (AI). Note the automated aligning of Doppler gate at an appropriate angle for the calculation of velocity time integral (VTI).

tricuspid regurgitation velocity. AI models were able to identify diastolic dysfunction (and its grading) comparable to that of human experts. AI models were able to detect diastolic dysfunction and its grade with accuracy of 0.9.[21]

The role of the right ventricle (RV) is often overlooked as passive conduit for LV filling. However, in critical care settings, various pathologies such as acute respiratory distress syndrome (ARDS), sepsis, pulmonary embolism, acute coronary syndrome, and acute cor pulmonale significantly impair RV function. RV functional assessment plays an important role in prognostication of pulmonary hypertension. 2D echo is the first method of choice of assessing RV function. However, irregular shape of RV (not fitting in to any particular geometrical shape) and absence of normative data make it a challenge to the treating physician. Cardiac magnetic resonance imaging (CMR) remains the gold standard for assessing RV functions. AI-derived parameters such as fractional area change (FAC), free wall strain (FWS), and tricuspid annular planar systolic excursion (TAPSE) had excellent sensitivity and negative predictive value (91% and 96%, respectively) for ruling out significant RV dysfunction (as defined by RV ejection fraction of less than 40% on CMR). AI-assisted RV assessment was comparable to that of expert sonographers and may serve as excellent screening tool to rule out RV dysfunction at bedside.[22] AI-derived models were able to predict postoperative RV failure following left ventricular assist devices (LVAD). These machine learning models that use preoperative echocardiograms outperform various clinical scoring systems.[23]

Assessment of inferior vena cava (IVC) dimensions helps the acute care physicians to guide the resuscitation. It can be used as both dynamic and static indices of fluid status assessment. It provides a rough estimate of right atrial pressure (RAP). As per guidelines, IVC diameter <2.1 cm and collapsibility >50% during inspiration suggest that RAP between 0.5 mm Hg and diameter >2.1 cm with <50% collapsibility correlates with RAP of 10–20 mm Hg.[24] In patients who are mechanically ventilated (without spontaneous respiratory effort and with tidal volume of 8 mL/kg), IVC distensibility index provides the dynamic index of fluid status.[25,26] SmartIVC (Mindray) or auto IVC (GE) **(Fig. 3)** provides automatic assessment of the IVC including the dynamic indices.

Coronary artery disease contributes to significant proportion of morbidity and mortality in cardiac critical care units. Echocardiography, by its ability to detect new onset regional wall motion abnormality (RWMA), offers low-cost, rapid, and point-of-care imaging tool in the diagnosis of myocardial infarction. However, detection of RWMA requires trained and experienced physicians. The availability of trained sonographers may not be always available, especially in resource-limited settings. Deep learning models and CNN facilitate the detection of RWMA with the area under the receiver operating characteristic (AUROC) of 0.85–0.90.[27] CNNs were able to detect

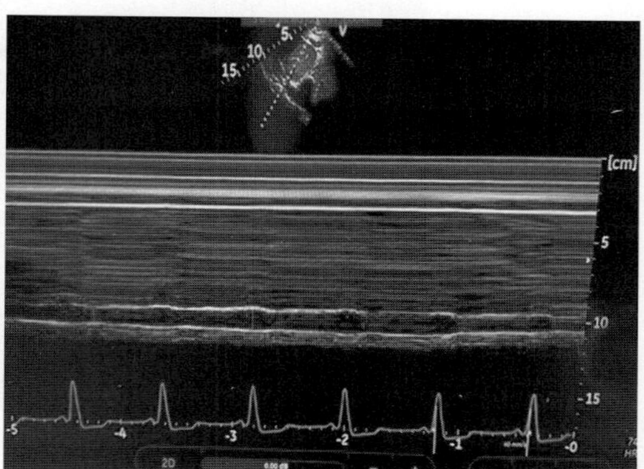

**Fig. 3:** AI-assisted tracing of inferior vena cava (IVC).

complex cardiovascular pathologies such as hypertrophic cardiomyopathy (HCM), amyloidosis, and pulmonary hypertension with reasonable accuracy (AUROC of 0.85–0.93).[11]

## ACKNOWLEDGMENT

We acknowledge Dr Poorna Pushkala Natarajan, MBBS, AB Internal Medicine, Cardiology and Advanced Heart Failure and Transplant Cardiology, for providing images from 4D vivid Iq machine.

## REFERENCES

1. Alsharqi M, Woodward WJ, Mumith JA, Markham DC, Upton R, Leeson P. Artificial intelligence and echocardiography. Echo Res Pract. 2018;5(4):R115-25.
2. Mayr A, Binder H, Gefeller O, Schmid M. The evolution of boosting algorithms. From machine learning to statistical modelling. Methods of Inf Med. 2014;53:419-27.
3. Barry T, Farina JM, Chao C-J, Ayoub C, Jeong J, Patel BN, et al. The Role of Artificial Intelligence in Echocardiography. J Imaging. 2023;9(2):50.
4. Qin C, Yao D, Shi Y, Song Z. Computer-aided detection in chest radiography based on artificial intelligence: a survey. Biomed Eng Online. 2018;17:113.
5. Horsch A, Hapfelmeier A, Elter M. Needs assessment for next generation computer-aided mammography reference image databases and evaluation studies. Int J Comput Assist Radiol Surg. 2011;6(6):749-67.
6. Almufleh A, Di Santo P, Marbach JA. Training Cardiology Fellows in Focused Cardiac Ultrasound. J Am Coll Cardiol. 2019;73:1097-1100.
7. Motazedian P, Marbach JA, Prosperi-Porta G, Parlow S, Di Santo P, Abdel-Razek O, et al. Diagnostic accuracy of point-of-care ultrasound with artificial intelligence-assisted assessment of left ventricular ejection fraction. NPJ Digit Med. 2023;6:201.
8. Kusunose K. Steps to use artificial intelligence in echocardiography. J Echocardiogr. 2021; 19(1):21-7.
9. Voelker R. Cardiac Ultrasound Uses Artificial Intelligence to Produce Images. JAMA. 2020;323(11):1034.
10. Narang A, Bae R, Hong H. Acquisition of diagnostic echocardiographic images by novices using a deep learning based image guidance algorithm. J Am Coll Cardiol. 2020;75:1564.
11. Zhang J, Gajjala S, Agrawal P, Tison GH, Hallock LA, Beussink-Nelson L, et al. Fully Automated Echocardiogram Interpretation in Clinical Practice. Circulation. 2018;138(16): 1623-35.
12. Knackstedt C, Bekkers SC, Schummers G, Schreckenberg M, Muraru D, Badano LP, et al. Fully Automated Versus Standard Tracking of Left Ventricular Ejection Fraction and Longitudinal Strain: The FAST-EFs Multicenter Study. J Am Coll Cardiol. 2015; 66(13):1456-66.
13. He B, Kwan AC, Cho JH, Yuan N, Pollick C, Shiota T, et al. Blinded, randomized trial of sonographer versus AI cardiac function assessment. Nature. 2023;616:520-4.
14. Parra V, Fita G, Rovira I, Matute P, Gomar C, Paré C. Transoesophageal echocardiography accurately detects cardiac output variation. Eur J Anaesthesiol. 2008;25(2):135-43.
15. Zhang Y, Wang Y, Shi J, Hua Z, Xu J. Cardiac Output measurement via echocardiography versus thermodilution: a systematic review and meta-analysis. PLoS ONE. 2019;14(10): e0222105.
16. Mercadal J, Borrat X, Hernández A, Denault A, Beaubien-Souligny W, González-Delgado D, et al.; Spanish Critical Care Ultrasound Network Group. A simple algorithm for differential diagnosis in hemodynamic shock based on left ventricle outflow tract velocity-time integral measurement: a case series. Ultrasound J. 2022;14(1):36.
17. Mika S, Gola W, Gil-Mika M, Wilk M, Misiołek H. Overview of artificial intelligence in point-of-care ultrasound. New horizons for

respiratory system diagnoses. Anaesthesiol Intensive Ther. 2024;56(1):1-8.

18. Kindermann M. How to diagnose diastolic heart failure: a consensus statement on the diagnosis of heart failure with normal left ventricular ejection fraction by the Heart Failure and Echocardiography Associations of the European Society of Cardiology. Eur Heart J. 2007;28(21):2686.
19. Hogg K, Swedberg K, McMurray J. Heart failure with preserved left ventricular systolic function; epidemiology, clinical characteristics, and prognosis. J Am Coll Cardiol. 2004;43:317-27.
20. Eisen LA, Davlouros P, Karakitsos D. Left ventricular diastolic dysfunction in the intensive care unit: trends and perspectives. Crit Care Res Pract. 2012;2012:964158.
21. Chen X, Yang F, Zhang P, Lin X, Wang W, Pu H, et al. Artificial Intelligence–Assisted Left Ventricular Diastolic Function Assessment and Grading: Multiview Versus Single View. J Am Soc Echocardiogr. 2023;36(10):1064-78.
22. Hsia BC, Lai A, Singh S, Samtani R, Bienstock S, Liao S, et al. Validation of American Society of Echocardiography Guideline-Recommended Parameters of Right Ventricular Dysfunction Using Artificial Intelligence Compared With Cardiac Magnetic Resonance Imaging. J Am Soc Echocardiogr. 2023;36(9):967-77.
23. Shad R, Quach N, Fong R, Kasinpila P, Bowles C, Castro M, et al. Predicting post-operative right ventricular failure using video-based deep learning. Nat Commun. 2021;12:5192.
24. Lang RM, Badano LP, Mor-Avi V, Afilalo J, Armstrong A, Ernande L, et al. Recommendations for Cardiac Chamber Quantification by Echocardiography in Adults: An Update from the American Society of Echocardiography and the European Association of Cardiovascular Imaging. J Am Soc Echocardiogr. 2015;28:1-39.
25. Feissel M, Michard F, Faller JP, Teboul JL. The respiratory variation in inferior vena cava diameter as a guide to fluid therapy. Intensive Care Med. 2004;30(9):1834-7.
26. Barbier C, Loubières Y, Schmit C, Hayon J, Ricôme JL, Jardin F, et al. Respiratory changes in inferior vena cava diameter are helpful in predicting fluid responsiveness in ventilated septic patients. Intensive Care Med. 2004;30(9):1740-6.
27. Lin X, Yang F, Chen Y, Chen X, Wang W, Chen X, et al. Echocardiography-based AI detection of regional wall motion abnormalities and quantification of cardiac function in myocardial infarction. Front Cardiovasc Med. 2022;9:903660.

CHAPTER 25

# Echocardiography in Cardiac Arrest

Nitin Rai

## INTRODUCTION

American Heart Association (AHA) reported Cardiac arrest occurrence affecting >300,000 population each year. Despite the best efforts in resuscitation mortality remains very high and <10% of patients survive to hospital discharge.[1] The use of echocardiography during cardiac arrest has been increasingly used in the past two decades. AHA has recommended point-of-care ultrasound (POCUS) to identify the reversible causes of cardiac arrest.[2] Many studies have demonstrated the benefits of echocardiography in the assessment of critically ill patients, especially during hemodynamic instability.

Advanced life support (ALS)-compliant echocardiography can be performed within the time frame dedicated for pulse check of the ALS algorithm allowing continuity of high-quality, uninterrupted cardiopulmonary resuscitation (CPR). This review focuses on the potential of echocardiography in diagnosing/identifying the cause of cardiac arrest during resuscitation, along with associated challenges that limit its wide-spread use in critically ill patients.

## BENEFITS OF ECHOCARDIOGRAPHY DURING CARDIOPULMONARY RESUSCITATION

Identifying the presence of contractility. The absence of blood pressure and palpable pulse can seem straightforward in diagnosing cardiac arrest. However, up to 45% of medical professionals are unable to accurately identify central pulses during CPR. Pulseless electrical activity (PEA) is accountable for approximately 50% of these presentations. PEA differs from asystole, as in PEA electrical cardiac activity is present which is expected to generate pulsatile circulation without a palpable pulse; whereas, in asystole, there is neither electrical cardiac activity nor a palpable pulse. Echocardiography in "true PEA" will demonstrate no detectable myocardial motion, whereas ECG will demonstrate myocardial activity. In "pseudo-PEA" the myocardium will demonstrate a very diminished myocardial motion with electrical activity on ECG. Both types of PEA are nonshockable rhythms warranting continued CPR. Echocardiography has the advantage of directly assessing cardiac contractility, thereby distinguishing true/pseudo-PEA and asystole from shockable rhythms.

In fact, a 2017 study has revealed that up to 10–35% of asystolic patients have a demonstrable cardiac contraction on POCUS examination. This differentiating carries a prognostic implication because patients having "pseudo-PEA" have higher survival rates compared to those with "true PEA."[3]

## Identifying the Causes

Identifying the cause of cardiac arrest is imperative for better outcomes. Causes such as hypoxia, hypothermia, and electrolyte disturbances can easily be diagnosed at the bedside using simple laboratory tests/arterial blood gas (ABG). Echocardiography can be helpful in identifying important reversible causes, such as hypovolemia, thrombosis [myocardial infarction (MI) and pulmonary embolism], and pericardial tamponade.

## HYPOVOLEMIA

Hypovolemia can result from trauma (blunt or penetrative), excessive blood loss (e.g., rupture of descending thoracic aorta or splenic artery aneurysm rupture in pancreatitis), or severe dehydration. Regardless of the cause of volume depletion, the need for early identification and aggressive resuscitation is warranted. During cardiac arrest, the hyperkinetic left ventricle is not appreciable, the diagnosis relies on visualizing the amount of blood volume inside the cardiac chambers since the blood loss is well correlated with left ventricular end-diastolic volume.[4] Hypovolemic results in a decrease in stressed volume with cardiac volumes and pressures usually low. It is characterized by the following findings on echocardiography:

- Small ventricular cavity with sometimes completely obliterated end-systolic cavity or "kissing ventricle" **(Figs. 1A and B)**.
- Small inferior and superior vena cava sizes with significant respiratory variation with mechanical ventilation **(Fig. 2)**.
- Left ventricle end-diastolic area <5.5 $cm^2/m^2$
- Low left heart filling pressures—low mitral E wave, low E/E′ ratio **(Figs. 3 and 4)**.
- Low aortic velocity time integral (VTI) and cardiac output **(Fig. 5)**

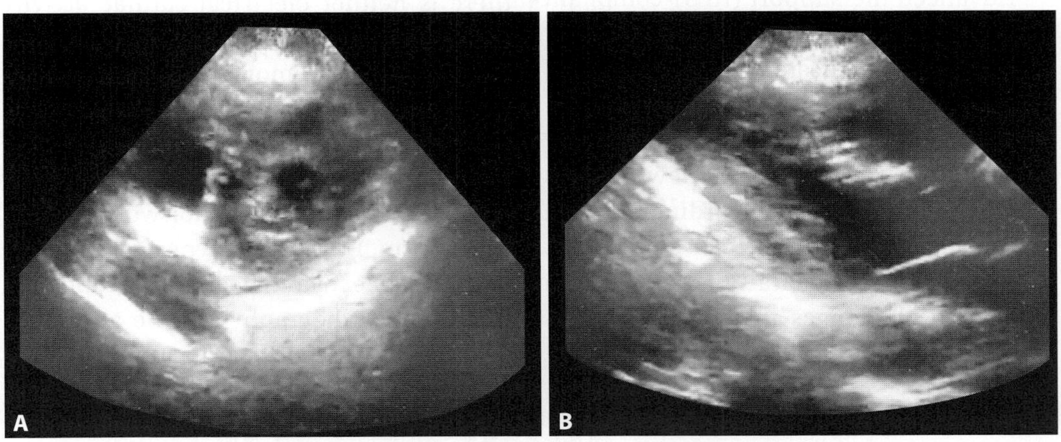


**Figs. 1A and B:** Para-sternal short and long axis view showing completely collapsed/kissing left ventricle cavity at end-systole.

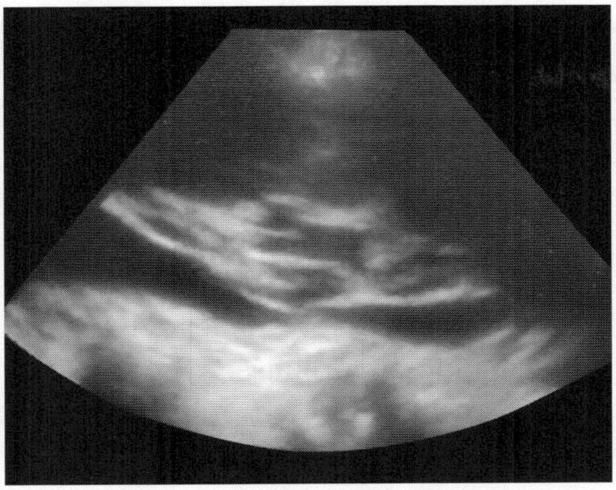

**Fig. 2:** Image from subcostal view showing collapsed inferior vena cava (IVC) indicating hypovolemia.

## PULMONARY EMBOLISM

Massive pulmonary embolism, occlusion of more than two-thirds of the pulmonary vascular bed is likely to cause cardiac arrest. Computed tomography pulmonary angiography (CTPA) is a modality of choice, but for unstable patients and during cardiac arrest, bedside two-dimensional (2D) echocardiography is a useful tool for diagnosing pulmonary embolism. Acute PE causes RV pressure overload and dysfunction, which is detected by echocardiography. However, a negative predictive

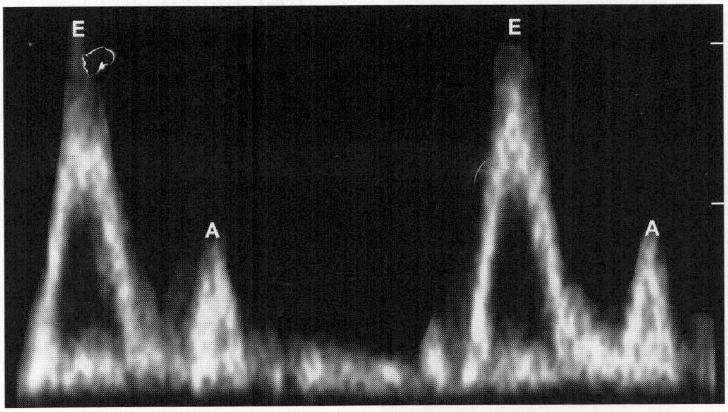


**Fig. 3:** Flow velocity across the mitral valve is examined in the apical four-chamber view (A4C) using pulsed Doppler. Normally, the peak E-wave velocity is between 0.6 and 0.8 m/s and it decreases significantly in hypovolemia.

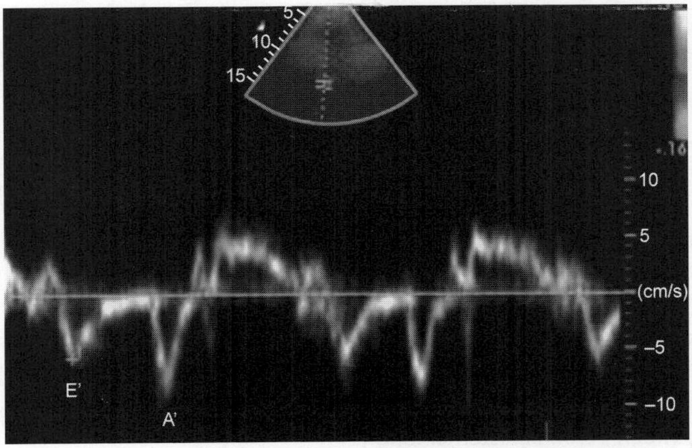


**Fig. 4:** E/E′ ratio is recorded with tissue Doppler sampling 1 cm below the mitral plane. The sample volume can be placed either medially or laterally. Normal E/E′ ratio is <15 and it is significantly decreased in hypovolemia.

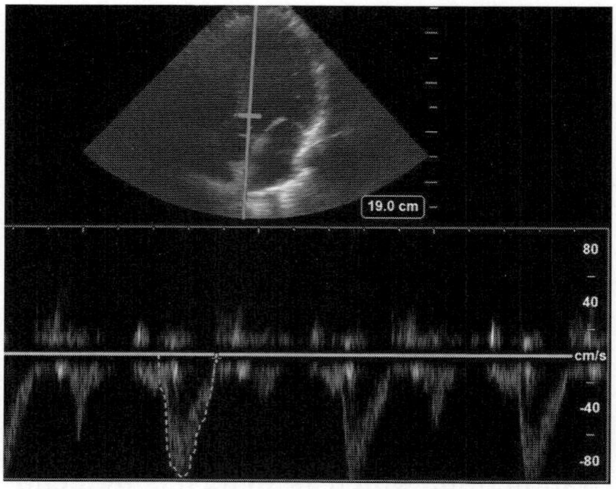


**Fig. 5:** VTI is obtained by using a pulsed wave doppler at the ventricle side of the LVOT approximately 1 cm from the valve in the apical 5-chamber view. Aortic VTI is <15 cm is found in hypovolemia. (LVOT: left ventricular outflow tract; VTI: velocity time integral)

**TABLE 1:** Various parameters on ECHO suggesting the presence of PE.

| | |
|---|---|
| Enlarged RV—in PLAX/A4C **(Figs. 6 and 7)** | Low sensitivity (approximately 25%) |
| Flattened interventricular septum **(Fig. 8)** | High sensitivity (81%), poor specificity (40%) |
| TAPSE <16 mm **(Fig. 9)** | Nonspecific cause of any RV dysfunction. *Only 72% sensitive and not 66% specific for pulmonary embolism* |
| Distended noncollapsing IVC | |
| McConnell's sign (akinetic free wall with hyperdynamic apex) | Low sensitivity (20%) high specificity (about 100%) |
| Clot visualization in RA, RV, or RVOT | Rare finding |
| 60:60 sign (pulmonary acceleration time <60 ms, RVSP <60 mm Hg) | High specificity (90%), low sensitivity (25%) |
| Systolic notching of the pulmonary artery ejection waveform | Difficult to visualize, need more training |

(A4C: apical four chamber; PLAX: parasternal long axis; RVSP: right ventricular systolic pressure; RVOT: right ventricular outflow tract; TAPSE: tricuspid annular plane systolic excursion)

value of 40–50% makes echocardiography an unreliable tool to rule out PE effectively.[5] On the other hand, signs of RV overload/dysfunction may also be observed in conditions other than PE (e.g., pulmonary hypertension). European Society of Cardiology (ESC) suggests TTE as the first-line investigation for suspected PE with hemodynamic compromise.

Signs of PE observed on transthoracic echocardiography (TTE) **(Table 1)**.[6]

## CARDIAC TAMPONADE

Cardiac tamponade is a common cause of PEA-associated cardiac arrest in trauma patients.[7] Fluid in the pericardial space **(Fig. 10)** causes pericardial pressures to exceed more than RV pressure causing impaired ventricular filling, decreasing cardiac output and eventually leading to cardiac arrest. During cardiac arrest the physiological signs of pericardial tamponade may not be appreciable, hence echocardiographic visualization of pericardial fluid should be performed to ascertain the cause of cardiac arrest. It must be noted that the rate of fluid accumulation is more important than the size of the tamponade as effusions of as little as 100 mL may result in cardiac arrest. Identification of pericardial effusion in a cardiac arrest situation mandates immediate drainage (pericardiocentesis). American Society of Echocardiography (ASE) and AHA recommend echocardiography-guided pericardiocentesis providing a high success rate (90%) and a low complication rate (1.2%).[8]

## MYOCARDIAL INFARCTION AND RELATED COMPLICATIONS

Myocardial infarction is a major cause of cardiac arrest. In the event of ongoing CPR, echocardiography is not very helpful as

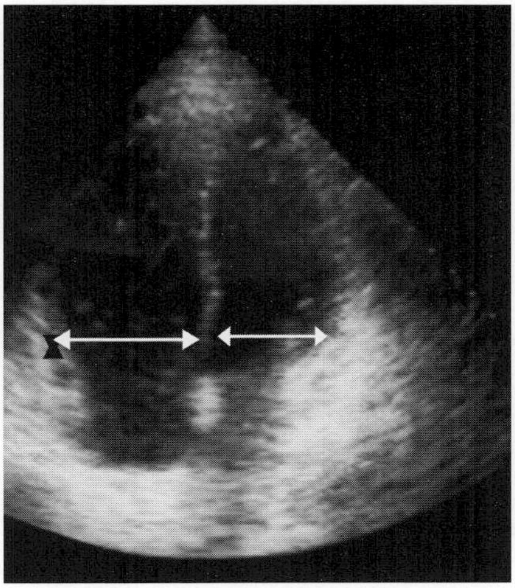

**Fig. 6:** Apical four-chamber view in pulmonary embolism showing marked right ventricular dilatation. (RV: right ventricular; LV: left ventricular) *Note:* The normal ratio of RV:LV diameter is <0.6. Here, the RV/LV ratio is >1, signifying significant right heart strain

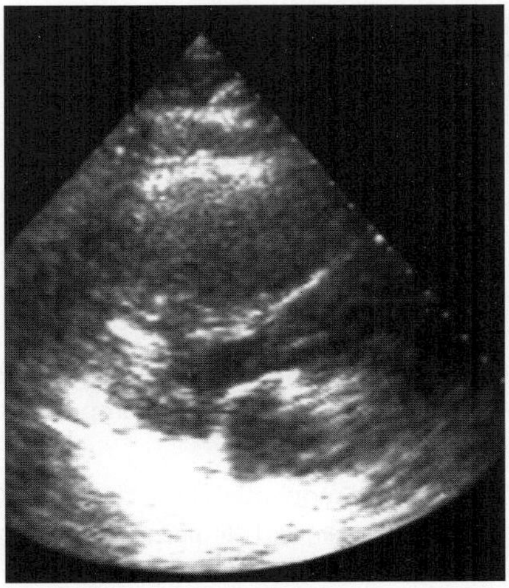

**Fig. 7:** Marked dilatation of right ventricular (RV) in parasternal long axis view.

regional wall motion abnormality is not detectable. Sometimes, severe left or right ventricular hypokinesia can be observed. Left ventricular free wall and septal rupture **(Fig. 11)** is detectable by echocardiography in 0.8–6.2% of patients after MI and results in sudden death due to tamponade.[4]

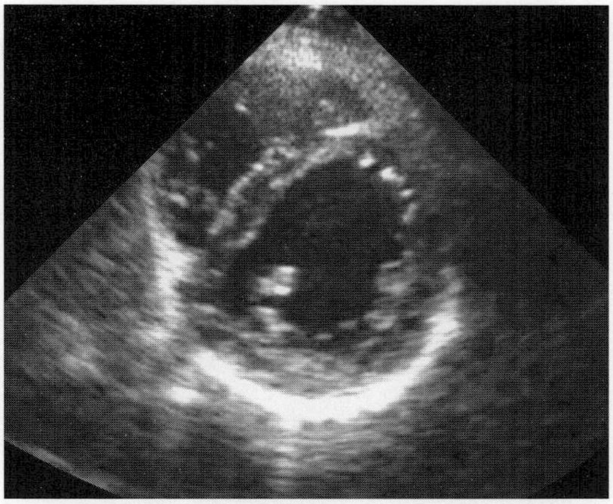

**Fig. 8:** Parasternal short axis view—pressure overload in pulmonary embolism produces a significant elevation of pressure in the subsequently, the right ventricle will push in on the septum in both systole and diastole causing the left ventricle to be D-shaped (D sign) throughout the cardiac cycles.

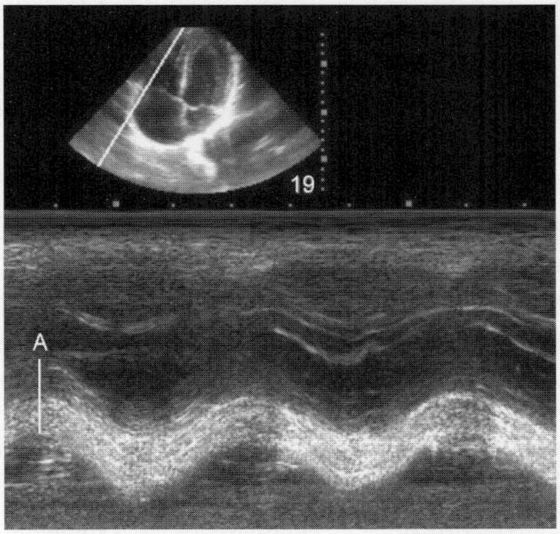


**Fig. 9:** Tricuspid annular plane systolic excursion (TAPSE) is measured by aligning an M-mode cursor parallel to the RV free wall at the point of junction with a tricuspid annulus in apical four-chamber view. Measurement <17 mm is considered abnormal.

## Protocol of a Focused Echocardiogram During Cardiac Arrest

It is imperative that echocardiographic assessment not interfere with the standard

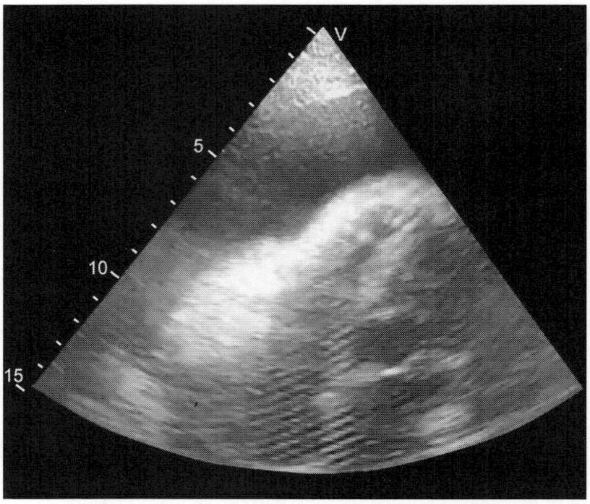


**Fig. 10:** Apical four-chamber (A4C) view identifying massive pericardial tamponade causing collapsed right ventricle resulting in cardiac arrest.

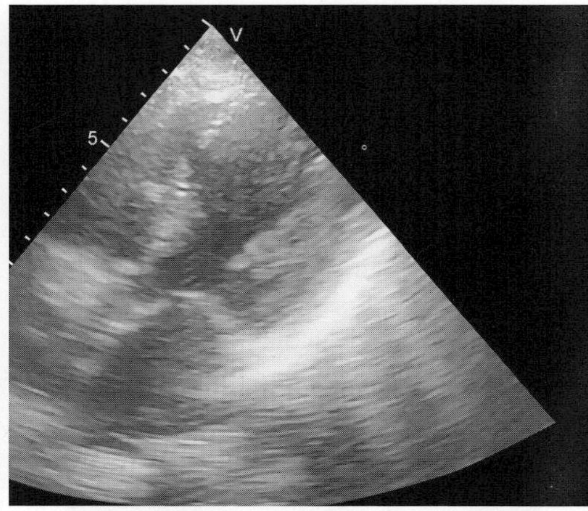


**Fig. 11:** Apical 4-chamber view showing ventricular septal rupture, a complication of myocardial infarction.

**TABLE 2:** Various focused echocardiography protocols for cardiac arrest.

| *Protocol* | *Focus area* | *Sequence* |
|---|---|---|
| Focused echocardiographic evaluation in resuscitation (Feer) | Cardiac | The 10-step algorithm, with four cyclical phases: preparation, image acquisition during pulse check (<10 s), resume CPR, image acquisition followed by necessary action |
| Focused echocardiographic entry Level (FeeL) | Cardiac | Same as above |
| Echocardiographic Assessment using a subcostal-only view in Advanced Life Support (eASy-ALS) | Cardiac, pulmonary, abdomen, and vascular | After an initial 2 minutes of CPR, a cardiac exam is performed from a subcostal view during sequential pulse checks (<10 s); additional images can be acquired from extracardiac locations during active CPR, without interfering with chest compressions |
| Cardiac Arrest Sonographic Assessment (CASA) | Cardiac, pulmonary, and abdomen | Evaluate for specific diagnoses in sequential pulse checks (<10 s): Tamponade, right heart strain, organized cardiac activity, lung, and abdominal ultrasound during active CPR |

Advanced Cardiovascular Life Support (ACLS) protocol. Many cardiac protocols have been proposed to operationalize an ideal echocardiographic approach during cardiac arrest. Every protocol for cardiac arrest described below has limitations, and randomized controlled trials are required recommending a universal methodology for routine implementation **(Table 2)**.

The following pointers should be followed while performing an echocardiography examination during CPR:

- In cardiac arrest scenarios, physicians trained in focused echocardiography should be the ones performing the procedure.

- It is recommended that CPR should proceed uninterrupted and echocardiographic imaging should be performed during the "pulse check" phase of CPR in no >10 seconds.[9]
- A timekeeper role is assigned who counts seconds out loud using a clock during CPR interruption for imaging.
- Detailed preparation should be done before pausing CPR for performing echocardiography. Preparation should include plugging in a device, setting the phased array probe to optimal depth/gain, sonographer optimally positioned with gel applied to the probe.
- Subcostal four-chamber view is the preferred point for imaging.

## Transesophageal Echocardiography during Cardiopulmonary Resuscitation

Sometimes TTE is not possible due to abdominal dressings, surgical drains, or poor acoustic window. In such situations, TEE may be a helpful tool if done by a qualified clinician. Unlike TTE, TEE does not mandate interrupting CPR. Also, TEE is safe and associated with shorter CPR pauses.[10] Disadvantages associated with TEE are the requirement for endotracheal intubation and the need for expert/trained personnel to perform the procedure.

### Time to incorporate echocardiography into ACLS?

Echocardiography during CPR is useful in differentiating asystole, PEA, and pseudo-PEA (a condition where no pulse is palpated but there are organized ventricular contractions when visualized echo). Patients with pseudo-PEA are associated with increased survival and return of spontaneous circulation when compared to a cardiac standstill, thereby hypothesizing the possibility of improved outcomes by continuing the CPR.[11]

This raises the question—"shall we consider the addition of echocardiography to ACLS algorithms for guiding the duration and futility of CPR?" However, the evidence is limited for the use of echocardiography as a prognostication tool during CPR and current literature remains inconclusive in recommending the role of echocardiography for deciding whether to halt or continue resuscitation.[12]

## CONCLUSION

Echocardiography may help in differentiating various shock etiologies, recognizing the causes of cardiac arrest, and understanding the different etiologies of nonshockable, life-threatening cardiac arrhythmias (true/pseudo-PEA and asystole) thereby expediting appropriate, quicker, and life-saving interventions. Various echocardiography protocols have been proposed for assessing the reversible causes of cardiac arrest without interrupting CPR. Though echocardiography is not very reliable in prognostication during CPR and is still not included in the ACLS algorithm, it is a useful adjunct in the decision to extend or terminate resuscitative efforts. Finally, randomized studies and universal protocols are necessary before echocardiography is added as a routine adjunct in algorithms involving CPR.

## REFERENCES

1. Patel K, Hipskind JE: Cardiac arrest. Treasure Island (FL): StatPearls Publishing; 2024.
2. Clattenburg EJ, Wroe P, Brown S, Gardner K, Losonczy L, Singh A, et al. Point-of-care ultrasound use in patients with cardiac arrest is associated with prolonged cardiopulmonary resuscitation pauses: a prospective cohort study. Resuscitation. 2018;122:65-8.

3. Rabiei H, Rahimi-Movaghar V. Application of ultrasound in pulseless electrical activity (PEA) cardiac arrest. Med J Islam Repub Iran. 2016;30:372.
4. Price S, Uddin S, Quinn T. Echocardiography in cardiac arrest. Curr Opin Crit Care. 2010; 16(3):211-5.
5. Konstantinides SV, Meyer G, Becattini C, Bueno H, Geersing GJ, Harjola VP, et al. 2019 ESC Guidelines for the diagnosis and management of acute pulmonary embolism developed in collaboration with the European Respiratory Society (ERS): The Task Force for the diagnosis and management of acute pulmonary embolism of the European Society of Cardiology (ECS). Eur Heart J. 2019;41(4):543-603.
6. Flower L, Olusanya O, Madhivathanan PR. The use of critical care echocardiography in peri-arrest and cardiac arrest scenarios: Pros, cons and what the future holds. J Intensive Care Soc. 2021;22(3):230-40.
7. Zafiropoulos A, Asrress K, Redwood S, Gillon S, Walker D. Critical care echo rounds: echo in cardiac arrest. Echo Res Pract. 2014;1(2): D15-21.
8. Labovitz AJ, Noble VE, Bierig M, Goldstein SA, Jones R, Kort S, et al. Focused cardiac ultrasound in the emergent setting: a consensus statement of the American Society of Echocardiography and American College of Emergency Physicians. J Am Soc Echocardiogr. 2010;23(12):1225-30.
9. Bolvardi E, Pouryaghobi SM, Farzane R, Chokan NM, Ahmadi K, Reihani H: The prognostic value of using ultrasonography in cardiac resuscitation of patients with cardiac arrest. Int J Biomed Sci. 2016;12(3):110-4.
10. Fair J 3rd, Mallin MP, Adler A, Ockerse P, Steenblik J, Tonna J, et al. Transesophageal Echocardiography During Cardiopulmonary Resuscitation Is Associated With Shorter Compression Pauses Compared With Transthoracic Echocardiography. Ann Emerg Med. 2019;73(6):610-6.
11. Gaspari R, Weekes A, Adhikari S, Noble V, Nomura JT, Theodoro D, et al. A retrospective study of pulseless electrical activity, bedside ultrasound identifies interventions during resuscitation associated with improved survival to hospital admission. A REASON Study. Resuscitation. 2017;120:103-7.
12. Reynolds JC, Issa MS, Nicholson TC, Drennan IR, Berg KM, O'Neil BJ, et al. Prognostication with point-of-care echocardiography during cardiac arrest: a systematic review. Resuscitation. 2020;152:56-68.

CHAPTER 26

# Echocardiography in Transplanted Heart

*Meera Rajeev, Sarvesh Pal Singh*

## INTRODUCTION

Echocardiography (ECHO) is a versatile bedside imaging modality that helps comprehensively evaluate the structure and function of the transplanted heart. Before performing ECHO, a physician should know certain aspects of the surgical technique used for heart transplantation (HT).

*Heart transplantation can be of two types:*
1. *Orthotopic HT (OHT):* When the recipient's heart is excised and the donor's is placed in the correct anatomical position
2. *Heterotopic HT:* When the donor's heart is placed in the right chest alongside the recipient's heart. The anastomosis allows blood to pass through either or both hearts.

*There are three major surgical techniques for OHT **(Figs. 1A to C)**:*
1. Biatrial technique involves attaching the donor heart to the recipient's atrial cuff, preserving portions of the recipient's left and right atria.[1]
2. Bicaval technique is characterized by two arterial, one left atrial, and two caval anastomoses, leaving the right atrium intact and only a small posterior part of the recipient's left atrial tissue between the pulmonary veins.[2]
3. Total orthotopic HT technique in which complete excision of the recipient's atria is undertaken. Ventricular as well as atrial orthotopic transplantation is performed.[3]

In these techniques, the biatrial technique was the first surgical approach used for OHT, and the bicaval technique is the most frequently used technique. Arterial connections are made in the ascending aorta and main pulmonary artery (PA).

In pediatric HT, the biatrial technique prevents pulmonary vein stenosis by avoiding pulmonary vein anastomosis. The bicaval technique is used in older children and adults.

Biatrial anastomosis will create an enlarged atrium with echodense suture lines, which can be mistaken for a thrombus. Pulmonary venous obstruction with echo-Doppler should be excluded in the immediate post-transplant period. In the bicaval technique, Doppler imaging should be done to rule out possible stenosis at the site of caval anastomosis. Superior vena cava (SVC) obstruction should be ruled out. Normal SVC waveform has an S and D wave. The loss of a biphasic pattern or an increase in the flow velocity of >1 m/s indicates obstruction.[4] Left-sided SVC should be looked for, and subsequent venous connection should be evaluated for obstruction.

The main PA should be looked at for stenosis. Branch PAs are used for anastomosis if native central PA is abnormal. Such anastomosis is prone to stenosis and is seen poorly by ECHO. In such cases, the presence

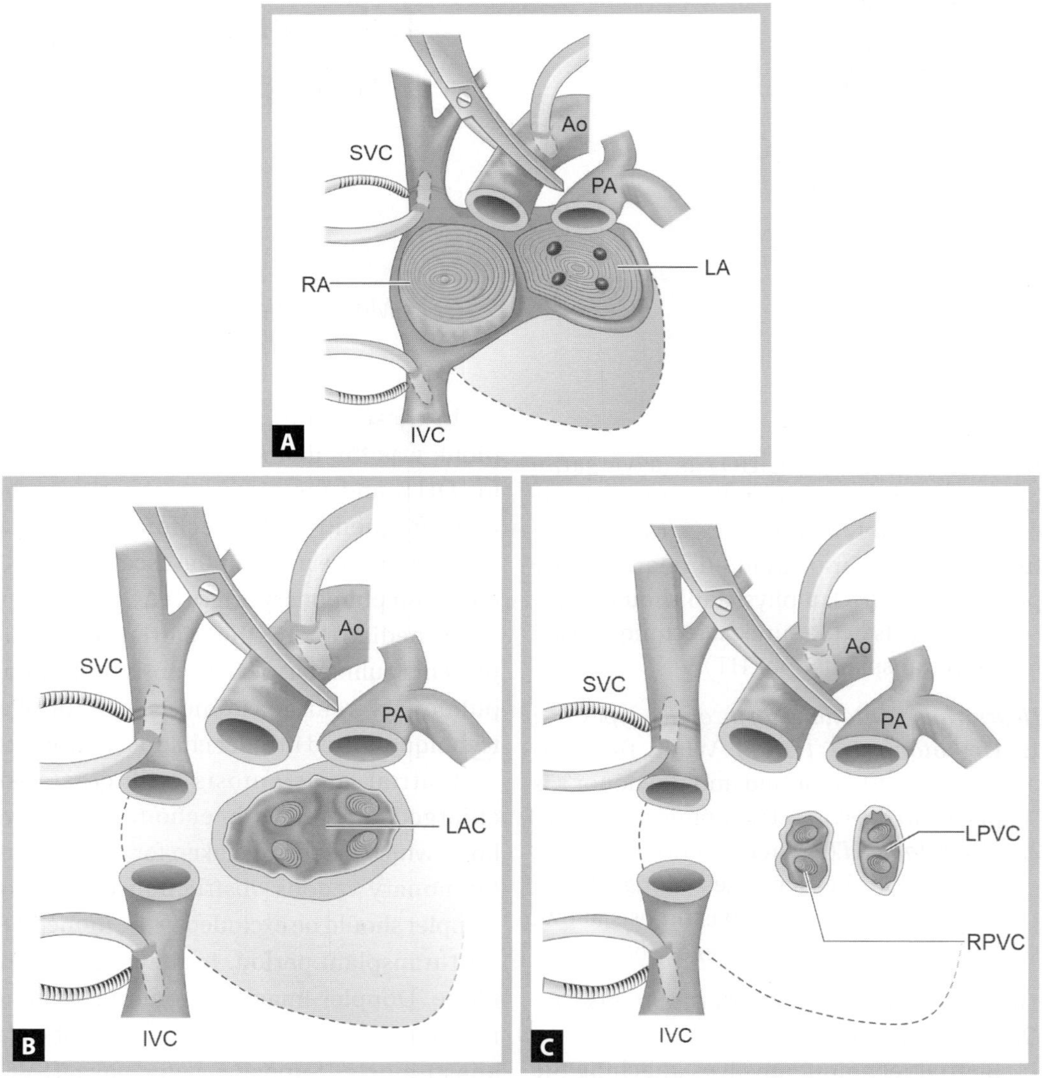


**Figs. 1A to C:** Three major surgical techniques for orthotopic heart transplantation: (A) Biatrial; (B) bicaval; and (C) total. (Ao: aorta; IVC: inferior vena cava; LA: left atrium; LAC: left atrial cuff; LPVC: left pulmonary veins cuff; PA: pulmonary artery; RA: right atrium; RPVC: right pulmonary veins cuff; SVC: superior vena cava)

of PA flow is confirmed indirectly by the presence of pulmonary venous flow. Aortic anastomosis is evaluated in the suprasternal long-axis (LAX) view. If there is native arch hypoplasia, arch reconstruction is required. The aorta should be evaluated for coarctation in such cases **(Figs. 2A and B)**.

## FUNCTIONAL IMAGING OF THE HEART

### What Changes Happen in a Transplanted Heart?

Graft physiology differs from a normal heart due to denervation and altered anatomy.

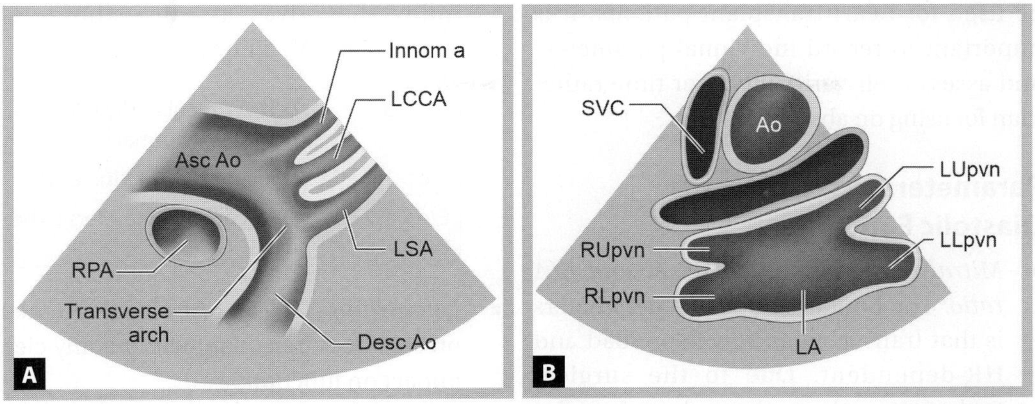


**Figs. 2A and B:** (A) Suprasternal short-axis view and (B) suprasternal aortic arch view—long-axis view. (Asc Ao: ascending aorta; Ao: aorta; Desc Ao: descending aorta; LA: left atrium; LCCA: left common carotid artery; LLpvn: left lower pulmonary vein; LSA: left subclavian artery; LUpvn: left upper pulmonary vein; RLpvn: right lower pulmonary vein; RPA: right pulmonary artery; RUpvn: right upper pulmonary vein; SVC: superior vena cava)

It also depends on the recipient's hemodynamic status. Often, there is a mismatch in the recipient cavity and donor heart size, leading to enhanced mobility and clockwise rotation in the recipient cavity. The atrial impulse originates from the donor atrium and is not controlled by the recipient's nervous system. The heart rate is almost fixed; therefore, heart transplant recipient's (HTR) cardiac output is preload dependent.[5]

Atrial morphology is altered in the biatrial technique, and the appearance of the snowman is seen in the apical four-chamber view. The bicaval technique preserves normal morphology and function, comparable to healthy control hearts. In both techniques, left atrial contractile reserve is markedly reduced compared with healthy controls. Atrial contribution to ventricular filling is reduced post-transplant due to surgical anastomosis. There will be added inflammatory edema related to ischemia-reperfusion injury, allograft ischemia time, surgery, and immune-mediated acute responses. Hence, in the initial period, there is a restrictive cardiac physiology, which, over time, progresses to a nonrestrictive physiology **(Table 1)**.[6]

**TABLE 1:** Anatomical imaging using TTE.

| *Structure* | *Echocardiographic view* |
|---|---|
| Right atrium | Apical 4C view |
| SVC | Suprasternal notch view |
| | Subcostal—coronal and sagittal views |
| IVC | Subcostal sagittal view |
| Left atrium | Apical 4C view |
| Pulmonary veins | Suprasternal SAX view |
| Ascending aorta | Suprasternal LAX view |
| Main pulmonary artery | Parasternal SAX view |
| | Parasternal LAX view |

(4C: four chamber; IVC: inferior vena cava; LAX: long-axis; SAX: short-axis; SVC: superior vena cava; TTE: transthoracic echocardiography)

## ECHOCARDIOGRAPHY EVALUATION OF DIASTOLIC FUNCTION

Evaluation of diastolic function is challenging as the most widely employed diastolic parameters are sensitive to heart motion and acoustic angle. Hence, normal values cannot be used for heart transplant patients. It is important to record individual parameters and assess their variability over time rather than focusing on absolute values.[5]

### Parameters Used to Assess Diastolic Function

- *Mitral inflow velocities—E, A, and E/A ratio:* The limitation of these parameters is that transvalvular flow is preload and HR-dependent. Due to the surgical technique, there is reduced atrial contribution for ventricular filling.

| ***Immediate post-transplant period*** | ***Later post-transplant period*** | ***After years of transplant*** |
|---|---|---|
| Restrictive filling pattern | Nonrestrictive filling pattern or delayed relaxation | Reduced atrial contribution to LV filling persists |
| Short IVRT, short DT, high peak E wave velocity, E/A ratio ≥2 | Prolonged IVRT, prolonged DT, decreased transmitral early filling velocities | E/A >2, LV filling pressures are low |

(DT: deceleration time; IVRT: isovolumic relaxation time; LV: left ventricular)

- *Tissue Doppler index-derived velocity (lateral and septal mitral annular velocity):* Both parameters have the limitation of exaggerated translational motion of the heart due to a mismatch of nonrecipient and clockwise rotation of the heart, which happens post-transplant. Lateral and septal annular e′ velocity increases over time, even though absolute values are lower than the normal population.
- *E/e′:* Transmitral velocities corrected for the influence of relaxation are a valuable index that gives an idea about left ventricular (LV) filling pressures.

| | |
|---|---|
| E/e′ <8 | Left ventricular (LV) filling pressure—normal |
| E/e′ >15 | LV filling pressure increased |
| E/e′ between 8 and 15 | Other echo parameters to be used |

- *Left atrium (LA) size:* Atrial enlargement present post-transplant without any clear impact on function.
- *Pulmonary vein velocities:* Not a valuable index of LV filling pressures.
- *Speckle tracking echocardiography (STE):* STE to determine global longitudinal strain (GLS) helps quantify ventricular function without the limitations of other methods, such as variability in measurements related to loading conditions, angle of image acquisition, regional wall motion abnormality (RWMA), and ventricular chamber geometry. It is an early marker of reduced myocardial function before measurable changes in other ECHO parameters occur. Altered LA and LV parameters correlate with LV filling pressures. Peak atrial longitudinal strain, peak atrial circumferential strain, GLS, and circumferential strain are used for serial monitoring.

## ECHOCARDIOGRAPHY EVALUATION OF SYSTOLIC FUNCTION (BOX 1)

### Assessment of Left Ventricular Systolic Function

After 3 months of HT, inflammatory edema and cell infiltration subside and the transplanted heart's LV mass and wall thickness generally normalize. If it persists beyond 3 months, it

**BOX 1:** Normal findings in a transplanted heart.

- Biatrial dilatation
- Hyperechogenic at biatrial anastomosis
- Pericardial effusion (small or loculated)
- Abnormal (in systole) or flat interventricular septal motion
- Decreased interventricular thickening
- Increased left ventricular (LV) posterior or septal thickness
- Increased LV mass or LV mass index
- Increased right ventricular (RV) dimensions and thickness
- Beat-to-beat variation in the mitral inflow pattern
- Mild pulmonic, tricuspid, or mitral regurgitation

can be due to acute rejection or hypertension secondary to the use of immunosuppressants. LV ejection fraction (LVEF) and regional wall motion (RWM) are preserved for most transplanted hearts for 10–15 years until coronary artery vasculopathy (CAV) sets in. Septal dyskinesias are frequent and common postheart transplants.[7]

## Assessment of Right Ventricular Systolic Function

Persistent high pulmonary pressures in the recipient cause right ventricular (RV) volume overload in the immediate post-transplant period, gradually decreasing over the first 3 months. The right ventricular systolic function assessed by tricuspid annular plane systolic excursion (TAPSE), RV fractional area change (RV FAC), TV S′ wave on tissue Doppler imaging (TDI), and GLS of RV free wall is lower than normal healthy hearts. The longitudinal parameters remain abnormal, do not normalize in follow-up, and are not sensitive markers to assess RV global systolic function.

## Valve Morphology and Function

In the early post-transplant period, mitral regurgitation (MR) and tricuspid regurgitation (TR) are common. MR occurs due to papillary muscle edema, which resolves over time. TR occurs due to the recipient's high pulmonary artery pressures (PAP). After 1 year of transplant, the most common valvular lesion is TR, the mechanism of which can be due to: (1) Persistent high PAP in the recipient; (2) enlargement of tricuspid annulus due to RV dilatation; (3) damage to valvular and subvalvular apparatus due to frequent endomyocardial biopsies (EMB); and (4) biatrial technique resulting in altered right atrial morphology and annulus dilatation.[8]

## Pericardium

Pericardial effusions (PE) are very common in the first year of follow-up. Small-to-moderate PE is present in 66% of post-HTRs at 3 months and 25% of patients at 6 months of follow-up.[9] Severe PE causing pericardial tamponade is rare and usually occurs due to an undersized heart for the recipient's body surface area. Frequent echocardiographic follow-up is required in such patients. New onset PE usually occurs post-HT due to RV perforation due to EMB, acute allograft rejection (AAR), infection, or a neoplasm.[10]

Echocardiography is an indispensable method of documenting biventricular systolic dysfunction, which is required to diagnose primary graft dysfunction (PGD) and monitor the effectiveness of therapy.

# ROLE OF ECHOCARDIOGRAPHY IN EVALUATING ACUTE GRAFT REJECTION

Acute allograft rejection occurs in 15% of HTRs during the first year. AAR presents with extremely variable clinical patterns, ranging from asymptomatic systolic dysfunction to cardiogenic shock. EMB is the current gold standard for diagnosing and grading rejection per the International Society for Heart and Lung Transplantation (ISHLT) guidelines. Due to sampling errors, histological false negatives can occur in 10–20% of HTRs. Transthoracic echocardiography (TTE) can be used as a screening and complementary tool to monitor acute graft rejection.

An early abnormality in patients with rejection is diastolic dysfunction. Myocardial edema (and later fibrosis) is caused by inflammation in response to an antigen-antibody reaction. Changes in myocardial echogenicity, LV mass, and wall thickness impair myocardial relaxation. The systolic function also decreases in acute rejections, and new-onset PE may occur. However, LV systolic function may not correlate with the severity of rejection on biopsy.

As the diastolic dysfunction progresses, the transmitral Doppler (TMD) shows a decreased isovolumic relaxation time (IVRT) and increased E velocity. However, reduced early and late diastolic peak mitral annulus (e′and a′) and lower systolic velocities (s′) on TDI correlate better with AAR episodes. The TDI is more sensitive in detecting rejection but with low specificity, as HTRs have abnormal diastolic function compared to normal hearts.

Considering rejection as a focal process, myocardial deformation imaging could identify small changes in myocardial function typical of acute rejection. Studies have shown that peak systolic GLS and strain rate are decreased in patients with acute rejection, as confirmed by EMB.[11] Regional strain and strain rate were reduced in the LV lateral wall but not in the septum in acute rejection. This occurs due to the paradoxical septal motion after all cardiac surgeries, including HT. The ISHLT guidelines do not specify the timings for echocardiographic evaluation or recommend ECHO as the alternative to serial EMB in rejection monitoring **(Box 2)**.

**BOX 2:** ECHO indicators of rejection.

- Progressive increase in wall thickness >4 mm (interventricular septum and posterior wall)
- Increased myocardial echogenicity
- Diastolic pattern indicating restriction
- New or increasing pericardial effusion
- New-onset MR or TR
- A more than 10% decrease in LVEF
- A more than 10% decrease in e′
- A 20% decrease in IVRT
- Dobutamine stress echo to detect allograft vasculopathy
- Speckle tracking global/regional strain is promising

(ECHO: echocardiography; IVRT: isovolumic relaxation time; LVEF: left ventricular ejection fraction; MR: mitral regurgitation; TR: tricuspid regurgitation)

A combination of two or more parameters may indicate rejection. These indicators can be absent even in a case of rejection, proven by biopsies.

## ROLE OF ECHOCARDIOGRAPHY IN THE EVALUATION OF CARDIAC ALLOGRAFT VASCULOPATHY

Chronic graft rejection manifests as coronary allograft vasculopathy (CAV). It is a diffuse process involving the epicardial vessels and the coronary microcirculation and has a multifactorial etiology. Due to the denervated heart, CAV progresses silently and manifests clinically as myocardial ischemia, LV dysfunction, heart failure, ventricular arrhythmias, or even sudden cardiac deaths.

Resting TTE is of limited use in diagnosing CAV. Systolic function is preserved even in advanced forms of CAV; hence, LVEF cannot detect it in HTRs. A RWMA can raise suspicion of CAV, but it is nonspecific. Worsening diastolic function during follow-up can also indicate CAV. Both systolic and diastolic parameters are not specific to detecting CAV, as they can also indicate AAR.

Hence, an invasive diagnostic approach such as coronary angiogram (CA) is required to detect CAV. Decreased absolute GLS is associated with CAV and coronary microcirculatory dysfunction.

The ISHLT guidelines recommend using dobutamine stress echocardiography (DSE) or treadmill stress echocardiography (TSE) for CAV detection in patients who cannot undergo repeated CAs. Because HTRs have a denervated heart and altered chronotropic response, exercise cannot act as an LV stressor. Hence, DSE is preferred over TSE. The accuracy of exercising ECHO may improve when combined with other techniques, such as myocardial strain analysis. For example, strain analysis may increase the sensitivity of DSE from 63% to 88% in the detection of CAV, a promising tool for further research.[12]

## REFERENCES


1. Lower RR, Shumway NE. Studies on orthotopic homotransplantation of the canine heart. Surg Forum. 1960;11:18-9.
2. Sievers HH, Weyand M, Kraatz EG, Bernhard A. An alternative technique for orthotopic cardiac transplantation, with preservation of the normal anatomy of the right atrium. Thorac Cardiovasc Surg. 1991;39:70-2.
3. Dreyfus G, Jebara V, Mihaileanu S, Carpentier AF. Total orthotopic heart transplantation: an alternative to the standard technique. Ann Thorac Surg. 1991;52:1181-4.
4. Appleton CP, Hatle LK, Popp RL. Superior vena cava and hepatic vein Doppler echocardiography in healthy adults. J Am Coll Cardiol. 1987;10:1032-9.
5. Sciaccaluga C, Fusi C, Landra F, Barilli M, Lisi M, Mandoli GE, et al. Diastolic function in heart transplant: From physiology to echocardiographic assessment and prognosis. Front Cardiovasc Med. 2022;9: 969270.
6. Nagueh SF, Smiseth OA, Appleton CP, Byrd BF, Dokainish H, Edvardsen T, et al. Recommendations for the evaluation of left ventricular diastolic function by echocardiography: an update from the American society of echocardiography and the European Association of Cardiovascular Imaging. J Am Soc Echocardiogr. 2016;29: 277-314.
7. Masarone D, Kittleson M, Gravino R, Valente F, Petraio A, Pacileo G. The Role of Echocardiography in the Management of Heart Transplant Recipients. Diagnostics (Basel). 2021;11:2338.
8. Bishawi M, Zanotti G, Shaw L, MacKenzie M, Castleberry A, Bartels K, et al. Tricuspid Valve Regurgitation Immediately After Heart Transplant and Long-Term Outcomes. Ann Thorac Surg. 2019;107:1348-55.
9. Ciliberto G, Anjos MC, Gronda E, Bonacina E, Danzi G, Colombo P, et al. Significance of pericardial effusion after heart transplantation. Am J Cardiol. 1995;76:297-300.
10. Al-Dadah AS, Guthrie TJ, Pasque MK, Moon MR, Ewald GA, Moazami N. Clinical course and predictors of pericardial effusion following cardiac transplantation. Transplant Proc. 2007;39:1589-92.
11. Marciniak A, Eroglu E, Marciniak M, Sirbu C, Herbots L, Droogne W, et al. The potential clinical role of ultrasonic strain and strain rate imaging in diagnosing acute rejection after heart transplantation. Eur J Echocardiogr. 2007;8:213-21.
12. Derumeaux G, Redonnet M, Mouton-Schleifer D, Bessou JP, Cribier A, Saoudi N, et al. Dobutamine stress echocardiography in orthotopic heart transplant recipients. VACOMED Research Group. J Am Coll Cardiol. 1995;25:1665-72.

CHAPTER 27

# Role of Echocardiography in Liver/Renal/Lung Transplantation

*Kulbhushan Saini, Arshdeep Singh, Ajay Singh*

## INTRODUCTION

The first organ transplant in India was done in 1970 and since then we have come a long way. Multiorgan system assessment of the recipient as well as a donor in living donor transplant is one of the most important prerequisites in organ transplant in order to ensure an optimal outcome for the recipient and also to avoid unnecessary wastage of organ transplant which is already scarce with a huge demand in both developing and developed nations.

Involvement of the cardiovascular system is well recognized in patients with liver, lung, and kidney diseases. Complications of the cardiovascular system account for considerable perioperative morbidity and mortality. Therefore, assessment of the cardiovascular system apart from heart transplant patients in other organ transplants is critical for the risk stratification and management of these patients.

Echocardiography is the primary noninvasive modality to assess the cardiovascular system. It is a versatile tool providing comprehensive information about cardiac structure and function. These examinations can be easily performed at the bedside and serially repeated without any patient discomfort.

In this chapter, we will be discussing in detail the role of echocardiography, the echocardiographic parameters used, and how echocardiography can be helpful in deciding further management and reducing the postoperative morbidity and mortality in patients of heart, liver, kidney, and lung transplant.

## ECHOCARDIOGRAPHY IN LIVER TRANSPLANT

Echocardiography plays an integral role in liver transplant patients both pre- and post-transplant. Cardiovascular diseases (CVDs) are one of the leading causes of mortality and morbidity postliver transplant. End-stage liver disease leads to hyperdynamic circulation imposing significant stress with elevated cardiac output, low peripheral vascular resistance, low effective blood volume, and arterial hypotension. This consequently results in ventricular systolic dysfunction and cardiomyopathy. Liver transplant may also unmask subclinical cirrhotic cardiomyopathy which manifests as heart failure events with patients showing signs of cardiovascular dysfunction in the first week after liver transplant.

Some baseline hemodynamic changes associated with end-stage liver disease (ESLD) are discussed underneath.

### Systemic Circulation

- *Plasma volume:* Increased
- *Total blood volume:* Increased
- *Noncentral blood volume:* Increased

- *Central blood volume:* Unchanged ↔ or decreased
- *Arterial blood pressure:* Unchanged ↔ or decreased
- *Systemic vascular resistance:* Decreased
- *Heart rate:* Increased
- *Cardiac output:* Increased

### Cardiac Hemodynamics

- *Left atrial (LA) volume:* Increased
- *LV volume:* Increased ↔
- *Right atrial (RA) volume:* Unchanged ↔ or increased ↓
- *RV volume:* Unchanged ↔ or increased ↓
- *RA pressure:* Unchanged ↔ or increased
- *RV end-diastolic pressure:* Unchanged ↔
- *Pulmonary capillary wedge pressure (PCWP):* Unchanged ↔
- *LV end-diastolic pressure:* Increased ↔

### Pulmonary Circulation

- *Pulmonary blood flow:* Increased
- *Pulmonary artery pressure:* Unchanged ↔ or increased
- *Pulmonary vascular resistance (PVR):* Unchanged ↔ or increased ↓

These hemodynamic changes reflect the complex alterations seen in ESLD, driven largely by alterations in volume status, systemic vasodilation, and changes in cardiac function. They contribute to the clinical manifestations and complications observed in patients with advanced liver disease.

## CARDIOVASCULAR CONCERNS IN PATIENTS FOR LIVER TRANSPLANT

### Left Ventricular Outflow Tract Obstruction and Hypertrophic Cardiomyopathy

- Patients with hypertrophic cardiomyopathy (HCM) and left ventricular hypertrophy (LVH) may develop dynamic left ventricular outflow tract obstruction (LVOTO).
- LVOTO is defined as an outflow tract gradient >36 mm Hg on preoperative dobutamine stress echocardiography (DSE).
- Management involves careful intraoperative monitoring, avoiding hypovolemia, tachycardia, and inotropic agents. Intraoperative TEE is crucial for continuous monitoring and management.

### Valvular Heart Disease

- Liver transplantation (LT) candidates may present with mitral regurgitation, tricuspid regurgitation, or both.
- While these conditions may not affect overall mortality, they can lead to intraoperative hypotension requiring vasopressor therapy.

### Portopulmonary Hypertension

- PPH is pulmonary arterial hypertension associated with portal hypertension, with or without cirrhosis.
- Screening with Doppler echocardiography is recommended for all LT candidates to assess for elevated pulmonary pressures.
- Right ventricle systolic pressure (RVSP) can be estimated using the peak tricuspid regurgitant velocity (TRV) and right atrial pressure (RAP).
- Right heart catheterization is recommended to confirm the diagnosis if RVSP is 45–60 mm Hg.

### Pericardial Effusion

- Up to 63% of LT candidates may have pericardial effusions, typically small and hemodynamically well tolerated.
- Regular monitoring is necessary to assess for changes in effusion size that may impact hemodynamics.

## Patent Foramen Ovale

- Echocardiography or color Doppler imaging is recommended to diagnose patent foramen ovale (PFO).
- Changes in intracardiac pressures during the perioperative period can lead to paradoxical emboli through the PFO.

These cardiovascular considerations are critical in the preoperative assessment and intraoperative management of patients undergoing LT, aiming to optimize outcomes and minimize perioperative complications.

The current recommendations for echocardiography in LT candidates, as outlined by the American Association for the Study of Liver Diseases (AASLD) and other guidelines, focus on several key aspects:

- *Routine TTE:*
  - TTE is recommended for all LT candidates to assess:
    - Chamber sizes
    - Hypertrophy
    - Systolic and diastolic function
    - Valvular function
    - LVOTO
- *Challenges in echocardiographic imaging in ESLD:*
  - Ascites, common in ESLD patients, can limit subcostal imaging and alter heart orientation in the thorax.
  - Off-axis views and unconventional imaging windows may be necessary due to ascitic fluid.
  - Ascites can also distort the contour of the left ventricle, potentially causing artifactual pseudodyskinesis of the posterior wall.
- *Assessment for coronary artery disease (CAD):*
  - LT candidates should undergo evaluation for CAD based on risk factors, such as:
    - History of smoking
    - Diabetes mellitus
    - Hypertension
    - Hyperlipidemia
    - Clinical or family history of heart disease
    - LVH
    - Age >50 years or >60 years (depending on guidelines)
- *DSE:*
  - DSE is recommended as an effective screening test for CAD in LT candidates.
  - Positive DSE results should prompt further evaluation with coronary angiography.

These recommendations underscore the importance of comprehensive cardiovascular assessment in LT candidates, aiming to identify and manage any cardiac conditions that could impact perioperative and postoperative outcomes. Echocardiography plays a crucial role in this assessment, providing valuable information on cardiac structure, function, and potential ischemic heart disease.

## Intraoperative Echocardiography for Liver Transplant

The American Association for the Study of Liver Diseases states that TEE should be used in all liver transplant candidates in order to assess chamber sizes, hypertrophy, systolic and diastolic function, valvular function, and left ventricle outflow tract obstruction. TEE during LT offers several benefits. It can guide targeted pharmacologic therapies for treatment of intraoperative hypotension, and mechanical circulatory support in cases of refractory cardiovascular collapse. Apart from being a cardiovascular monitoring tool it also can identify graft hepatic vein or inferior vena cava (IVC) stenosis, which may require immediate intervention.

## ECHOCARDIOGRAPHY IN RENAL TRANSPLANT

### Cardiovascular Disease and Mortality

- CVD is a leading cause of morbidity and mortality in patients with end-stage kidney failure, both before and after transplantation.
- CVD accounts for 30% of mortality in patients with functioning allografts, with the highest rates occurring in the peritransplantation period.

### Challenges in Cardiac Evaluation

- Accurate and effective cardiac evaluations are challenging due to:
  - The large size of the target population.
  - The high prevalence of CVD.
  - Extended waiting periods between initial evaluation and transplantation surgery.

There are at least four distinct clinical guidelines addressing the preoperative cardiac evaluation of renal transplant candidates:

1. American College of Cardiology (ACC)/ American Heart Association (AHA) 2007 Guidelines on perioperative cardiovascular evaluation and care for noncardiac surgery.
2. Kidney Disease Outcomes Quality Initiative Clinical Practice Guidelines for Cardiovascular Disease in Dialysis Patients (KDOQI)
3. Report of the Lisbon Conference on the Care of the Kidney Transplant Recipient (Lisbon)
4. The Evaluation of Renal Transplant Candidates, which appeared in a journal published by the American Society of Transplantation (AST).

## CARDIOVASCULAR CONCERNS IN PATIENTS FOR RENAL TRANSPLANT

### Coronary Artery Disease

- *Atherosclerotic CAD:* A major concern in the chronic kidney disease (CKD) population, often emphasized due to its prevalence and impact on morbidity and mortality.
- *Coronary artery calcification:* Common in advanced CKD, linked to the abnormal metabolic environment of CKD rather than traditional atherosclerotic processes.

### Left Ventricular Hypertrophy

- Highly prevalent in renal transplant candidates.
- *Uremic cardiomyopathy:* This encompasses LVH, LV systolic dysfunction, and LV dilation, all contributing to the cardiovascular burden in CKD patients.

### Cardiac Valvular Disease

- Patients may present with various forms of valvular disease, necessitating thorough evaluation.
- *Common valvular issues:* These can include mitral regurgitation, aortic stenosis, and other valve dysfunctions.

### Systematic Approach to Pretransplant Cardiac Screening

#### *Comprehensive Cardiac Evaluation*

- Assessment of chamber sizes, ventricular function, and valvular function through routine echocardiography.
- Stress testing (e.g., DSE) for CAD detection.
- Coronary angiography for patients with positive stress test results or significant risk factors.

### Specific Conditions

- *LVH:* Assessment of LV mass and function to identify uremic cardiomyopathy.
- *Valvular disease:* Detailed evaluation to determine the presence and severity of any valvular abnormalities.

### Pulmonary Hypertension

Screening for elevated pulmonary pressures due to its impact on transplantation outcomes.

## Clinical Implications

- *Risk stratification:* Identifying high-risk patients to optimize perioperative management and improve post-transplant outcomes.
- *Interventional planning:* Deciding on the need for interventions such as revascularization and valve repair/replacement prior to transplantation.
- *Post-transplant monitoring:* Continuous monitoring of cardiac function and addressing any complications promptly.

# CURRENT RECOMMENDATIONS FOR ECHOCARDIOGRAPHY IN RENAL TRANSPLANT CANDIDATES

## Guidelines and Recommendations

### Initial Screening

The National Kidney Foundation (NKF)/KDOQI "Clinical Practice Guidelines for Cardiovascular Disease in Dialysis Patients" recommends performing a resting echocardiogram for all patients at the initiation of dialysis, ideally within 1–3 months after achieving dry weight. This is Level of Evidence A recommendation, indicating the strongest level of evidence.

### Purpose of Echocardiography

- *Detection of LVH and enlargement:* Identifies significant LVH and abnormalities in other cardiac chambers.
- *Valvular abnormalities:* Detects conditions, such as mitral stenosis, aortic stenosis, and valvular calcification.
- *PH:* Assesses for elevated pulmonary artery pressure which is associated with adverse post-transplant outcomes.

### Serial Echocardiography

- Important for monitoring known aortic stenosis to determine the timing for aortic valve replacement prior to transplantation.
- Essential for evaluating the progression of PH, which may necessitate further investigations such as sleep studies for obstructive sleep apnea and right heart catheterization.

### Diastolic Dysfunction

- Common in early ESRD with preserved systolic function. Diastolic dysfunction is associated with perioperative cardiopulmonary events in patients undergoing surgery.
- The E/E' ratio (early transmitral flow velocity to early diastolic velocity of the mitral annulus) is a reliable indicator of diastolic function and LV filling pressure, useful for predicting in-hospital major cardiovascular complications postkidney transplantation.

### Prognostic Information

- Echocardiographic findings at rest and after stress provide significant prognostic information for long-term mortality in CKD patients.

- A strong relationship exists between left ventricular ejection fraction (LVEF) and outcomes, underscoring the importance of identifying and correcting any reversible causes of poor LVEF before transplantation.

## Clinical Implications

- *Early detection:* Early echocardiographic evaluation helps in the timely identification of cardiac abnormalities, facilitating appropriate interventions.
- *Monitoring and management:* Regular monitoring through serial echocardiography allows for the assessment of disease progression and the effectiveness of therapeutic interventions.
- *Predictive value:* Echocardiographic parameters, especially the E/E' ratio and LVEF, are valuable for risk stratification and predicting post-transplant outcomes.
- *Interventional planning:* Findings guide preoperative planning and management, ensuring that patients are in optimal cardiac health before undergoing renal transplantation.

In summary, echocardiography is a critical tool in the cardiovascular evaluation of renal transplant candidates, aiding in the detection, monitoring, and management of cardiac conditions to improve transplantation outcomes.

# ECHOCARDIOGRAPHY IN LUNG TRANSPLANT

## Introduction

Lung transplantation is the definitive treatment for end-stage lung disease that is refractory to guideline-directed medical therapy. PH is a serious complication of advanced lung disease and is associated with a worse prognosis.

## Role of Echocardiography

As part of the preoperative workup for lung transplant patients, investigation of cardiac function with echocardiography is crucial. Echocardiography helps in the assessment of cardiac function, identifying any cardiac issues that could pose a risk during or after the transplant.

## Preoperative Phase

### *Assessment of Cardiac Function*

- Evaluate left and RV function.
- Assess for the presence of PH.
- Identify valvular heart disease or structural abnormalities.
- Measure chamber sizes and wall thicknesses.

### *Risk Stratification*

- Based on the severity of disease, presence of end-organ damage, and ease of control with standard therapies.
- Patients with moderate or severe ventricular systolic dysfunction are often excluded from lung transplantation due to higher perioperative risk.

### *Hemodynamic Assessment*

- Determine pulmonary artery pressure and RAP.
- Estimate the PVR using Doppler echocardiography.

## Intraoperative Phase

### *Monitoring Cardiac Function*

- Continuous intraoperative monitoring of ventricular volumes and function.
- Assessing for dynamic changes in cardiac output and filling pressures.

### *Guidance for Management*

- Guidance for volume resuscitation and the use of vasopressor therapy.
- Monitoring for signs of right heart failure or other complications during surgery.

## ROLE OF PREOPERATIVE ECHOCARDIOGRAPHY

Assessing abnormal diastolic function through preoperative echocardiography is crucial as it is linked to increased cardiovascular comorbidity. Studies have shown that mortality rates are higher in hospitalized patients with LVEFs of <39%. The association between echocardiographic markers of abnormal relaxation and decreased survival, even in patients with no history of congestive heart failure (CHF), highlights the importance of echocardiography in identifying individuals at risk of adverse outcomes. Furthermore, many lung transplant candidates are excluded based on systolic dysfunction; hence, evaluating isolated diastolic dysfunction is essential in identifying those at high risk for complications.

### Right Heart Catheterization versus Echocardiography

Right heart catheterization remains the gold standard for assessing PH in clinical practice. Numerous studies have compared Doppler echocardiography with Swan–Ganz catheterization measurements. These studies have generally found that hemodynamic data obtained via echocardiography, such as estimations of RAP, pulmonary artery systolic pressure, PCWP, cardiac output, and PVR, correlate well with values from invasive catheterization. However, echocardiography has limitations, particularly in patients with advanced lung disease, where it often inaccurately estimates systolic pulmonary artery pressure, leading to the overdiagnosis of PH. Therefore, echocardiography should complement rather than replace invasive catheterization as a cardiac assessment tool.

### Role of Intraoperative Transesophageal Echocardiography

Lung transplantation is a complex surgery involving the vascular anastomosis of the donor and recipient pulmonary arteries, as well as the anastomosis of the donor pulmonary vein cuff to the recipient's left atrium. Any obstruction in these anastomoses can lead to severe complications, such as PH, RV dysfunction, hypotension, hypoxemia, primary graft dysfunction, and eventually allograft failure and death.

Despite its critical role, the use of intraoperative TEE in lung transplantation holds only a class IIb recommendation from the American Society of Echocardiography, and there are no specific guidelines from the Society of Cardiovascular Anesthesiologists.

Intraoperative TEE allows for the rapid diagnosis of vascular anastomotic complications, facilitating timely surgical corrections that would otherwise be delayed, potentially leading to postoperative graft failure. Both pulmonary artery and pulmonary vein cuff anastomoses should be evaluated with 2D TEE and Doppler echocardiography after the reperfusion of the allograft. Postclosure, these anastomoses should be reassessed to identify any compression of the pulmonary vein cuff due to allograft-recipient thorax size mismatch, which can also result in graft failure.

Beyond detecting anastomotic issues, TEE offers significant benefits for hemodynamic monitoring and guiding fluid resuscitation. Unlike conventional invasive monitors such as the pulmonary artery catheter, which provide only numerical measures,

TEE can diagnose a failing RV, offering a more comprehensive assessment during lung transplantation.

## CONCLUSION

Echocardiography is a cornerstone of perioperative management in transplantation. Its ability to provide detailed, real-time information on cardiac structure and function significantly enhances the safety and efficacy of the procedure. Mastery of echocardiographic techniques and interpretation is essential for anesthesiologists involved in transplant surgeries, ensuring optimal outcomes for patients undergoing this life-saving operation.

CHAPTER 28

# Optimizing Patient Outcomes in ECMO Therapy: The Role of Echocardiography

*Velmurugan Selvam, Shrikanth Srinivasan*

## INTRODUCTION

Echocardiography (ECHO) has become a valuable tool in managing patients on extracorporeal membrane oxygenation (ECMO), providing critical insights into cardiac function and hemodynamics that are vital for guiding therapeutic decisions.

Extracorporeal membrane oxygenation is a life-saving intervention used for critically ill patients, experiencing severe cardiac and/or respiratory failure that does not respond to conventional treatments. Utilizing transthoracic echocardiography (TTE) or transesophageal echocardiography (TEE), clinicians can assess ventricular function, detect structural abnormalities, and identify complications that may arise during ECMO therapy. This dynamic imaging modality allows for precise evaluation of hemodynamic parameters, guiding decisions on cannula placement, ECMO flow adjustments, and weaning strategies.

For intensivists, mastering ECHO in the context of ECMO is crucial for delivering high-quality care. Integrating ECHO into ECMO management enhances diagnostic accuracy, informs therapeutic interventions, and ultimately improves patient outcomes. This chapter aims to provide a comprehensive overview of the applications, techniques, and benefits of ECHO in ECMO management, equipping clinicians with the knowledge to effectively utilize this powerful tool in caring for critically ill patients.

## BASICS OF EXTRACORPOREAL MEMBRANE OXYGENATION

Extracorporeal membrane oxygenation is a life-saving technique used in patients with severe cardiac or respiratory failure who are unresponsive to conventional therapies. There are two primary types of ECMO:

1. *Veno-arterial (VA) ECMO:*
   a. Provides both cardiac and respiratory support
   b. Indicated in cases of severe cardiac failure, such as cardiogenic shock or cardiac arrest
   c. Cannulation involves the drainage of blood from the venous system and returning oxygenated blood to the arterial system.
2. *Veno-venous (VV) ECMO:*
   a. Provides respiratory support only
   b. Indicated in severe respiratory failure, such as acute respiratory distress syndrome (ARDS)
   c. Cannulation involves the drainage and return of blood to the venous system.

Understanding the ECMO circuit (**Figs. 1A to C**), which includes the pump,

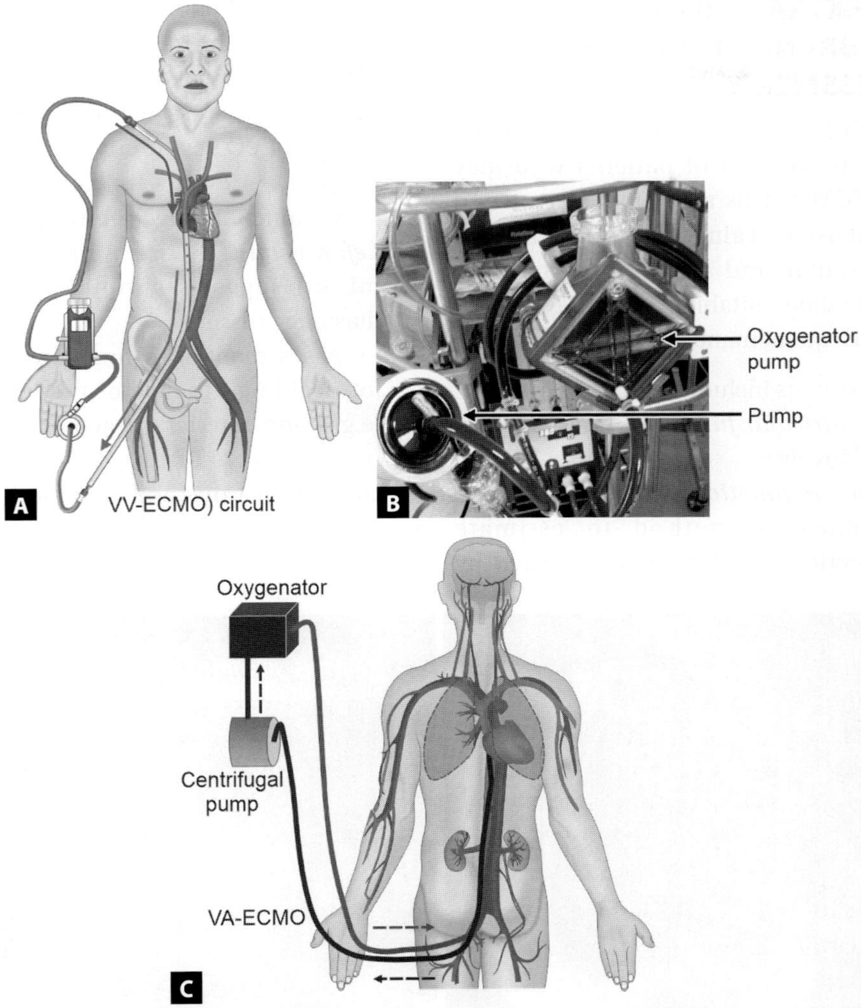


**Figs. 1A to C:** Veno-arterial (VA) and veno-venous (VV) extracorporeal membrane oxygenation (VV-ECMO) circuit.

oxygenator, and cannulas, is essential for effective echocardiographic assessment and management.

## ECHOCARDIOGRAPHY: AN ESSENTIAL TOOL

Echocardiography, utilizing TTE and TEE modalities, is invaluable in the intensive care unit (ICU) for patients on ECMO. Its real-time imaging capabilities allow for dynamic assessment of cardiac structure and function, guiding critical management decisions.

## ADVANTAGES OF TRANSTHORACIC ECHOCARDIOGRAPHY

- Noninvasive and repeatable at the bedside
- Provides detailed anatomical and functional information
- Essential for monitoring and troubleshooting ECMO-related complications.

## PRE-EXTRACORPOREAL MEMBRANE OXYGENATION ASSESSMENT

The pre-ECMO assessment is a critical phase in the management of patients who may require ECMO. This assessment involves a comprehensive evaluation of the patient's cardiovascular and respiratory status to determine their suitability for ECMO and to guide subsequent management.

Key assessments include:

- *Left ventricular function:* Assessment of the LV involves:
    - *Global function:* Measured by the Simpson's method to estimate ejection fraction (EF), S′ wave by tissue Doppler imaging (TDI) at mitral annulus and velocity time integral in left ventricular outflow tract (LVOT).
    - EF <20%, S′ wave velocity by <6 cm/s and LVOT velocity–time integral (VTI) <10 cm/s indicates severe LV dysfunction (**Figs. 2A to C**).
- *Left atrium (LA) size:* A dilated LA (>28 mL/m) suggests chronically elevated diastolic pressures.

Assessment of LV functions is crucial for deciding the type of ECMO support [e.g., veno-arterial extracorporeal membrane oxygenation (VA-ECMO) for combined cardiac and respiratory failure].

- *Right ventricular function:* Evaluation of right ventricular size and function,

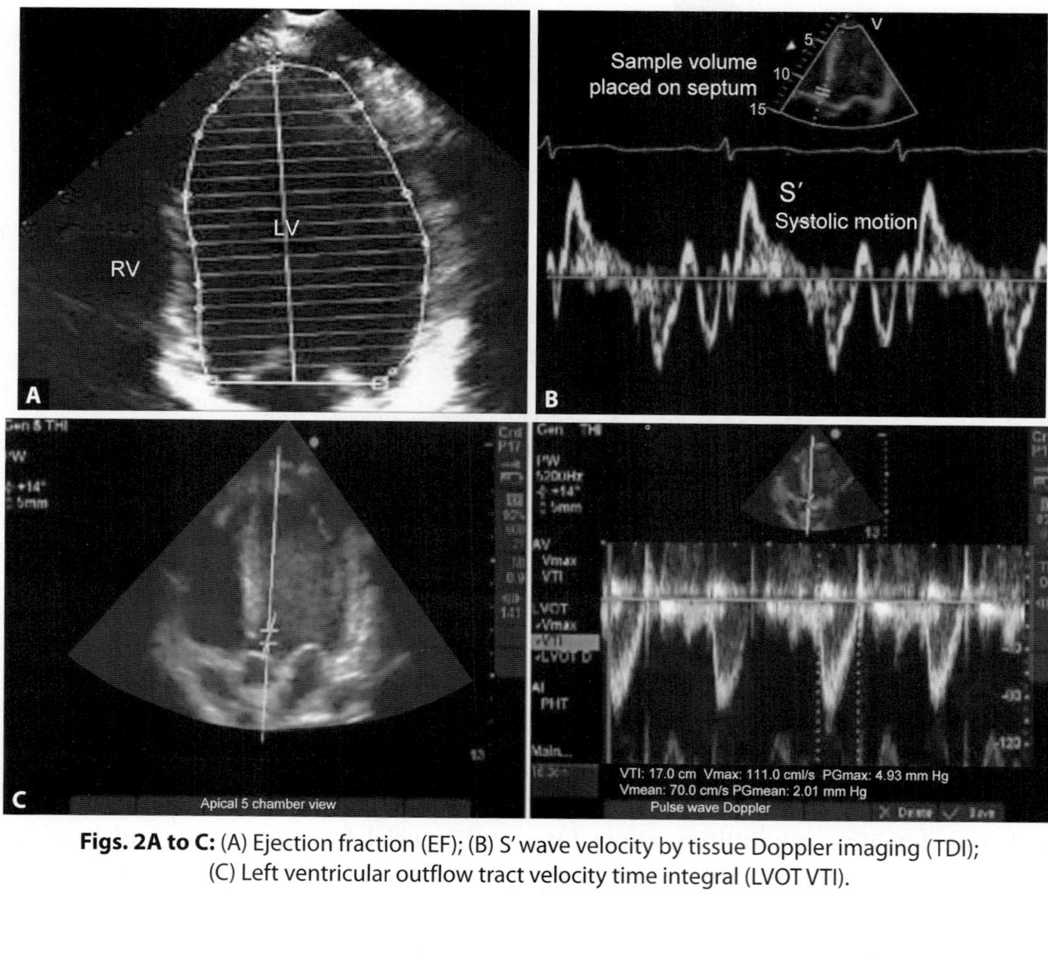


**Figs. 2A to C:** (A) Ejection fraction (EF); (B) S′ wave velocity by tissue Doppler imaging (TDI); (C) Left ventricular outflow tract velocity time integral (LVOT VTI).

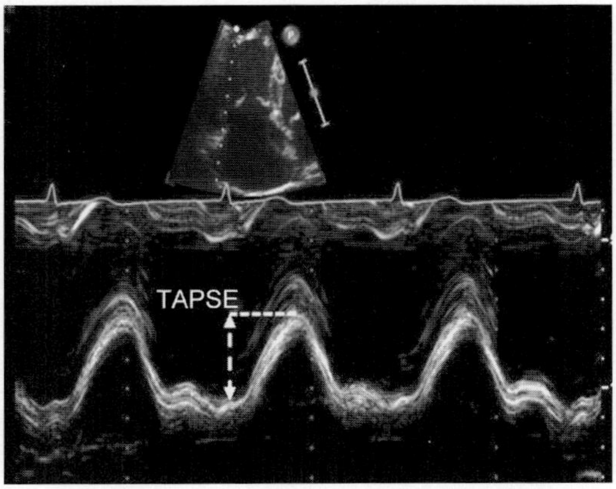


**Fig. 3:** Tricuspid annular plane systolic excursion (TAPSE).

including parameters such as tricuspid annular plane systolic excursion (TAPSE) **(Fig. 3)**, tricuspid annular systolic peak velocity (S′) assessed using TDI, and fractional area change (FAC), is essential as right ventricular failure can significantly impact ECMO outcomes. The right ventricular systolic pressure can be estimated using the simplified Bernoulli equation by measuring the peak velocity of the tricuspid regurgitation (TR) jet.

$$[\Delta P = 4 \times (\text{peak TR velocity})^2]$$

Echocardiography also helps in identifying structural heart diseases or anomalies that may influence ECMO candidacy.

- *Valvular assessment:* Echocardiography (TTE or TEE) is valuable for detecting important valvular conditions before starting ECMO.
  - *Aortic regurgitation:* It can worsen with VA-ECMO, leading to LV dilation, pulmonary edema, and subendocardial ischemia.
  - *Mitral regurgitation:* It causes increased pulmonary edema and requires evaluation to determine if surgical intervention is necessary.
- *Intracardiac shunts:* An atrial septal defect or patent foramen ovale (PFO) may not impact oxygenation significantly during ECMO but could cause complications during weaning due to potential right-to-left shunting.
- *Aortic dissection:* It must be ruled out as it can cause hemodynamic instability and is a relative contraindication for VA-ECMO.

Establishing baseline echocardiographic measurements is crucial for monitoring the patient's progress and response to ECMO therapy. Baseline data provide reference points for assessing the effectiveness of ECMO and for making necessary adjustments during treatment.

## ROLE OF ECHOCARDIOGRAPHY IN EXTRACORPOREAL MEMBRANE OXYGENATION CANNULA INSERTION AND POSITION CONFIRMATION

By providing real-time visualization and detailed assessment, ECHO enhances the accuracy and safety of ECMO cannulation procedures. Its use in both cannula insertion and position confirmation ensures that the cannulas are optimally placed, flow dynamics are appropriate, and any complications are promptly addressed.

### Extracorporeal Membrane Oxygenation Cannula Insertion

During ECMO cannulation, ECHO, including TTE and TEE, is employed to guide the insertion process with precision. The main benefits of using ECHO during cannula insertion include:

*Visualizing vascular structures:* ECHO helps in identifying and delineating the vascular structures, ensuring that the guide wire and subsequently, the cannula is inserted into the correct vessel and reduces the risk of vascular injury and ensures proper access and avoids malposition.

- *Guiding cannula placement:* Real-time imaging allows clinicians to monitor the advancement of the cannula, ensuring it follows the intended path and reaches the target location.
- *Minimizing complications:* Echocardiographic guidance helps in avoiding complications such as arterial perforation, improper cannula positioning, or insertion-related trauma. This is particularly important in patients with challenging anatomy or in emergency situations.

### Cannula Position Confirmation

After the cannula is inserted, confirming its correct position is essential to ensure effective ECMO support. ECHO provides detailed images that are crucial for this verification:

- *Assessing cannula tip position:* ECHO allows for the visualization of the cannula tips within the heart and major vessels. Proper positioning is essential for effective drainage and return of blood.
    - *For VV-ECMO:*
        - Superior vena cava (SVC) cannula (return)—SVC–RA junction
        - Inferior vena cava (IVC) cannula (drain)—just before hepatic vein drain into IVC
        - IVC cannula (return)—into RA
    - *For VA-ECMO:*
        - Venous drainage is similar to VV-ECMO—positioned at the IVC-RA junction.
        - Return cannula—inserted through the femoral artery, with the tip at iliac artery or bifurcation of distal aorta.
- *Monitoring flow dynamics:* ECHO helps in assessing the flow dynamics within the cannulas, ensuring there are no obstructions, kinks, or malposition that could impair ECMO function. Adequate venous drainage and arterial return are verified through dynamic imaging.
- *Detecting and managing complications:* ECHO can detect complications such as cannula malposition, kinking, or migration. Early detection allows for prompt intervention to correct these issues, maintaining the efficacy and safety of ECMO support.

## ROLE OF ECHOCARDIOGRAPHY IN EXTRACORPOREAL MEMBRANE OXYGENATION MONITORING

Echocardiography is an indispensable tool in the intra-ECMO monitoring of patients, providing continuous, real-time insights into cardiac function and hemodynamics that are crucial for guiding therapeutic decisions and optimizing patient outcomes.

### Right Ventricular Assessment in Veno-venous Extracorporeal Membrane Oxygenation

In patients on veno-venous extracorporeal membrane oxygenation (VV-ECMO), the primary focus is on the assessment of the right ventricle (RV) due to its critical role in pulmonary circulation and oxygenation:

- *Right ventricular size and function:* Right ventricular size should be measured at end diastole using a focused apical four-chamber view. TAPSE, right ventricular TDI S′ and FAC **(Fig. 4)** should be assessed to measure right ventricular systolic function.
- *Tricuspid regurgitation velocity:* This is used to estimate systolic pulmonary artery pressure (sPAP) in the absence of pulmonary stenosis.

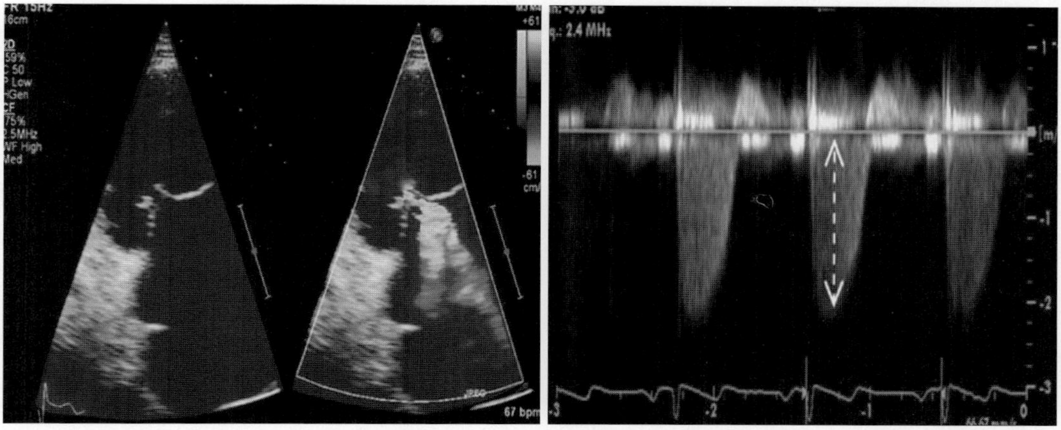

**Fig. 4:** Tricuspid regurgitation (TR) gradient and systolic pulmonary artery pressure (sPAP) measurement.

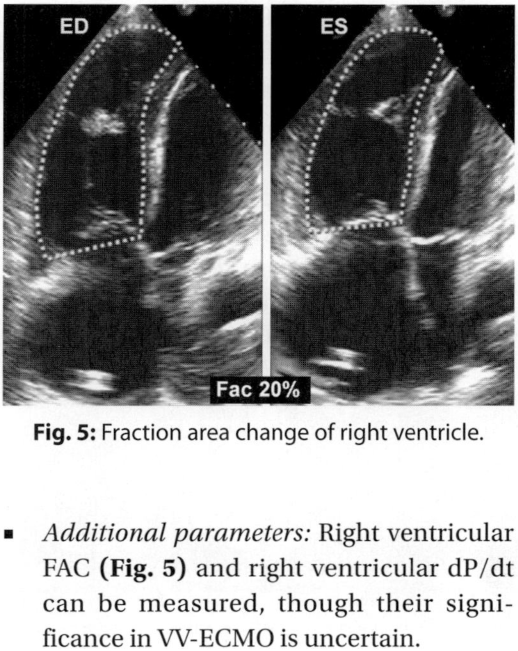


**Fig. 5:** Fraction area change of right ventricle.

- *Additional parameters:* Right ventricular FAC **(Fig. 5)** and right ventricular dP/dt can be measured, though their significance in VV-ECMO is uncertain.

## Comprehensive Cardiac Assessment in Veno-arterial Extracorporeal Membrane Oxygenation

Veno-arterial extracorporeal membrane oxygenation supports both cardiac and respiratory functions, necessitating a thorough assessment of both the LV and RV:

- *Left ventricular size and function:* LV cavity size is critical, with increasing dimensions indicating possible intracardiac blood flow stasis. Parameters such as visual estimation of LV size and ejection fraction (EF), Simpson's biplane EF, TDI to measure lateral mitral annular peak systolic velocity (TDI lat S′), and mitral regurgitation (MR) dP/dt should be assessed.
- *Aortic and LV outflow tract VTI:* It is obtained using continuous and pulse wave Doppler, and these measurements provide insights into the flow dynamics and help guide therapeutic interventions.
- Right ventricular *assessment:* The approach for right ventricular assessment in VA-ECMO mirrors that in VV-ECMO, focusing on size, systolic function, and TR velocity.

# ROLE OF ECHOCARDIOGRAPHY IN DETECTION AND MANAGEMENT OF COMPLICATIONS

Echocardiography plays a crucial role in the early detection and management of complications during ECMO. Among the key complications are:

- *Ventricular distension:* Particularly common in VA-ECMO, ventricular distension— especially of the LV **(Fig. 6)**—can occur due to inadequate ejection.

  Echocardiography is vital for the early identification of ventricular distension, which allows for timely interventions such as venting procedures or adjustments in ECMO flow rates. It helps in detecting the underlying causes of ventricular overdistension, such as increased afterload, aortic regurgitation, left ventricular dysfunction, and fluid overload, thereby guiding prompt corrective actions **(Fig. 6)**.

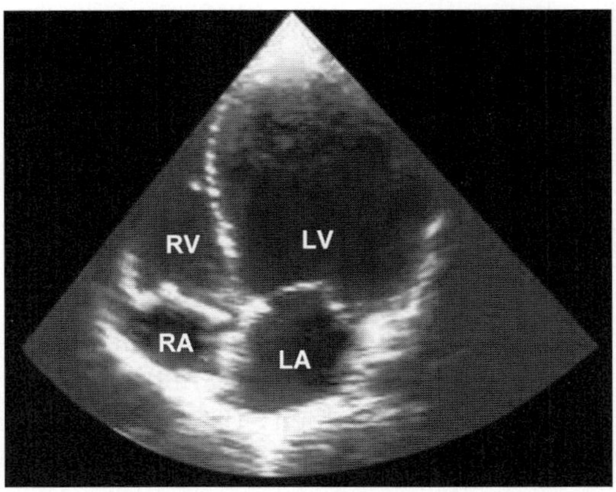


**Fig. 6:** Dilated left ventricle (LV).

- *Cardiac tamponade:* This life-threatening condition involves the accumulation of fluid in the pericardium, leading to decreased cardiac output and potential hemodynamic collapse. ECHO is essential for the prompt diagnosis of cardiac tamponade, enabling timely pericardiocentesis to prevent hemodynamic instability and collapse **(Fig. 7)**.
- *Thrombus formation:* ECMO patients are at significant risk for thrombus formation due to the large cannulas used, which can lead to thrombosis or venous and arterial obstruction. ECHO can detect intracardiac and extracardiac thrombi early, facilitating prompt anticoagulation management or surgical intervention if necessary. Both TTE and TEE are employed to detect these issues, with TEE generally offering superior spatial

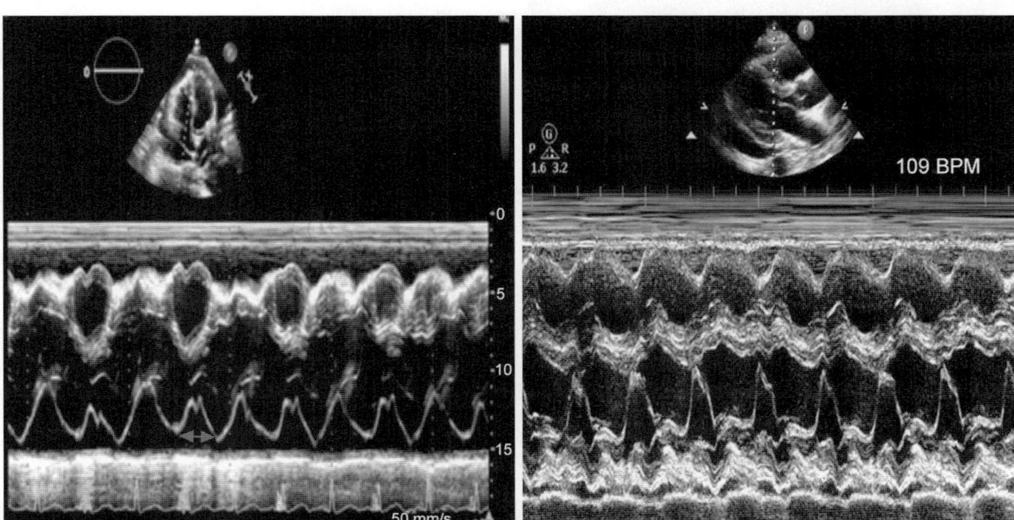


**Fig. 7:** Right atrial (RA) and right ventricular (RV) collapse of cardiac tamponade.

resolution, making it more effective for identifying thrombi in cannulas and cardiac chambers.

Continuous echocardiographic assessment is crucial for adjusting ECMO flow rates to ensure adequate perfusion and oxygenation while avoiding complications. This dynamic adjustment is essential for maintaining hemodynamic stability and ensuring the effectiveness of ECMO therapy.

## ROLE OF ECHOCARDIOGRAPHY IN WEANING FROM EXTRACORPOREAL MEMBRANE OXYGENATION

Echocardiography is also instrumental in the decision-making process regarding the weaning of patients from ECMO. It provides detailed assessments of cardiac function and hemodynamic stability, helping to determine the appropriate timing for reducing ECMO support and eventual decannulation. Weaning from VV-ECMO focuses mainly on assessing oxygen levels and lung compliance. This process involves gradually lowering the gas flow in the ECMO circuit while transitioning back to standard lung protective ventilation, rather than reducing the blood flow within the ECMO circuit. In contrast, weaning from VA-ECMO is a more variable process due to the lack of standardized protocols, leading to different approaches across medical centers.

This procedure is typically initiated when there are clear signs of cardiac recovery, such as enhanced ventricular contractility. In practice, ECMO flows are incrementally reduced under stringent hemodynamic and echocardiographic monitoring, generally to levels between 1 and 1.5 L/min. However, predicting successful weaning remains challenging until ECMO support is fully withdrawn, as residual right ventricular dysfunction may not be apparent.

Currently, there are no internationally recognized echocardiographic protocols to guide VA-ECMO weaning, resulting in varied methods across centers.

Key indicators for successful weaning include:

- Left ventricular ejection fraction (LVEF) of 20–25%
- Aortic VTI of at least 12 cm
- TDI lateral S′ wave velocity of at least 6 cm/s.
- It is also crucial to confirm the absence of left ventricular dilation or significant pericardial effusion.

Monitoring right ventricular size and function, along with serial assessments of sPAP, can provide valuable insights into the heart's response to changing respiratory dynamics. Measurements of TAPSE and right ventricular TDI S′ are especially useful for tracking right ventricular recovery, with serial evaluations offering more comprehensive data than single measurements.

The dynamic nature of echocardiographic imaging allows for real-time feedback on the patient's response to various interventions, including inotropic support, fluid management, and adjustments in ECMO settings. This real-time monitoring ensures that clinicians can make informed, timely decisions to optimize patient care continuously.

## ADVANTAGES OF TEE OVER TTE IN MANAGING EXTRACORPOREAL MEMBRANE OXYGENATION PATIENTS

- *Superior image quality:* High-resolution images: TEE provides clearer, more detailed images due to the proximity of the esophagus to the heart, allowing for better visualization of cardiac structures.

- *Enhanced visualization of cardiac structures:*
  - *Posterior structures:* TEE excels in visualizing posterior cardiac structures, such as the left atrium and mitral valve, which are often difficult to see with TTE.
  - *Valvular function:* TEE offers superior assessment of valvular function, including detecting subtle valvular regurgitation and stenosis.
- *Better assessment of cardiac thrombi:* Intracardiac pathology: Superior in identifying intracardiac thrombi, masses, and septal defects
- *Guidance for ECMO cannula placement:*
  - *Precise placement:* It helps in accurate placement and verification of ECMO cannulas, reducing the risk of malposition.
  - *Detection of complications:* It identifies complications such as cannula migration, kinking, or thrombosis.
- *Useful in challenging patient populations:* Poor acoustic windows: It overcomes limitations of TTE in patients with poor acoustic windows, such as those with obesity, emphysema, or mechanical ventilation.

## CONCLUSION

Echocardiography (ECHO) is essential in managing patients on ECMO, providing real-time visualization of cardiac function that enables the detection of complications and guides precise interventions. It helps optimize ECMO settings, tailor treatments to individual patient needs, and facilitate the weaning process by assessing cardiac recovery. Overall, ECHO's noninvasive, real-time insights significantly enhance patient care and outcomes, and its role in ECMO management will continue to grow with advancements in technology and expertise.

## FURTHER READING


1. Bailleul C, Aissaoui N. Role of echocardiography in the management of veno-arterial extra-corporeal membrane oxygenation patients. J Emerg Crit Care Med. 2019;3:25.
2. Douflé G, Roscoe A, Billia F, Fan E. Echocardiography for adult patients supported with extracorporeal membrane oxygenation. Crit Care. 2015;19:326.
3. Hussey PT, von Mering G, Nanda NC, Ahmed MI, Addis DR. Echocardiography for extracorporeal membrane oxygenation. Echocardiography. 2022;39(2):339-70.
4. Kapoor PM. Echocardiography in extracorporeal membrane oxygenation. Ann Card Anaesth. 2017;20:S1-3.
5. Kapoor PM. Role of echocardiography in ECMO. Qatar Med J. 2017;2017(1).
6. Platts DG, Sedgwick JF, Burstow DJ, Mullany DV, Fraser JF. The role of echocardiography in the management of patients supported by extracorporeal membrane oxygenation. J Am Soc Echocardiogr. 2012;25:131-41.
7. Victor K, Barrett NA, Gillon S, Gowland A, Meadows CIS, Ioannou N. Critical care echo rounds extracorporeal membrane oxygenation. Echo Res Pract. 2015;2(2):D1-11.

CHAPTER 29

# Comprehensive Echocardiography in Management of Trauma

*Kapil Dev Soni*

## INTRODUCTION

Trauma patients may present with varying severity and often transit through different phases—initial shock, which could be hemorrhagic or nonhemorrhagic, followed by complications such as sepsis and septic shock. Frequently, underlying comorbidities, including cardiac problems and medications, further confound the response to shock and modify the fluid therapy and response. A clinician encounters numerous challenges when managing major trauma patients. Rapid identification of the cause of shock during resuscitation is paramount, as is the detection of cardiac injury and cardiac tamponade. Understanding the baseline status of cardiac function, particularly the impact of preexisting cardiac comorbidities, becomes fundamental in modifying the management strategy during a state of shock in addition to ruling out direct cardiac injury. In the later phases of treatment, additional challenges arise as complications such as acute respiratory distress syndrome (ARDS), sepsis, septic shock, deep vein thrombosis (DVT), and pulmonary embolism (PE) that can all exert direct or indirect effects on cardiac function.

Echocardiography is an essential tool for evaluating shock in trauma patients. The ability of transthoracic echocardiography (TTE) to provide actionable information during different stages of shock management is vital. During the initial presentation of patients with hemorrhagic shock, TTE can help quantify cardiac reserves, assess cardiac dysfunction, and evaluate the response to fluid therapy. Direct cardiac injury, during initial stages, can go unnoticed even with a thorough examination. Echocardiography elucidates any direct cardiac injury. The presence of cardiac tamponade is established with the help of echocardiography during the Extended Focused Assessment with Sonography for Trauma (EFAST), an adjunct to the primary survey. Furthermore, during the development of sepsis physiology, echocardiography helps identify hypovolemia, vasoplegia, and fluid responders.

Following key echocardiographic parameters are essential to measure while performing cardiac examination. The aim is to identify left ventricle dysfunction—systolic and diastolic, Right ventricular (RV) dysfunction, identification of regional wall and valvular abnormalities.

Key measurements during hemorrhagic shock include:

- Left ventricular (LV) dimensions
- Ejection fraction
- LV contractility
- Velocity time integral (VTI)
- LV filling pressure

- Mitral valve abnormalities
- Mitral annular plane systolic excursion (MAPSE)
- Fractional area change (FAC)
- E-point septal separation (EPSS)
- Right ventricle (RV) dimensions
- Tricuspid annular plane systolic excursion (TAPSE)
- Tricuspid annular peak systolic velocity (TAPSV)
- Tricuspid regurgitation (TR) jet evaluation
- Pulmonary artery pressure estimations [pulmonary arterial systolic pressure (PASP), mean pulmonary arterial pressure (MPAP), pulmonary capillary wedge pressure (PCWP), and pulmonary acceleration time (PAcT)]

Specific scenarios of trauma patient management during which echocardiography is particularly useful.

## EVALUATION AND MANAGEMENT OF HYPOVOLEMIC SHOCK

Trauma patients commonly present with hypovolemic state due to hemorrhage, often complicated by nonhemorrhagic etiologies as well such as cardiogenic or obstructive component. Also, due to intense inflammation following major trauma, large amounts of fluid can get sequestered in third space, thus leading to intravascular hypovolemia.

Evaluating the magnitude of hypovolemia and response to fluid therapy during shock is crucial. Though the primary goal of management of hemorrhagic shock remains control of hemorrhage, the intravenous fluids are administered empirically in conjunction with identifying source of bleed and stopping the hemorrhage. The degree of hypovolemia and response can vary substantially between patients depending on injury severity, patterns of injury, and preexisting comorbidities. Therefore, individualized fluid therapy is essential once the fluids are initiated empirically. The echocardiography assessment provides baseline assessment of cardiac contractility, filling pressures, and overall status. All the basic views of heart—parasternal long axis, parasternal short axis, apical four-chamber, and subcostal views—are obtained for precise estimation of hypovolemia.

Findings suggestive of hypovolemia include **(Fig. 1)**:

- *Underfilled left ventricle during end-diastole:* The cardiac chambers appear small and left ventricle diastolic area is significantly reduced.
- Kissing left ventricle walls during mid-systole-hyperdynamic left ventricle contractility due to reduced preload
- *Low-VTI and low-cardiac output:* Exaggerated respiratory variations are observed in aortic VTI due to variation in venous return because of heart–lung interaction physiology.

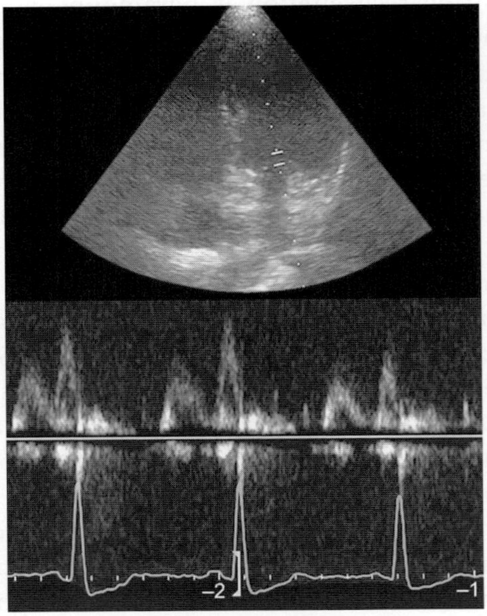


**Fig. 1:** Hypovolemia.

- *Inferior vena cava (IVC) collapse:* The IVC diameter is small and often collapsing with phases of respiration.
- *Low mitral E-wave velocity (<0.8 m/s):* Reflecting reduced LV filling due to hypovolemia
- *Shortened mitral E-wave velocity deceleration time:* Less than 180 m/s.
- Low E/e′ ratio on flow Doppler and tissue Doppler, suggesting low left atrial pressure

## IDENTIFICATION AND MANAGEMENT OF DIRECT CARDIAC INJURY

Early identification of cardiac injury in polytrauma patients is paramount as it can complicate hemorrhagic shock. Cardiac injury is suspected based on the pattern of injuries and mechanism of trauma. The presentation is often subtle and can lead to missed injury. Initial symptom varies from chest pain, shortness of breath to altered sensorium due to frank hypotension and arrhythmia. The presence of unexplained tachycardia and hypotension should raise suspicion of cardiac injury in patient of chest trauma. Failure to immediately identify cardiac in the setting of hemorrhagic shock can be life threatening. Though initial computed tomography (CT) scan reveals associated cardiac injury, TTE is used as an initial screening aid. Abnormal findings on TTE and electrocardiogram (ECG), in conjunction with CT scans, often confirm the presence of direct cardiac injury or hemopericardium.

Cardiac injuries vary from simple contusions to wall ruptures, commonly involving the RV and atria due to anterior location. In a study, the incidence ranged from 17% to 32% for the RV and from 8% to 65% for the right atrium. In severe cases, cardiac rupture may occur, resulting in cardiac tamponade, a medical emergency. Symptoms of cardiac rupture include sudden hemodynamic instability and shock. The mechanisms underlying cardiac ruptures include the sudden compression of the heart within the thoracic cavity or a rapid increase in intra-abdominal pressures. Less commonly, blunt cardiac trauma can result in valvular disruption, which leads to heart murmurs and symptoms of heart failure, such as dyspnea and pulmonary crackles. Septal rupture might not produce immediate symptoms but can manifest later with heart failure. Blunt and penetrating injuries can impact cardiac valves, resulting in valvular regurgitation, with an increased risk in the presence of preexisting valvular lesions. Penetrating injuries frequently lead to valve perforations, typically affecting the tricuspid valve more than the mitral valve. Blunt trauma commonly causes rupture of the chordae tendineae and tears in the papillary muscles. Aortic valve injury, often associated with sternal trauma or sudden deceleration, presents as aortic valve regurgitation. Penetrating injuries can also lead to aneurysm formation followed by clot formation in the long term.

Following are the common findings on echo examination suggestive of direct cardiac injury:

- *Increased echogenicity within the walls of cardiac chambers:* Suggestive of myocardial contusion
- Regional wall motion abnormalities
- Global LV dysfunction
- *Valvular regurgitations:* Suggestive of valve injuries and chordae tendineae ruptures
- Septal perforations and valve disruptions visualized directly on echocardiography
- The presence of echo-free space between pericardium and epicardium: Suggestive of hemopericardium.

## Hemopericardium and Cardiac Tamponade

Cardiac tamponade is a medical emergency. Hemopericardium, the collection of blood in the pericardial space, can cause tamponade physiology, evident as shock and distended neck veins. Its identification is essential during the initial presentation after major trauma. Failure to identify obstructive shock due to cardiac tamponade leads to blunted or no response to fluid therapy and can result in fluid overload condition, further complicating the management. Both blunt and penetrating injuries are linked to the occurrence of hemopericardium, though penetrating mechanisms are more frequently associated. Bleeding can originate from vessels, myocardium, or the pericardial cavity. Typically, the volume of fluid around the heart is less than 10 mL.

Echocardiographic signs of tamponade include **(Fig. 2)**:

- *Right atrial systolic collapse:* Early sign of cardiac tamponade
- *Right ventricular diastolic collapse:* Specific sign of cardiac tamponade
- *Increase ventricular interdependence:* Doppler signs of increased respiratory flow variations in the inflow velocities of the mitral and tricuspid valves, acting as an indicator of pulsus paradoxus.
- *Pericardial effusion:* The presence of pericardial effusion as echo-free space in both anterior and posterior aspect of the heart can be detected in cardiac tamponade.
- *Plethoric IVC:* The IVC often appears distended with minimal respiratory fluctuation, indicating increased central venous pressure.

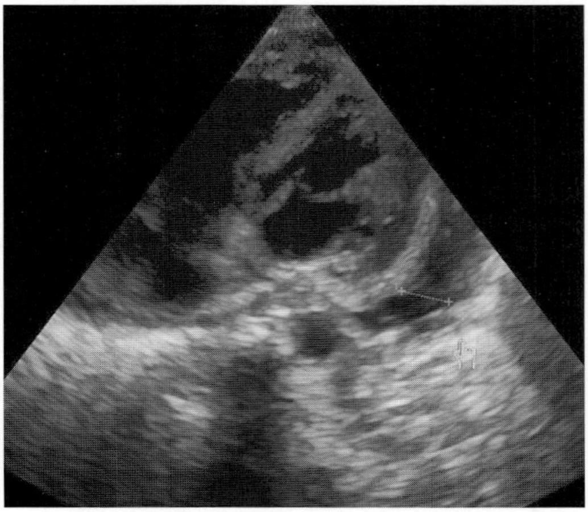

**Fig. 2:** Cardiac tamponade.

Pericardiocentesis serves as a temporizing measure to evacuate pericardial fluid in tamponade and alleviate cardiogenic shock. The catheter is typically inserted directly into the pericardial cavity under ultrasound guidance and can drain fluid intermittently. Surgical exploration is often warranted following pericardiocentesis, particularly if there is recurrent accumulation of blood.

## THORACIC AORTA INJURIES

Thoracic aortic injury, often resulting from sudden deceleration, can lead to dissections. Direct blunt trauma to the thorax can also precipitate aortic dissection, particularly at the junction of the aortic isthmus and the ligamentum arteriosum. Depending on the anatomical location of the dissection, various classification schemes are employed to categorize the injury and guide management. The clinical presentation of aortic dissection following blunt chest trauma is often subtle and may lead to unrecognized injury. However, given the high-risk mechanism of injury and associated patterns of trauma, a heightened index of suspicion should be maintained. Prompt diagnosis and appropriate intervention are critical to mitigate the morbidity and mortality associated with this potentially life-threatening complication of blunt thoracic trauma.

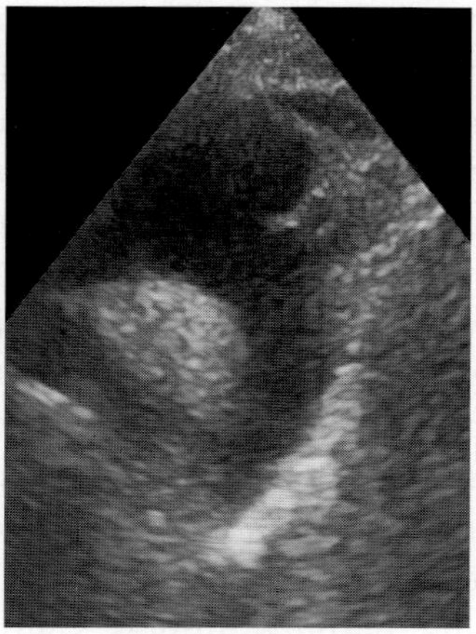

**Fig. 3:** Aortic injury.

Though the gold standard for diagnosing dissections is CT aortography, transesophageal echocardiography (TEE) has shown similar accuracy in studies with high sensitivity and specificity. Moreover, it enables rapid bedside evaluation of suspected thoracic aortic injury with direct visualization.

Findings on TEE suggestive of thoracic aortic injury are **(Fig. 3)**:

- *The presence of intimal flap:* Suggestive of aortic dissection
- Aortic wall hematoma
- The presence of pseudoaneurysm
- Caliber or contour changes of aorta—dilation or narrowing.

The role of TTE is limited for bedside evaluation of thoracic aortic injury and may miss intramural hematoma or the extent of dissection.

## OTHER TRAUMA SCENARIOS WHERE ECHOCARDIOGRAPHY CAN BE USEFUL

### Fat Embolism

Fat embolism commonly occurs within 24–72 hours of posttrauma, especially in young patients with long bone or pelvic fractures undergoing transportation or surgical procedure. The presentation includes sudden oxygen desaturation, dyspnea, altered sensorium, and occasionally hemodynamic instability. Both TTE and TEE can detect echogenic material within the right atrium during acute episodes. TEE studies have identified fat embolism in 41% of cases, involving long bone surgeries with surgical fixations. The fat appears echogenic and varies in diameter from 1 to 10 mm. Fat embolism can also lead sudden increased pulmonary pressures and RV dysfunction evident as paradoxical interventricular septal movement. Intraoperative TEE offers real-time visualization of fat during acute episodes and serves as a monitoring tool for orthopedic procedures associated with a high risk of fat embolism.

### Deep Vein Thrombosis

To mitigate the risk of perioperative thromboembolism, screening echocardiography is often performed. There are multiple risk factors for DVT following trauma. A transition from a hypocoagulant to a hypercoagulant state often increases the likelihood of thrombosis. Ultrasound is commonly employed to exclude thrombosis in major vessels. The presence of spontaneous echo contrast in vessels and cardiac chambers indicates the presence of thrombi, thus increased risk.

### Head injury–induced Sympathetic Surge

Though infrequent, takotsubo cardiomyopathy (TCM), also known as "stress cardiomyopathy", has been reported in patients with various acute neurological conditions, including traumatic brain injury (TBI). It typically develops 1–5 days after acute insult due to intense sympathetic surge following severe TBI. It is characterized by typical regional wall motion abnormalities evident on echocardiography. The clinical significance of TCM in TBI is uncertain, with some research indicating it may not correlate with substantial myocardial dysfunction or adverse outcomes. Nevertheless, timely identification of TCM is crucial for guiding proper management and monitoring of affected patients.

Limitations of echocardiography in settings of Trauma:

- *Inability to detect myocardial edema without wall motion abnormalities:* Minor cardiac injury resulting in only myocardial edema cannot be detected by 2D echocardiography. These are frequently missed.
- *Dependence on acoustic windows:* Often in case of chest injury, the presence of associated pneumothorax and subcutaneous emphysema preclude optimized image acquisition, thus limiting the comprehensive echo examination.
- *Lack of sensitivity for minor conduction abnormalities:* Echocardiography may lack the sensitivity required to detect minor conduction abnormalities or arrhythmias associated with blunt cardiac injury. As a result, these subtle electrical disturbances might go unnoticed.
- *Operator dependence:* The accuracy of echocardiographic findings in trauma patients hinges significantly on the proficiency and expertise of the operator conducting and interpreting the examination. Operators with less experience may overlook or misinterpret critical findings.

Overall, comprehensive echocardiographic evaluation in trauma patients is crucial for accurate diagnosis and management of shock and associated cardiac injuries.

CHAPTER 30

# Echocardiography in Neurocritical Care

*Kiran Jangra, Gyaninder Pal Singh*

## CASE

A 14-year-old male, with no known comorbidities, underwent surgery for craniopharyngioma. He developed diabetes insipidus on postoperative day 1, which was being managed with free fluid replacement and subcutaneous desmopressin injections guided by water deficit, urine output, and clinical parameters. On postoperative day 13, the patient developed severe vasospasm involving the right supraclinoid internal carotid artery and M1 segment of the middle cerebral artery. In an attempt to increase blood pressure for treating vasospasm, he developed sudden dyspnea, tachypnea, and oxygen desaturation (arterial blood oxygen saturation of 80–85% on room air), suggestive of severe pulmonary edema.

Under normal circumstances, the cause of pulmonary edema in such cases is considered as fluid overload. In the current case, echocardiography revealed a severely depressed ejection fraction **(Fig. 1A)**, suggestive of neurogenic myocardial dysfunction secondary to severe vasospasm. The peculiar nature of neurogenic dysfunction is that it resolves **(Fig. 1B)** when intracranial pathology is resolved.

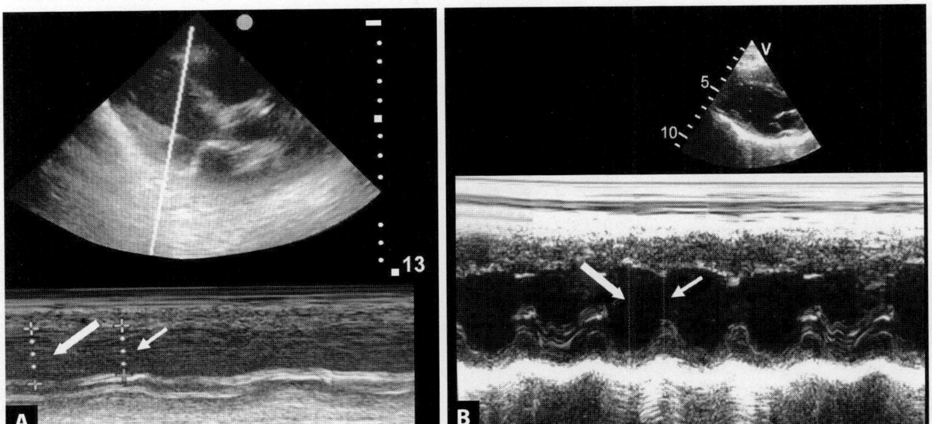


**Figs. 1A and B:** Parasternal long-axis view with M-mode at midventricular level shows left ventricular contractility. (A) The difference of the left ventricular internal diameter during diastole (big white arrow) and systole (small white arrow) in minimal suggesting severely reduced contraction with ejection fraction of 10–15%; (B) The left ventricular internal diameter in systole (small white arrow) is smaller than the diastole (big white arrow), suggesting a normal ejection fraction after resolution of neurogenic myocardial dysfunction.

## INTRODUCTION

The brain–heart interaction is an interesting domain in neurologically ill patients in perioperative and intensive care unit (ICU) setup. Acute intracranial insults such as subarachnoid hemorrhage (SAH), traumatic brain injury (TBI), strokes (ischemic or hemorrhagic), central nervous system (CNS) infections, vasospasm, seizures, or psychogenic stress may result in transient myocardial dysfunction.[1-7] Sudden onset of neurological complications such as vasospasm can cause myocardial motion abnormalities. The myocardial involvements vary from mild electrocardiographic (ECG) changes to malignant arrhythmias and myocardial dysfunction on echocardiography. The echocardiographic involvements are also known as stress-induced cardiomyopathy, neurogenic stunned myocardium, or neurogenic stress cardiomyopathy (NSC).[8-10]

The echocardiographic changes are seen in 12–20% of cases after SAH.[11] The pattern of echocardiographic changes includes left ventricular (LV) regional wall motion abnormalities (RWMA) (basal/mid-ventricular or apical dysfunction), apical ballooning or apical sparing, and global hypokinesia **(Fig. 2A)**. Apical ballooning is also known as "takotsubo cardiomyopathy (TTC)", "broken heart syndrome", or stress cardiomyopathy **(Fig. 2B)**. It may also be seen in severe psychological or physical stresses.

## CENTRAL CONTROL OF CARDIOVASCULAR SYSTEM

The CNS has a significant influence on controlling the cardiovascular system (CVS). The sympathetic nervous system increases heart rate and contractility, while the parasympathetic system slows down and decreases sympathetic system activity. The imbalance in these two systems leads to NSC. CVS receives the parasympathetic innervations through vagus nerves, sympathetic innervations through the middle cervical sympathetic ganglion, and stellate ganglion. The parasympathetic innervations are mainly present in the atrial myocardium, sinoatrial (SA) node, and atrioventricular (AV) nodes, but the ventricles are devoid of it.[12] The right vagus nerve preferentially supplies the SA node and controls heart rate, while the left vagus predominantly

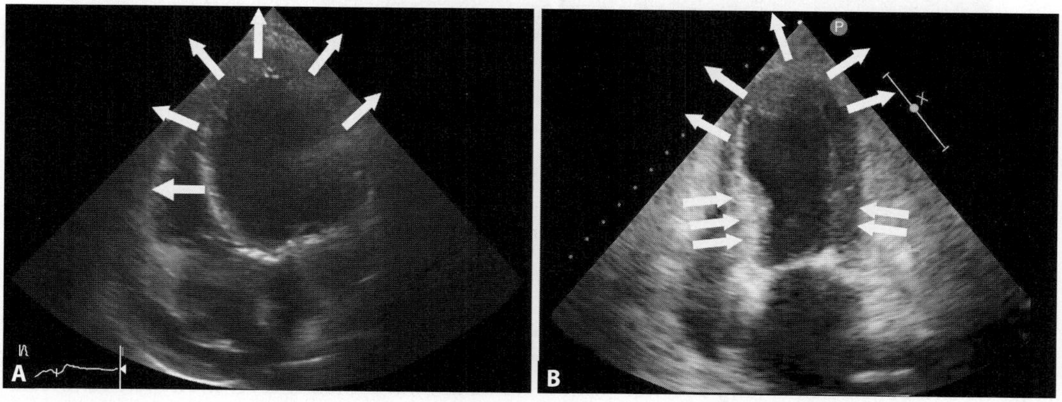

**Figs. 2A and B:** Apical 4-chamber view in ventricular systole showing: (A) Rounding of the left ventricle (white arrows) giving it a globular appearance, known as global hypokinesia; and (B) Ballooned out apex (white outward arrows) and hypercontraction of basal segment (white inward arrows), known as apical ballooning or takotsubo cardiomyopathy.

controls the AV node.[13,14] These asymmetrical innervations may explain the laterality of NSC in human and animal studies.[15] An organized intrinsic cardiac plexus is formed by parasympathetic and sympathetic fibers that are considered major targets of CNS outflow. The neurological insults cause malfunctioning of central autonomic nuclei and thus cause autonomic imbalances.[16,17]

## NEUROGENIC VERSUS ISCHEMIC CARDIAC DYSFUNCTION

A major difference between the myocardial injury due to ischemic insult and NSC is the pattern of myocardial involvement. Ischemic heart diseases compromise a particular vascular territory, while NSC follows cardiac nerve innervation. In NSC, the RWMA extends beyond a single vascular territory, e.g., apical ballooning (TTC), indicating vulnerability of the apex to the catecholamine-induced toxicity due to a larger proportion of $\beta_2$- than $\beta_1$-adrenergic receptors.[8,18-20] Other authors have also observed "apex sparing" with the basal and mid-ventricular RWMA, probably due to the lesser number of sympathetic nerve terminals at the apex.[21,22] These patients may develop sudden cardiac death perioperatively or in the ICU.[8,23]

## CLINICAL APPLICATION OF ECHOCARDIOGRAPHY IN NEUROINTENSIVE CARE

Besides the usual role of echocardiography as a tool for the management of critical patients in the ICUs, the specific applications in neurointensive care are:

- To detect neurogenic myocardial dysfunction
- To differentiate between neurogenic or cardiogenic pulmonary edema
- Transthoracic and transesophageal echocardiography have been used for managing fluid therapy.
- To titrate inotropic support for various conditions, such a blood pressure augmentation during vasospasm in SAH raised intracranial pressure (ICP).
- In head injury patients, to rule out associated myocardial contusion/injury, aortic injuries. In hemodynamically unstable trauma victims, e-FAST (Extended Focused Assessment with Sonography in Trauma) examination is done to rule out bleeding in the thorax and abdomen.
- To rule out head injury associated NSC and neurogenic pulmonary edema in trauma victims

## BRAIN ECHOGRAPHY[24]

In the neurointensive care units, besides echocardiography, the role of ultrasonography for brain (brain echography) is growing fast. Brain echography has emerged as a useful noninvasive bedside tool to monitor intracranial pressure, blood flow and visualize intracranial structures, vessels, and brain lesions. Brain echography is performed using a phased array probe on the temporal bone and other natural windows including orbital and foramen magnum. The presets are set at abdominal for parenchymal study and transcranial Doppler for vascular study. It provides important information about ICP, cerebral perfusion pressure (CPP), blood flow velocities, mass lesion, midline shift, hematoma, and hydrocephalous **(Figs. 3A to D)**. In patients with cranial defects such as craniectomy parenchymal details are better visualized **(Figs. 4A and B)**.

Color duplex provides details about vascular anatomy and helps in the diagnosis of vascular stenosis, vasospasm, cerebral blood

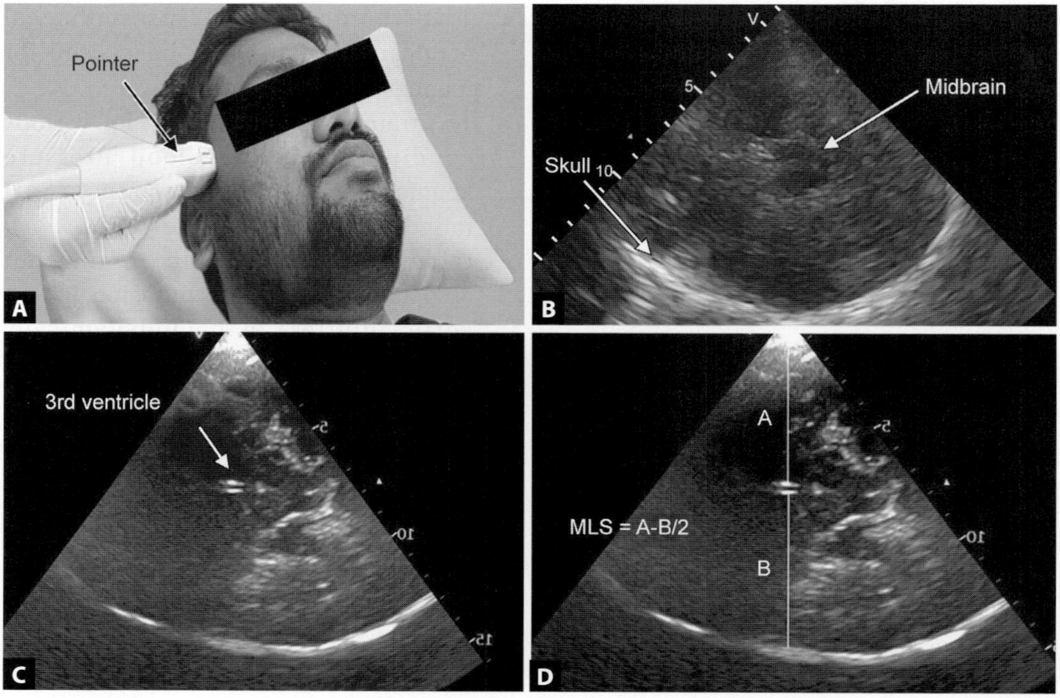


**Figs. 3A to D:** (A) The probe placement in the orbitomeatal line with the pointer facing anteriorly; (B) The first image acquired to ensure correct insonation, the butterfly shape structure is the midbrain (white arrow); (C) Image acquired by tilting the probe by 10–20° toward the vertex. Two parallel lines in the center correspond to the midbrain (white arrow); (D) Midline shift (MLS) is calculated by measuring the distance of midbrain lines on both sides and dividing their difference by two.

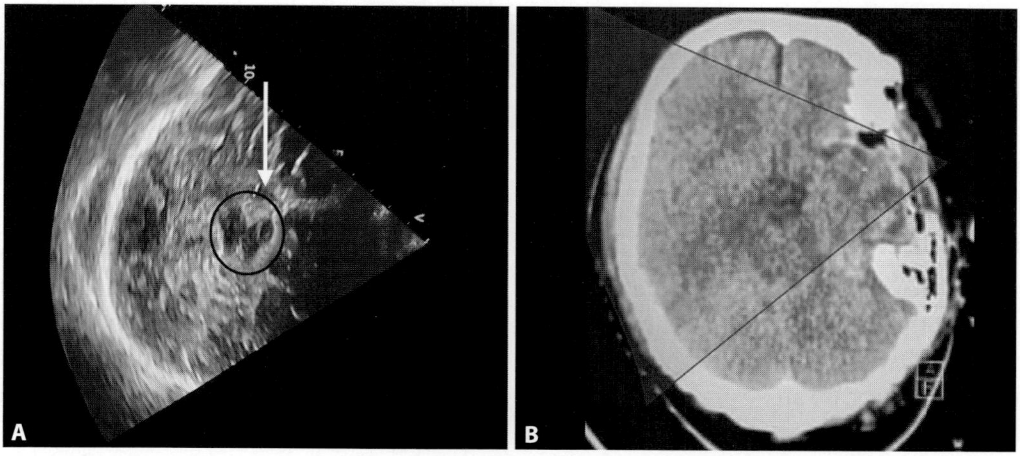

**Figs. 4A and B:** Postcraniectomy scans of same patient at the midbrain level. (A) Sonographic image at midbrain (black circle) showing large hypoechoic area underneath the probe (white arrow) suggestive of edema; (B) Corresponding computed tomographic scan.

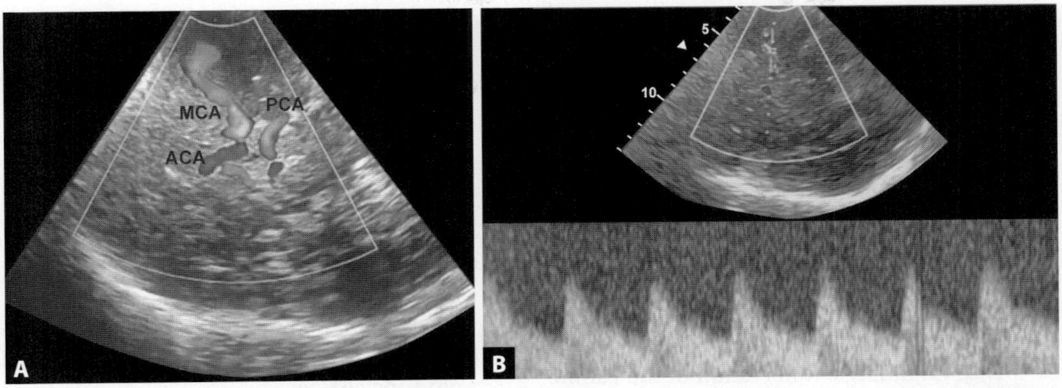


**Figs. 5A and B:** Color Doppler applied at midbrain level showing: (A) Components of the circle of Willis; (B) Pulse wave Doppler at MCA showing flow velocities. (ACA: anterior cerebral artery; MCA: middle cerebral artery; PCA: posterior cerebral artery)

supply, circulatory arrest, and much more **(Figs. 5A and B)**. It is an evolving field and may replace the need for repeated computed tomography (CT) scans as it is a bedside tool and can be performed repeatedly.

## CONCLUSION

Intense brain–heart interactions are widely recognized in association with severe brain injury and are commonly seen in neurointensive care setups. One should have a high level of suspicion for neurogenic cardiac dysfunction, and a timely diagnosis should be made so that secondary brain insult can be avoided. More aggressive management of brain pathology reverses the cardiac changes. So, serial monitoring of the heart with echocardiography is important for better management and to achieve good neurological outcomes.

## REFERENCES


1. Banki NM. Acute neurocardiogenic injury after subarachnoid hemorrhage. Circulation. 2005;112:3314-9.
2. Banki N, Kopelnik A, Tung P, Lawton MT, Gress D, Drew B, et al. Prospective analysis of prevalence, distribution, and rate of recovery of left ventricular systolic dysfunction in patients with subarachnoid hemorrhage. J Neurosurg. 2006;105:15-20.
3. Riera M, Llompart-Pou JA, Carrillo A, Blanco C. Head injury and inverted Takotsubo cardiomyopathy. J Trauma. 2010;68:E13-5.
4. Yoshimura S, Toyoda K, Ohara T, Nagasawa H, Ohtani N, Kuwashiro T, et al. Takotsubo cardiomyopathy in acute ischemic stroke. Ann Neurol. 2008;64:547-54.
5. Gelow J, Kruer M, Yadav V, Kaul S. Apical ballooning resulting from limbic encephalitis. Am J Med. 2009;122:583-6.
6. Stollberger C, Huber JO, Enzelsberger B, Finsterer J. Fatal outcome of epileptic seizure-induced Takotsubo syndrome with left ventricular rupture. Eur J Neurol. 2009;16:e116-7.
7. Reddy A, Thappa P, Jangra K, Dhandapani S, Sihag BK. Neurogenic myocardial dysfunction post craniopharyngioma resection: A diagnostic dilemma. Paediatr Anaesth. 2024;34:178-81.
8. Lee VH, Oh JK, Mulvagh SL, Wijdicks EF. Mechanisms in neurogenic stress cardiomyopathy after aneurysmal subarachnoid hemorrhage. Neurocrit Care. 2006;5:243-9.
9. Banki NM, Zaroff JG. Neurogenic cardiac injury. Curr Treat Options Cardiovasc Med. 2003;5:451-8.

10. Nguyen H, Zaroff JG. Neurogenic stunned myocardium. Curr Neurol Neurosci Rep. 2009;9:486-91.
11. Jangra K, Grover VK, Bhagat H, Bhardwaj A, Tewari MK, Kumar B, et al. Evaluation of the Effect of Aneurysmal Clipping on Electrocardiography and Echocardiographic Changes in Patients With Subarachnoid Hemorrhage: A Prospective Observational Study. J Neurosurg Anesthesiol. 2017;29:335-40.
12. Kent KM, Epstein SE, Cooper T, Jacobowitz DM. Cholinergic innervation of the canine and human ventricular conducting system. Circulation. 1974;50:948-55.
13. Martin P. The influence of the parasympathetic nervous system on atrioventricular conduction. Circ Res. 1977;41:593-9.
14. Yoon BW, Morillo CA, Cechetto DF, Hachinski V. Cerebral hemispheric lateralization in cardiac autonomic control. Arch Neurol. 1997;54:741-4.
15. Osteraas ND, Lee VH. Neurocardiology. Handb Clin Neurol. 2017;140:49-65.
16. Pereira VH, Cerqueira JJ, Palha JA, Sousa N. Stressed brain, diseased heart: a review on the pathophysiologic mechanisms of neurocardiology. Int J Cardiol. 2013;166:30-7.
17. Barron SA, Rogovski Z, Hemli J. Autonomic consequences of cerebral hemisphere infarction. Stroke. 1994;25:113-6.
18. Dec GW. Recognition of the apical ballooning syndrome in the United States. Circulation. 2005;111:388-90.
19. Kopelnik A, Zaroff J. Neurocardiogenic injury in neurovascular disorders. Crit Care Clin. 2006;22:733-52.
20. Paur H, Wright PT, Sikkel MB, Tranter MH, Mansfield C, O'Gara P, et al. High levels of circulating epinephrine trigger apical cardio depression in a beta2-adrenergic receptor/Gi-dependent manner: a new model of Takotsubo cardiomyopathy. Circulation. 2012;126:697-706.
21. Kline RC, Swanson DP, Wieland DM, Thrall JH, Gross MD, Pitt B, et al. Myocardial imaging in man with I-123 meta-iodobenzyl guanidine. J Nucl Med. 1981;22:129-32.
22. Khush K, Kopelnik A, Tung P, Banki N, Dae M, Lawton M, et al. Age and aneurysm position predict patterns of left ventricular dysfunction after subarachnoid hemorrhage. J Am Soc Echocardiogr. 2005;18:168-74.
23. Bybee KA, Prasad A. Stress-related cardiomyopathy syndromes. Circulation. 2008;118:397-409.
24. Robba C, Goffi A, Geeraerts T, Cardim D, Via G, Czosnyka M, et al. Brain ultrasonography: methodology, basic and advanced principles and clinical applications. A narrative review. Intensive Care Med. 2019;45:913-27.

CHAPTER 31

# Training and Competency in Intensive Care Unit Echocardiography

*Mohd. Luqman, Srikant Behera*

## EDUCATION AND CERTIFICATION PROGRAMS

### INTRODUCTION

Echocardiography in the intensive care unit (ICU) is an essential tool used globally for patient management. The type and extent of echocardiography performed depend on various factors, including the healthcare provider's competency.

### TYPES OF ECHOCARDIOGRAPHY (FIG. 1)

- *Basic screening echocardiography:* Initial assessment to provide rapid insights into cardiac function
- *Advanced echocardiography:* Comprehensive evaluation using transthoracic echocardiography (TTE) and transesophageal echocardiography (TEE).[1-3]

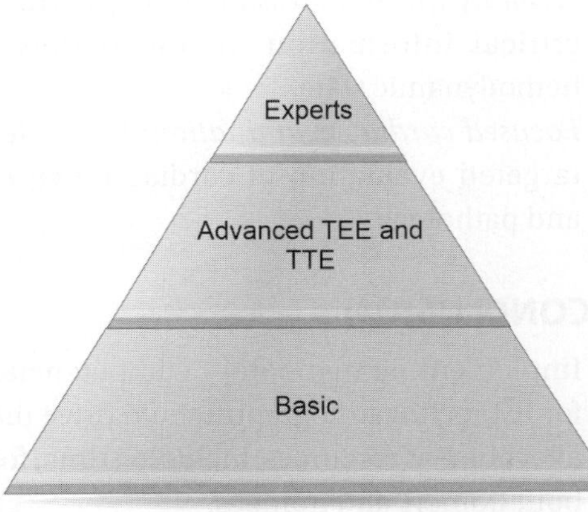


**Fig. 1:** Different levels of working with echocardiography in ICU. These levels can act as milestones for a physician in the pursuit of skill enhancement. (ICU: intensive care unit; TEE: transesophageal echocardiography; TTE: transthoracic echocardiography)

- The perceived importance of bedside ICU echocardiography among intensive care physicians underscores the need for structured training and certification.

### TRAINING AND CERTIFICATION

- Multiple training and certification pathways exist to equip healthcare providers with the necessary skills for ICU echocardiography.
- ICU echocardiography is a core component of point-of-care ultrasound (POCUS) and requires established training programs for intensivists to develop the required competencies.

### BARRIERS TO IMPLEMENTATION

- *Inadequate training:* Lack of sufficient training programs hinders the widespread adoption of ICU echocardiography.
- *Absence of formal qualifications:* The lack of recognized qualifications prevents standardization and acceptance.
- *Mentorship challenges:* Difficulty in finding suitable mentors for hands-on training impedes skill development.[4]

## IMPORTANCE OF STANDARDIZATION

- Patient safety mandates the establishment of standardized care protocols in the ICU.
- Best practice expectations should be well-defined and reproducible to ensure consistency and safety.

## BENEFITS OF INTENSIVE CARE UNIT ECHOCARDIOGRAPHY

- *Hemodynamic assessment:* It provides critical information on the patient's hemodynamic state.
- *Focused cardiac examination:* It enables targeted evaluation of cardiac function and pathology.[5]

## CONCLUSION

- Implementing mandatory competencies for ICU echocardiography could drive the allocation of resources, including time, for both trainers and trainees.
- Ensuring proper training and certification pathways would enhance the quality of care provided to ICU patients and improve overall outcomes.

By addressing the barriers and emphasizing the need for standardized training, ICU echocardiography can be more effectively integrated into routine intensive care practice, ultimately benefiting patient care.

## SCOPE AND PRACTICE OF INTENSIVE CARE MEDICINE

Intensive care medicine deals with a wide array of critically ill patients from post-operative cardial surgical/neurosurgical/oncosurgery patients to medical patients as stroke, poisoning, pancreatitis, pneumonia, geriatric, etc. As an intensivist, echocardiography now forms an important part of the scope of practice for the intensivists as core training for the unit.

## BENEFIT VERSUS RISK

Intensive care unit echocardiography has been proved to be a useful tool for assessment of acute hemodynamics and ruling out a cardiac lesion such as regional wall motion abnormality (RWMA), tamponade, shunting of blood flow, and left ventricular (LV)/right ventricular (RV) ejection fraction.

To ensure patient safety and accurate interpretation of echocardiography studies in the ICU, a standardized protocol is essential. Misinterpretation and incorrect reporting can lead to inappropriate treatment decisions and potential patient harm.

## IMPORTANCE OF STANDARDIZED PROTOCOLS

- *Prevention of misinterpretation:* Standardized protocols help prevent incorrect interpretation of echocardiography studies.
- *Consistency in reporting:* It ensures that echocardiographic findings are reported consistently and accurately, reducing the risk of miscommunication and errors.

## RISKS OF TRANSESOPHAGEAL ECHOCARDIOGRAPHY

- Transesophageal echocardiography, while valuable, carries procedural risks, including but not limited to:
  - *Damage to teeth:* Risk of dental trauma during probe insertion
  - *Injury to pharynx and esophagus:* Potential for erosions, bleeding, or even rupture[6]
  - *Gastric injury:* Risk of burns or other injuries to the stomach

- These risks necessitate that ICU personnel performing TEE are highly trained and skilled.

## TRAINING AND SKILL DEVELOPMENT

- *Comprehensive training:* Those working in ICUs must undergo thorough training to handle echocardiography equipment and interpret results accurately.
- *Certification and competency:* Formal qualifications and certifications should be mandated to ensure that healthcare providers have the necessary expertise.
- *Mentorship:* Access to experienced mentors is crucial for hands-on training and skill refinement.

## STANDARDS

- *International guidelines:* Multiple international organizations have produced recommendations, accreditation statements, and guidelines for ICU echocardiography practices and training.[7-15]
- *Consistency with national and international bodies:* Achieving consistency with national and international intensive care organizations and related medical bodies is fundamental for any policy matter.
- *Reflecting institutional or regional aspirations:* Guidelines developed for trainees or trainers can reflect specific institutional or regional aspirations, ensuring they are tailored to local needs and resources.

## TRAINING

- *Knowledge and practical skills:* Training standards include both the acquisition of theoretical knowledge and practical bedside skills.
    - *Log books:* Trainees should maintain detailed log books documenting their echocardiography practice.
    - *Image acquisition:* Skills in acquiring high-quality echocardiographic images are essential.
    - *Discussion and feedback:* Participation in continuing medical education (CME) activities, seminars, and subsequent discussion sessions is crucial for ongoing learning and improvement.
- *Varied training methods:* There are various methods for fellows and trainees to achieve competency in ICU echocardiography, including:
    - *Hands-on training:* Practical experience under the supervision of experienced mentors
    - *Formal education:* Participation in structured educational programs and workshops
    - *Peer learning:* Collaborative learning with peers and senior colleagues
- *Minimum standards:* The minimum standards for training are established by international intensive care organizations, along with advice from regional experts. These standards ensure that all trainees receive a comprehensive education and are adequately prepared for clinical practice.

## REINVENTING THE TRAINING PARADIGM IN INTENSIVE CARE UNIT ECHOCARDIOGRAPHY

### Classical Training Approach

- *Professional societies:* Traditional thinking suggests that professional societies publish protocols and run training programs for colleagues. These centralized courses often include a hands-on or face-to-face component to ensure practical skill acquisition.

- *Centralized training:* Centralized training aims to provide consistent point-of-care ultrasound (POCUS) training and address the lack of local trainers. The expectation is that trained individuals will become the next generation of trainers, disseminating their knowledge locally.
- *Limited success:* However, only a small proportion of those who start their accreditation journey complete it. Despite a decade of competency definitions by societies, the expected result of widespread dissemination of training has not been achieved.[16]

## Decentralization Approach

- *Local courses:* There is a need for a paradigm shift from a top-down approach to a bottom-up approach. Instead of societies providing centralized courses, they should enable the running of more local courses.
- *Enabling local training:* The role of societies should focus on empowering and facilitating local trainers to conduct courses. This approach can help overcome barriers such as travel constraints, time commitments, and accessibility issues.[4]
- *Increased participation:* Decentralizing training can increase participation and completion rates by making courses more accessible and tailored to the needs of local healthcare providers.
- *Building local expertise:* By fostering local expertise and training hubs, the knowledge and skills necessary for ICU echocardiography can be more widely disseminated and sustainably maintained within communities.

Advantages and disadvantages of centralized versus local courses are summarized in **Table 1**.

## Education Programs

- *Medical college and residency:* The first process of starting basic principles of ultrasound and echocardiography are invariably introduced in medical college and residency programs.
- *Superspeciality and fellowships:* Critical care super speciality and fellowships often include dedicated training in echocardiography, with hands-on experience and interactive lectures.
- *Workshops and certificate courses:* Various professional societies offer workshops and courses. Examples include:
    - *Indian Society of Echocardiography* (ISE) courses
    - *American Society of Echocardiography* (ASE) courses

**TABLE 1:** Advantages and disadvantages of centralized versus local courses.

| | ***Centralized courses*** | ***Local courses*** |
|---|---|---|
| *Advantages* | Availability of experts | • Promoting local expertise<br>Tailored to local needs |
| | Global standardization | Availability of courses |
| *Disadvantages* | • Increased pool of trainers not certain<br>• Sustainability | • Need for "train the trainers" course<br>• Difficult quality control |
| | Environmental impact (transportation accounts for the majority of workshop carbon footprint) | |

- *Society of Critical Care Medicine* (SCCM) courses
- *European Society of Intensive Care Medicine* (ESICM) courses
- *Focused Intensive Care Echocardiography* (FICE) training program in the UK

- *Online resources:* Online courses and virtual simulators are increasingly used to provide training in echocardiography. For example, USG 123, etc.

## Certification Programs

*Basic and advanced level certifications: Various organizations offer certifications*:

- *National Board of Echocardiography (NBE):* It provides certification examinations such as the Examination of Special Competence in Adult Echocardiography (ASCeXAM) and Critical Care Echocardiography Board Exam (CCEeXAM).
- *Indian Association of cardiothoracic Anaesthesiologist (IACTA):* It offers certification in transesophageal echocardiography FTEE.
- *European Association of Cardiovascular Imaging (EACVI):* It offers certification in transthoracic and transesophageal echocardiography.
- *ASE:* It provides certification for specific competencies through the Certification Board of Cardiovascular Computed Tomography (CBCCT) and others.
- *FICE Accreditation:* In the UK, the FICE program provides a structured pathway for achieving competency in ICU echocardiography.

## Equipment

Adequate training in all levels of ICU echocardiography is not possible without standard echocardiographic equipment, which should reflect established ICU echocardiography practice and training requirements. Ultrasound machine with a cardiac probe is sufficient for basic screening. However, advanced screening requires proper equipment. The recommendations for ICU echocardiography equipment need to be developed as done in the expert committee for one part of world.[1,17]

# QUALITY ASSURANCE AND CONTINUING EDUCATION

Ongoing participation in professional development activities associated explicitly with ICU echocardiography is mandatory for all levels of training whether basic or advanced.

## QUALITY ASSURANCE

- *Competency assessment:* Regul r assessments through direct observation, image review, and written tests
- *Performance metrics:* Monitoring the accuracy of echocardiographic interpretations and the impact on clinical outcomes
- *Peer review:* Regular peer review of studies performed by practitioners to ensure adherence to standards
- *Accreditation of units:* Units performing echocardiography may seek accreditation from bodies recognized in the field, which ensures adherence to best practices and guidelines.

## CONTINUING EDUCATION

- *Continuing medical education:* Ongoing participation in CME activities, including attending conferences, workshops, and online courses.
- *Simulation training:* Use of simulation centers to practice advanced skills and handle complex cases

- *Case reviews and morbidity and mortality (M&M) conferences:* Regular case reviews and M&M conferences to discuss diagnostic challenges and improve practice
- *Guidelines and updates:* Staying current with guidelines and updates from professional societies such as ASE, EACVI, and SCCM
- *Research and publications:* Encouraging involvement in research and publications to contribute to the evolving field of ICU echocardiography
- *Mentorship and teaching:* Senior clinicians mentoring junior staff and participating in teaching activities to disseminate knowledge

Overall, ensuring proficiency in ICU echocardiography involves a combination of structured education, certification, quality assurance measures, and a commitment to ongoing learning and professional development.

## CONCLUSION

Standardizing training in ICU echocardiography is essential for ensuring competency, improving patient safety, and delivering high-quality care. The introduction of protocols and training guidelines provides a structured pathway for achieving these goals. By adopting a decentralized training approach, professional societies can empower local trainers, making training more accessible and effective. This literature serves as a valuable guide for trainees and trainers, helping to shape the future of ICU echocardiography practice.

## REFERENCES


1. Nanjayya VB, Orde S, Hilton A, Yang Y, Costello C, Evans J, et al. Levels of training in critical care echocardiography in adults. Recommendations from the College of Intensive Care Medicine Ultrasound Special Interest Group. Australas J Ultrasound Med. 2019;22(1):73-9.
2. McLean A, Yastrebov K. Echocardiography training for the intensivist. Crit Care Resusc. 2007;9:320-2.
3. Yang Y, Royse C, Royse A, Williams K, Canty D. Survey of the training and use of echocardiography and lung ultrasound in Australasian intensive care units. Crit Care. 2016;20:339.
4. Zawadka M, Wong A, Janiszewska A, Sanfilippo F, La Via L, Sobieraj P, et al. Critical care echocardiography: barriers, competencies and solutions. A survey of over 600 participants. Anaesthesiol Intensive Ther. 2023;55(3):158-62.
5. Vignon P. What is new in critical care echocardiography? Crit Care. 2018;22:40.
6. Hilberath JN, Oakes DA, Shernan SK, Bulwer BE, D'Ambra MN, Eltzschig HK. Safety of transesophageal echocardiography. J Am Soc Echocardiogr. 2010;23:1115-27.
7. British Society of Echocardiography. Accreditation in critical care echocardiography. Information pack. British Society of Echocardiography; 2017.
8. European Society of Intensive Care Medicine. (2017). European diploma in advanced critical care echocardiography. [online] Available from https://www.esicm.org/education/edec-2/ [Last accessed September, 2024]
9. Expert Round Table on Echocardiography in ICU. International consensus statement on training standards for advanced critical care echocardiography. Intensive Care Med. 2014;40:654-66.
10. Expert Round Table on Ultrasound in ICU. International expert statement on training standards for critical care ultrasonography. Intensive Care Med. 2011;37:1077-83.
11. Price S, Via G, Sloth E, Guarracino F, Breitkreutz R, Catena E, et al. Echocardiography practice, training and accreditation in the intensive care: document for the World Interactive Network Focused on Critical Ultrasound (WINFOCUS). Cardiovasc Ultrasound. 2008;6:49.

12. Arntfield RT, Millington SJ, Ainsworth CD, Arora RC, Boyd J, Finlayson G, et al. Canadian recommendations for critical care ultrasound training and competency for the Canadian Critical Care Society. Can Respir J. 2014;21:341-5.
13. Mayo PH, Beaulieu Y, Doelken P, Feller-Kopman D, Harrod C, Kaplan A, et al. American College of Chest Physicians/La Société de Réanimation de Langue Française statement on competence in critical care ultrasonography. Chest. 2009;135:1050-60.
14. Díaz-Gómez J, Frankel H, Hernandez A. National certification in critical care echocardiography: its time has come. Crit Care Med. 2017;45:1801-4.
15. Oren-Grinberg A, Talmor D, Brown S. Focused critical care echocardiography. Crit Care Med 2013;41:2618-26.
16. Flower L, Dempsey M, White A, Sanfilippo F, Olusanya O, Madhivathanan PR. Training and accreditation pathways in critical care and perioperative echocardiography. J Cardiothorac Vasc Anesth. 2021; 35:235-47.
17. Costello C, Yastrebov K, Yang Y, Hilton A, Vij S, Orde S. Minimum standards for ultrasound equipment in intensive care. Recommendations from CICM Ultrasound Special Interest Group. Australas J Ultrasound Med. 2017;20:41-6.

CHAPTER 32

# Flowchart of Echo Approach in Shock Differentiation, Acute Dyspnea, Acute Chest Pain, and Deresuscitation

*Anant Vikram Pachisa*

## SHOCK ETIOLOGY DIFFERENTIATION (FLOWCHART 1)

**Flowchart 1:** Differentiation of shock with echocardiography.

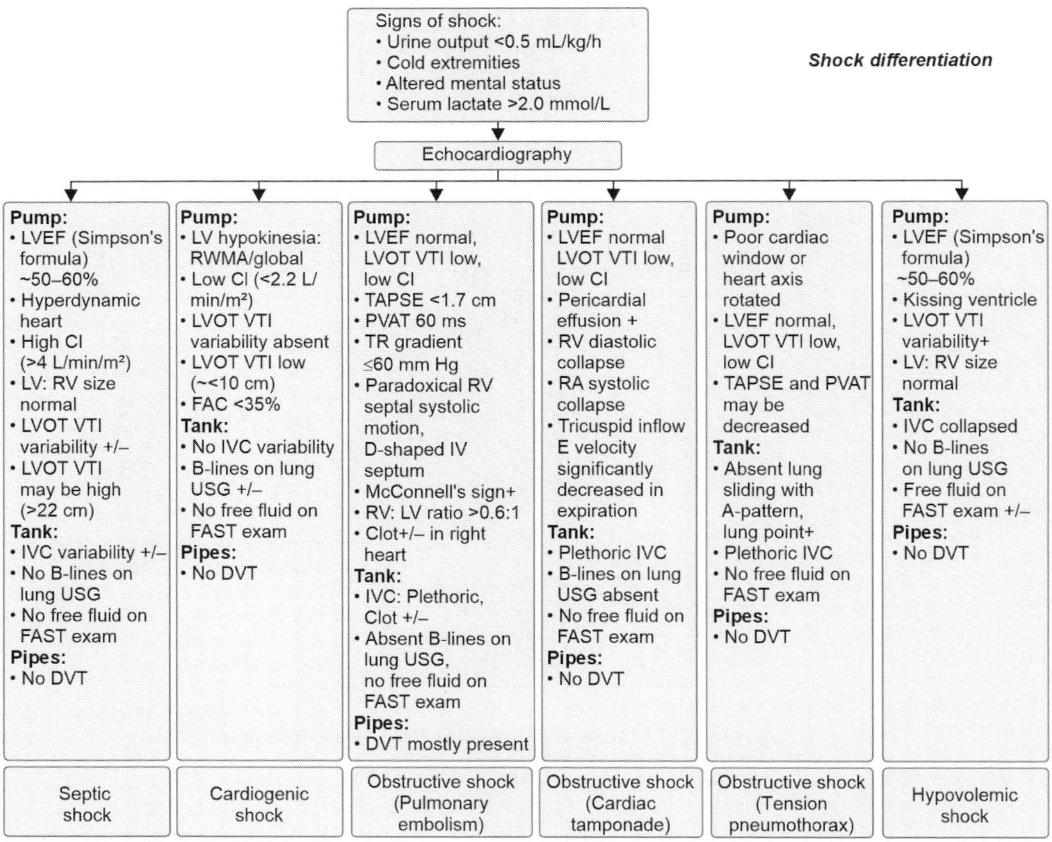


(CI: cardiac index; DVT: deep vein thrombosis; FAC: fractional area change; FAST: focused assessment with sonography in trauma; IV: interventricular; IVC: inferior vena cava; LV: left ventricle; LVEF: left ventricular ejection fraction; LVOT VTI: left ventricular outflow tract-velocity time integral; PVAT: pulmonary valve acceleration time; TAPSE: tricuspid annular plane systolic excursion; RA: right atrium; RV: right ventricle; RWMA: regional wall motion abnormality; TR: tricuspid regurgitation; USG: ultrasonography)

## DIFFERENTIATING ETIOLOGY OF ACUTE ONSET DYSPNEA (FLOWCHART 2)

**Flowchart 2:** Evaluation of acute onset dyspnea with echocardiography.

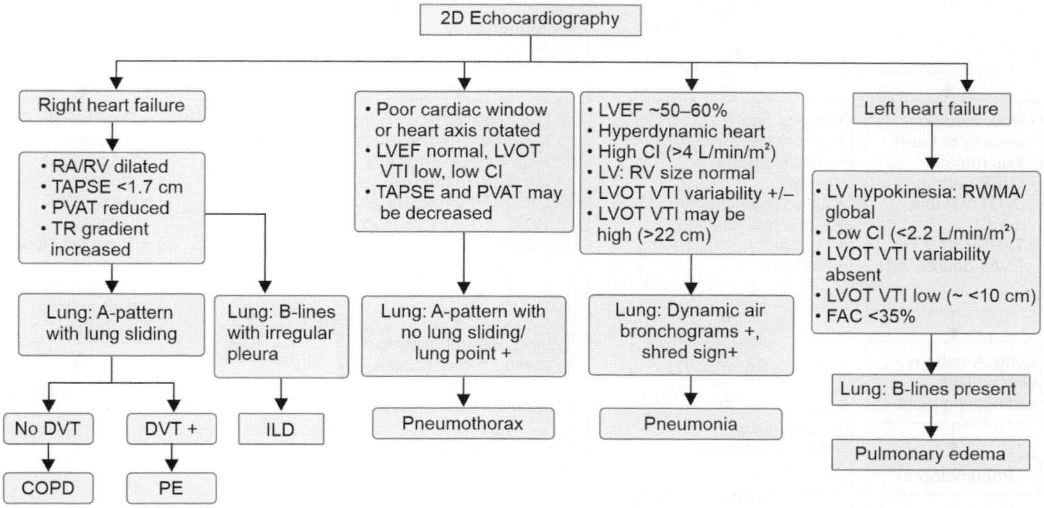


(CI: cardiac index; COPD: chronic obstructive pulmonary disease; DVT: deep vein thrombosis; FAC: fractional area change; FAST: focused assessment with sonography in trauma; ILD: interstitial lung disease; IV: interventricular; IVC: inferior vena cava; LV: left ventricle; LVEF: left ventricular ejection fraction; LVOT VTI: left ventricular outflow tract-velocity time integral; PE: pulmonary embolism; PVAT: pulmonary valve acceleration time; TAPSE: tricuspid annular plane systolic excursion; TR: tricuspid regurgitation; RV: right ventricle; RA: right atrium; RWMA: regional wall motion abnormality)

## DIFFERENTIATING CAUSES OF ACUTE CHEST PAIN (FLOWCHART 3)

**Flowchart 3:** Evaluation of acute onset chest pain with echocardiography.

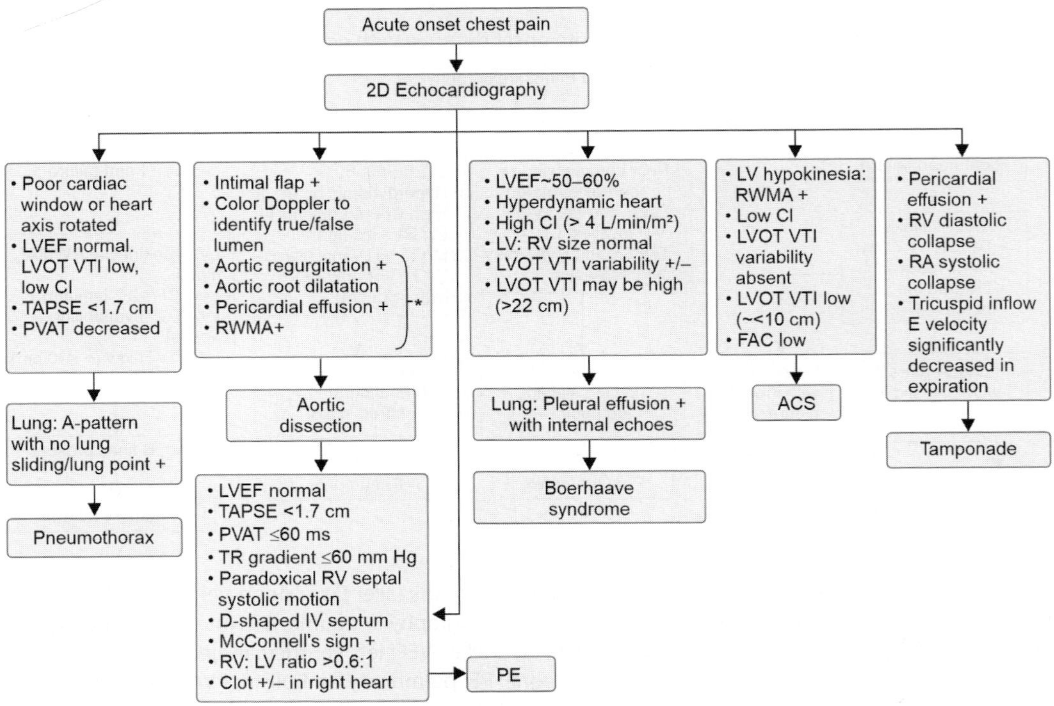


*Seen with type a aortic dissection.

(FAC: fractional area change; DVT: deep vein thrombosis; IV: interventricular; IVC: inferior vena cava; LVEF: left ventricular ejection fraction; LV: left ventricle; LVOT VTI: left ventricular outflow tract-velocity time integral; FAST: focused assessment with sonography in trauma; PVAT: pulmonary valve acceleration time; TAPSE: tricuspid annular plane systolic excursion; TR: tricuspid regurgitation; RV: right ventricle; RA: right atrium; RWMA: regional wall motion abnormality)

## ROLE OF POCUS IN DERESUSCITATION (FLOWCHART 4)

**Flowchart 4:** Deresuscitation with the help of echocardiography.

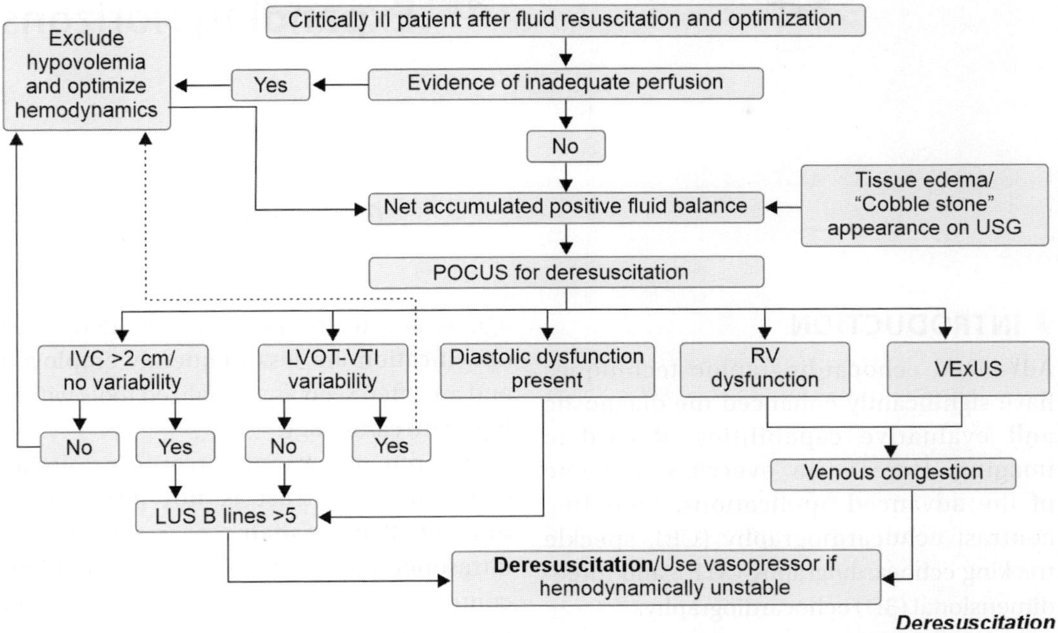


(IVC: inferior vena cava; LUS: lung ultrasound; LVOT VTI: left ventricular outflow tract-velocity time integral; RV: right ventricle, VExUS: venous excess ultrasound)

CHAPTER 33

# Advanced Echocardiography in Intensive Care Unit: Expanding Horizons

*Gourav Mittal, Puneet Khanna*

## INTRODUCTION

Advanced echocardiographic techniques have significantly enhanced the diagnostic and evaluative capabilities of cardiac imaging. Here is an overview of some of the advanced applications, including contrast echocardiography (CE), speckle tracking echocardiography (STE), and three-dimensional (3D) echocardiography.

## CONTRAST ECHOCARDIOGRAPHY

Contrast echocardiography is a well-known technique for assessing various cardiac structures and functions. In intensive care unit (ICU) settings agitated saline and similar large-sized air bubble contrast agents are commonly used. However, advanced agents and techniques for left-sided heart opacification are less frequently employed and are often seen as specialized tools within high-end cardiology.

Despite common perceptions, using ultrasound contrast is not particularly difficult. It necessitates a strong grasp of ultrasound physics, familiarity with modern contrast agents, proficiency with advanced ultrasound scanners, and regular hands-on practice. This chapter aims to demystify CE and provide intensive care physicians, trained in advanced echocardiographic techniques, with the essential knowledge to incorporate this valuable method into their routine clinical practice. Types of contrast used in echocardiography are discussed in **Flowchart 1**.

**Flowchart 1:** Types of contrast used in echocardiography.

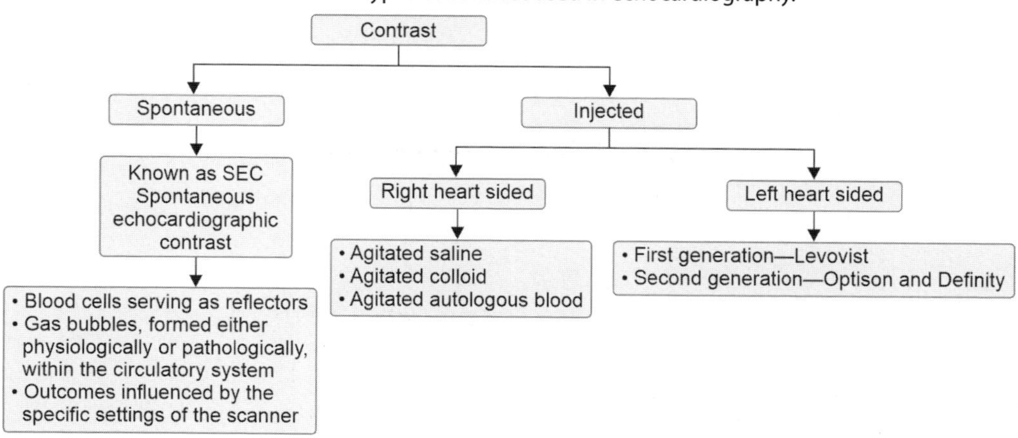

**Q1. What does the presence of spectral signify and how to differentiate it from pseudospec?**

Spectral appears as a smoke pattern on two-dimensional (2D) echocardiography and indicates sluggish blood flow, suggesting a propensity for a prothrombotic state. The presence of SPEC should prompt a thorough search for thrombus, especially in the left side of the heart, where the risk of systemic embolization is highest, a diagnosis that is challenging in critically ill patients. Two key indicators of true SPEC are very slow swirling velocity and smoke density.

However, it is important to differentiate true SPEC from pseudo-SPEC, which can sometimes result from machine artifacts rather than patient pathology. When SPEC is observed, it is essential to check for risk factors of a prothrombotic state, such as low cardiac output, regional wall motion abnormalities, and low ventricular function.

**Q2. How agitated contrast (saline and blood) is prepared?**

**Ans.**

- Connect two 10 mL syringes with a three-way stopcock **(Fig. 1)**
- Vigorously exchange 7–8 mL of isotonic saline and 1–2 mL of air between the syringes (indicated by arrows), mixing them to form fine bubbles.

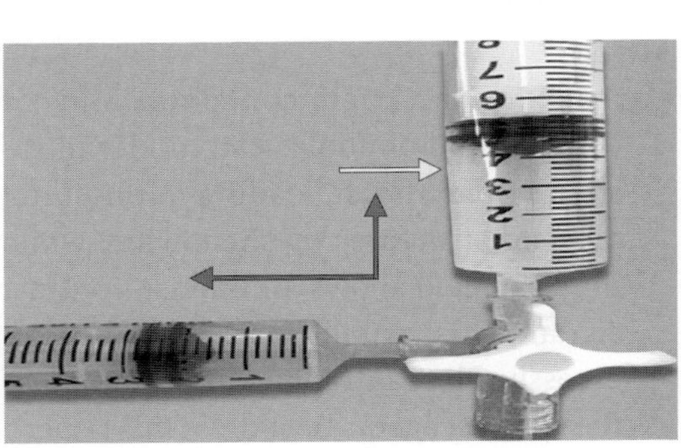

**Fig. 1:** Preparation of agitated saline.

- The mixture will appear slightly "milky" in the syringe (arrow).
- Promptly inject this mixture into the venous system, as the small air bubbles are very unstable and will quickly merge into a larger bubble.
- For optimal results, inject the mixture into a larger vein near the scanning area.

**Q3. Enlist the indications of right-sided contrast echo in critically ill patients.**

**Ans.**

- *Interatrial shunt detection:* For detection of a right-to-left shunt, the pressure in the right-sided heart chambers must briefly exceed that in the left-sided chambers, allowing bubbles to pass through the septal defect. In typical settings, patients may perform a Valsalva maneuver or cough to create this pressure differential. However, ICU patients often cannot cooperate and are usually on mechanical ventilation. In such cases, increasing positive end-expiratory pressure (PEEP) to 20 $H_2O$ or using inspiratory breath-hold techniques, with ventilator adjustments, can achieve the necessary pressure increase in the right atrium.
- *Ventricular shunt detection:* This method is particularly useful for patients with significant pulmonary hypertension, extremely high PEEP, severely failing left ventricles, or those using mechanical ventricular assist devices. These conditions can reduce end-diastolic left ventricular pressure below diastolic right ventricular pressure.
- *Differential diagnosis of hypoxemia:* CE helps identify shunts and other abnormalities, aiding in the differential diagnosis of hypoxemia.
- *Enhancements in Doppler signal:* Enhancing the Doppler signal is particularly useful for accurately measuring

the tricuspid regurgitation signal to determine right heart systolic pressures.

- *Procedural assistance:* CE confirms needle or catheter placement during invasive procedures, such as central line insertions and pericardial or pleural drainage.
- *Right-sided contrast and extracorporeal membrane oxygenation (ECMO):* It is used to diagnose venous admixture bypassing the oxygenator in ECMO patients. Ideally, agitated contrast should be filtered out by the oxygenator; if it appears in the right atrium, it indicates venous admixture.

**Q4. What are the risks involved while using an agitated contrast medium?**

**Ans.**

If agitated bubbles go into the systemic circulation through large intracardiac or transpulmonary shunts, they may transiently block brain capillaries, potentially causing ischemic strokes or transient ischemic attacks, though such occurrences are rare. Consequently, the benefits of identifying a possible intracardiac right-to-left shunt must be balanced against the risk of cerebral microvascular occlusion, particularly if the shunt is significant. It is essential to carefully evaluate the neurological status of patients before and after administering right-sided contrast, especially when a right-to-left shunt is detected, while also considering the practical limitations within the intensive care setting.

**Q5. Enlists indications of manufactured contrasts used for CE.**

**Ans.**

According to the ASE and the ESC, and recognized by regulatory authorities such as the United States Food and Drug Administration (US FDA) and TGA, the indications for using manufactured contrast agents in CE include:

- *Left ventricular opacification (LVO):*
  - Evaluation of left ventricular ejection fraction (LVEF)
  - Both rest and stress echocardiography
- *Ventricular morphological evaluation:*
  - Identification of apical hypertrophic cardiomyopathy (HCM)
  - Detection of noncompaction cardiomyopathy
  - Evaluation of pseudoaneurysm formation
- *Right ventricular opacification:*
  - Enhanced definition of the right ventricular free wall
  - Assessment of right ventricular (RV) function
- *Assessment of cardiac masses:*
  - Evaluation of intraventricular masses (thrombus, etc.)
  - Assessment of intra-atrial masses
  - Identification of large vessel masses
  - Diagnosing among abscess cavities and blood-filled defects
- *Other applications:*
  - Enhancement of spectral Doppler signals
  - Use in 3D echocardiography
  - Off-label use for perfusion imaging, as no agent is currently approved for this purpose

**Q6. What are the artifacts observed while performing contrast echo and how one can rectify them?**

**Ans.**

- *Attenuation:* High concentrations of contrast microbubbles can hinder ultrasound penetration, leading to obscured far-field structures by shadowing, while the near field shows an intense contrast signal. This usually occurs due to an excessive dose or rapid administration of the contrast agent. To address this issue:
  - Reduce the contrast dose

- Decrease the administering rate
- Apply color Doppler
- Wait when bolus was used, as the concentration shall diminish over time.

- *Swirling:* Swirling happens when bubbles are destroyed by long exposure to USG energy. This can generally be resolved by:
  - Adjusting the transmit power.
  - Revarying the dose of the contrast agent.
  - Administering low mechanical index (MI) imaging modalities to minimize contrast swirling.
- *Blooming:* Spectral blooming can occur when using contrast agents to enhance spectral Doppler signals, resulting in an artifact when the Doppler signal is excessively strong. This issue can be mitigated by:
  - Ensuring the contrast concentration is not very high.

Reducing the Doppler gain significantly compared to what is typically used for noncontrast Doppler imaging.

### *Speckle Tracking Echocardiography*

Speckle tracking echocardiography involves analyzing the frame-by-frame movement of grayscale "speckles" (or "kernels") within the myocardium's image. These speckles are natural ultrasound artifacts and do not correspond to actual myocardial structures. They are produced by interferences from scattered ultrasound wave reflections from closely spaced small reflectors that cannot be individually distinguished on the ultrasound image.

Speckle tracking echocardiography is a semiautomated postprocessing technique, meaning that the analysis is performed on stored images. This method measures the deformation of speckles relative to one another, known as "strain." The strain offers an estimate of contractile function: The closer the speckles move toward each other, the better the contractile function. Strain values are negative because they represent relative deformation (i.e., the movement of one speckle compared to another). Thus, a more negative strain value indicates greater deformation and better systolic function.

**Q7. Enlist the advantages and disadvantages of STE.**

**Ans.**

*Advantages of Speckle Tracking Echocardiography*

- *Angle-independent:* Provides accurate measurements regardless of the angle of insonation.
- *Enhanced detection:* Can identify cardiac dysfunctions that are not visible with standard echocardiography.
- *Accuracy:* Comparable to gold-standard imaging techniques such as MRI.
- *Differentiation:* Can distinguish between passive (tethering) and active myocardial movement.
- *Comprehensive analysis:* Capable of describing additional cardiac motions, including torsion, dyssynchrony, and diastolic function.

*Disadvantages of Speckle Tracking Echocardiography*

- *Time-consuming:* Requires significant time to perform the analysis.
- *Learning curve:* Takes time to learn and master the technique.
- *Specific imaging needs:* Requires specific imaging techniques to obtain accurate results.
- *Frame rate sensitivity:* Low frame rates must be avoided to ensure accuracy.

- *Limited research in critically ill:* Fewer studies have been conducted in critically ill patients.
- *Validated parameters:* Only longitudinal strain is currently validated for clinical use.
- *Full myocardial view:* The entire myocardium view must be visualized throughout the cardiac cycle.
- *Invalidated information:* A wealth of information, such as right ventricle and atrial analysis, has not been validated.
- *Clinical relevance:* The clinical significance of all measured parameters has not been fully investigated.

**Q8. Briefly explain the terminology used in STE.**

**Ans.**

- *Strain (S):*
  - *Definition:* The relative deformation between groups of speckles (or kernels) as they come together.
  - *Value:* Negative; a more negative value indicates greater deformation and better systolic function.
  - *Note:* This is the most validated term in speckle tracking.
- *Strain rate (SR):*
  - *Definition:* The rate of deformation.
  - *Measurement:* Strain/second.
  - *Note:* Generally considered little influenced by the cardiac load.
- *Strain rate early relaxation (SRe):*
  - *Definition:* The rate at which speckles move apart after contraction.
  - *Purpose:* May be used as a measure of relaxation or diastolic function.
  - *Note:* Currently supported by limited data.
- *Time to peak strain:*
  - *Definition:* The time difference for individual segments to reach peak strain.
  - *Purpose:* Used to assess dyssynchrony.
- *End-systolic strain:*
  - *Definition:* The strain value measured at the end of systole.
  - *Purpose:* Indicates effective systolic function.
- *Postsystolic peak strain:*
  - *Definition:* Strain measured after the closure of the atrioventricular (AV) valve.
  - *Purpose:* Reflects noneffective systolic function.
- *Longitudinal strain:*
  - *Definition:* Measures deformation in the base-to-apex direction.
- *Global longitudinal strain:*
  - *Definition:* Average strain from A4C, 2-C, and three-chamber views.
  - *Purpose:* Provides an overall assessment of left ventricular systolic function.
- *Bullseye plot:*
  - *Definition:* A graphical representation of global longitudinal strain (GLS).
- *Circumferential strain:*
  - *Definition:* Assesses deformation in the short-axis view around the circular direction.
- *Radial strain:*
  - *Definition:* Measures myocardial deformation in the short-axis view toward the center (inward deformation).
- *Twist:*
  - *Definition:* The angular difference between apical rotation (anticlockwise in apex view) and basal rotation (clockwise) at systole.
- *Torsion:*
  - *Definition:* Normalized twist.
- *Untwist:*
  - *Definition:* Diastolic angular difference between apical and basal rotation.
  - *Note:* Relatively load-independent parameter for diastolic function.

**Q9. Application and evidence in critically ill patients.**

**Ans.**

*Septic Shock*

- *Sensitivity:* STE can detect both left ventricular (LV) and right ventricular (RV) strain more sensitively than conventional echocardiography.
- *Study findings:* Orde et al. studied sixty patients with septic shock, revealing LV impairment in 69% of cases (compared to 33% with LV-EF changes) and RV impairment in 72% of cases (compared to 32% with RV dysfunction in normal echo).[1]
- *Mortality marker:* A GLS impairment of ≥–13% is a strong indicator of ICU mortality.[2]

*Acute Heart Failure*

- *Prognostic value:* Impaired systolic strain, particularly GLS, serves as an independent predictor of adverse outcomes in heart failure (HF) patients and is more accurate than LV-EF.[3]
- *Multicenter study:* In a study of 147 HF patients with reduced LV-EFs, clinical events occurred in 20% during 12 months. GLS showed the highest prognostic value with a sensitivity of 73% and specificity of 83% at a cutoff of –7%.[4]
- *Sensitivity to loading conditions:* STE is highly sensitive to cardiac loading conditions, making it valuable for assessing LV strain in the American College Health Foundation (ACHF) for treatment.

*Myocarditis*

- *Diagnostic aid:* STE provides significant diagnostic value in acute myocarditis (AM), particularly in patients with preserved EF, providing better sensitivity for detecting regional LV dysfunction compared to routine echocardiography.[5-7]
- *Correlation with lymphocytic infiltrates:* Longitudinal myocardial deformation abnormality usually correlates significantly with lymphocytic infiltrates.[8]

*Takotsubo Cardiomyopathy*

- *Pattern description:* STE can characterize the typical pattern of LV dysfunction in Takotsubo cardiomyopathy (TC), showing apical dyskinesis, attenuated longitudinal strain in mid-ventricular segments, and hyperkinesis at the base.
- *Comparative study:* A study using 2DSTE compared myocardial function in TC and acute anterior myocardial infarction (MI), finding lower radial and longitudinal strains in TC and lower GLS and LV-EF values in TC patients compared to MI patients.[9]

*ST-Elevation Myocardial Infarction*

- *Early dysfunction identification:* GLS and regional longitudinal strain (RLS) can detect early myocardial dysfunction and myocardial scar in STEMI patients with preserved LVF.
- *Study findings:* Cimino et al. investigated twenty STEMI patients treated with PCI, finding that GLS before coronary intervention predicts complications.[10,11]

*Non-ST Elevation Myocardial Infarction*

- *Rapid Assessment Tool:* STE can quickly and sensitively identify NSTEMI patients who may benefit from urgent revascularization. It detects microvascular obstruction and impaired function of subendocardial fibers before wall-motion abnormalities become apparent.[12,13]

*Patients Undergoing Mechanical Ventilation*

- *PEEP effects:* In critically ill patients on mechanical ventilation with positive end-expiratory pressure (PEEP), left atrial (LA), right atrial (RA), and RV GLS acutely decrease with increasing PEEP, while LV strain does not change. This suggests that reduced cardiac output with higher PEEP is related to preload rather than contractility.

- *Influence of high PEEP:* High PEEP can differentially affect STE variables, particularly at elevated PEEP levels.

## THREE-DIMENSIONAL ECHOCARDIOGRAPHY

Real-time 3D echocardiography enables single- or multibeat acquisition of pyramidal datasets during a breath-hold, eliminating the need for offline reconstruction. This imaging technique offers several key advantages:

- *Enhanced accuracy and reproducibility:* Improves the precision and consistency of chamber volume measurements by removing the requirement for geometric modeling and minimizing false values associated with foreshortened A4C.
- *Comprehensive visualization:* Offers detailed imaging of cardiac valves and congenital abnormalities, enhancing diagnosis and treatment planning.
- *Guidance for interventions:* Assists in guiding interventions for structural heart diseases by providing a clearer and more detailed view of the heart's anatomy.

## CLINICAL APPLICATIONS

### Direct and Automated Evaluation

- *Direct evaluation:* Facilitates automated assessment of chamber volumes, bypassing the need for modeling.
- *Accuracy improvement:* Mitigates the negative impact of foreshortened apical views, leading to more precise and reproducible measurements of LV and RV volumes and EF compared to traditional 2D echo.

### Assessment of Regional Wall Motion Abnormalities

- *Detection of IHD:* Enables objective detection of ischemia both at rest and during stress testing.
- *Systolic dyssynchrony:* Allows for the systolic dyssynchrony objective quantification, which helps guide resynchronization therapy in congestive heart failure (CHF) patients.

### Evaluation of Valve Lesions

- *Size and morphology:* Directly assesses the size of the vena contracta.
- *Volumetric quantification:* Provides detailed volumetric measurements of mitral valve MV and tricuspid valve (TV) lesions.

### Guidance of Interventional Procedures

- *Procedure guidance:* Assists in guiding interventions for structural heart diseases.
- *3D printing:* Facilitates the use of 3D printing for personalized presurgical planning.

### Automated Stroke Volume Measurement

*AI integration:* Employs artificial intelligence to automate stroke volume measurements from basic apical four-chamber images, streamlining the process and enhancing accuracy.

## LIMITATIONS

### Temporal Resolution Constraints

- *Current limitations:* The temporal resolution is limited by the sampling rates, which range from 10 to 20 volumes per second.

- *Troubleshooting:* Researchers suggest acquiring sample volumes over multiple heartbeats and using the electrocardiographic signal to "reorder" the samples. This method can achieve higher frame rates with existing technology, but it assumes periodic heart motion from beat to beat. This approach may be less applicable to patients with variable R-R intervals, such as those with atrial fibrillation and frequent premature atrial complexes.

## Validation and Applicability

*Need for further studies:* Although this technique shows potential for improving real-time 3D assessment of valvular function, additional studies are needed to validate its effectiveness and reliability in clinical settings.

## REFERENCES

1. Orde SR, Pulido JN, Masaki M, Gillespie S, Spoon JN, Kane GC, et al. Outcome prediction in sepsis: speckle tracking echocardiography based assessment of myocardial function. Crit Care. 2014;18(4):R149.
2. Chang W-T, Lee W-H, Lee W-T, Chen PS, Su YR, Liu PY, et al. Left ventricular global longitudinal strain is independently associated with mortality in septic shock patients. Intensive Care Med. 2015;41(10):1791-9.
3. Cho GY, Marwick TH, Kim HS, Kim MK, Hong KS, Oh DJ. Global 2-dimensional strain as a new prognosticator in patients with heart failure. J Am Coll Cardiol. 2009;54(7):618-24.
4. Mignot A, Donal E, Zaroui A, Reant P, Salem A, Hamon C, et al. Global longitudinal strain as a major predictor of cardiac events in patients with depressed left ventricular function: a multicenter study. J Am Soc Echocardiogr. 2010;23(10):1019-24.
5. Friedrich MG, Sechtem U, Schulz-Menger J, Holmvang G, Alakija P, Cooper LT, et al. Cardiovascular magnetic resonance in myocarditis: a JACC white paper. J Am Coll Cardiol. 2009;53(17):1475-87.
6. Khoo NS, Smallhorn JF, Atallah J, Kaneko S, Mackie AS, Paterson I. Altered left ventricular tissue velocities, deformation and twist in children and young adults with acute myocarditis and normal ejection fraction. J Am Soc Echocardiogr. 2012;25(3):294-303.
7. Sturmberger T, Niel J, Aichinger J, Ebner C. Acute myocarditis with normal wall motion detected with 2D speckle tracking echocardiography. Echo Res Pract. 2016;3(1):K15-9.
8. Escher F, Kasner M, Kühl U, Heymer J, Wilkenshoff U, Tschöpe C, et al. New echocardiographic findings correlate with intramyocardial inflammation in endomyocardial biopsies of patients with acute myocarditis and inflammatory cardiomyopathy. Mediators Inflamm. 2013;2013:875420.
9. Heggemann F, Hamm K, Kaelsch T, Sueselbeck T, Papavassiliu T, Borggrefe M, et al. Global and regional myocardial function quantification in Takotsubo cardiomyopathy in comparison to acute anterior myocardial infarction using two-dimensional (2D) strain echocardiography. Echocardiography. 2011;28(7):715-9.
10. Cimino S, Canali E, Petronilli V, Cicogna F, De Luca L, Francone M, et al. Global and regional longitudinal strain assessed by two-dimensional speckle tracking echocardiography identifies early myocardial dysfunction and transmural extent of myocardial scar in patients with acute ST-elevation myocardial infarction and relatively preserved LV function. Eur Heart J Cardiovasc Imaging. 2013;14:805-11.
11. Woo JS, Kim WS, Yu TK, Ha SJ, Kim SY, Bae JH, et al. Prognostic value of serial global longitudinal strain measured by two-dimensional speckle tracking echocardiography in patients with ST-segment elevation myocardial infarction. Am J Cardiol. 2011;108(3):340-47.

12. Bergerot C, Mewton N, Lacote-Roiron C, Ernande L, Ovize M, Croisille P, et al. Influence of microvascular obstruction on regional myocardial deformation in the acute phase of myocardial infarction: a speckle-tracking Echocardiography study. J Am Soc Echocardiogr. 2014;27(1):93-100.
13. Caspar T, Samet H, Ohana M, Germain P, El Ghannudi S, Talha S, et al. Longitudinal 2D strain can help diagnose coronary artery disease in patients with suspected non-ST-elevation acute coronary syndrome but apparent normal global and segmental systolic function. Int J Cardiol. 2017;236:91-4.

CHAPTER 34

# Transesophageal Echocardiography in the Intensive Care Unit

*Meera Rajeev, Sarvesh Pal Singh*

## INTRODUCTION

Cardiac point-of-care ultrasound done at the bedside is common in all intensive care units (ICUs). According to the American Society of Echocardiography, it is not possible to obtain adequate images for decision-making via standard transthoracic echocardiography (TTE) in 30% of critically ill patients[1] due to the presence of invasive mechanical ventilation, external dressings, and limited mobility which contribute to poor image acquisition. However, by eliminating these factors, transesophageal echocardiography (TEE) can significantly improve patient outcomes. A recent study observed that adding TEE to TTE in critically ill patients led to a new diagnosis or a change in management about 45% of the time,[2] highlighting the significant impact of TEE on patient care.

### Q1. How does an intensivist transesophageal echocardiography examination differ from a cardiologist transesophageal echocardiography?

**Ans.** All intensivists should be skilled in critical care echocardiography (CEE), a standard part of critical care training. However, to truly make a difference in patient care, it is crucial for intensivists to strive for competence in advanced CCE, which includes critical care TEE. Advanced CCE differs in many ways from cardiology-based echocardiography, and the more competent an intensivist is in this area, the more they can contribute to improved patient outcomes.

- The intensivist performs it at the patient's bedside during the active process of diagnosis and management of cardiovascular instability. This unique role means the clinician decides what examination component is relevant within the clinical context, integrating the findings into an immediate clinical management plan in ways different from the consultative cardiology echocardiographer. This underscores the value and integral role of the intensivist in the patient's care.
- It is also used as a hemodynamic monitoring tool by performing sequential examinations on patients on mechanical ventilation to assess the efficacy and tolerance of therapeutic changes. Hence, intensivists should be competent enough to use echocardiography as a sequential assessment tool. Mastering image acquisition and subsequent image interpretation knowledge of essential aspects of pathophysiological function is important.

## TRAINING IN ADVANCED TRANSESOPHAGEAL ECHOCARDIOGRAPHY

Effective training programs should be implemented depending on faculty preferences, local resource availability, and learner preferences. Faculty should be skilled and recognized with a formal certification by a national authority or a critical care society established nationally or internationally. As per the American Society of Echocardiography, a minimum of 35 full TEE studies should be done as part of advanced CCE training in which a significant proportion of case studies should be performed in critically ill patients.[3] Competence in critical care TEE is an important component of advanced CCE. Hence, the TEE probe is an essential requirement in all ICUs. Competence in image acquisition and interpretation of 2D TEE views is an important part of advanced CCE training.

## TRANSESOPHAGEAL ECHOCARDIOGRAPHY PROBE INSERTION

A TEE probe is inserted in the esophagus, similar to an orogastric tube. Before insertion, a thorough oral cavity examination must be done to rule out any loose tooth or any other obvious abnormalities. A dental guard should always be used to minimize the risk of dental trauma and probe damage. The probe control lock should always be neutral and never engaged during probe placement or manipulation. However, slight anteflexion of the tip with the control wheel may be helpful during insertion. A generous amount of lubrication should be applied to the probe before placement in the oropharynx. The probe should never be forced if met with resistance. Jaw lifting is done with the left hand, and the probe is inserted with the right hand. The probe is held between the index finger and thumb in a pen-holding fashion. A constant gentle pressure is applied while inserting the probe, and a loss of resistance is felt when the larynx and cricopharyngeal muscle are passed—an excessive extension of the head and neck results in increased resistance while advancing the probe. Direct laryngoscopy may also be used. The examination should be performed to minimize overall probe manipulation, including minimizing the number of times the probe is advanced and withdrawn.

*Terminology to describe probe manipulations* ***(Fig. 1)***:

- Withdraw
- Advance
- Anterior-anteflexion
- Posterior-retroflexion
- Flex to right
- Flex to left
- Transesophageal echocardiography probe control (**Figs. 2A to D**)
- Anteflexion and retroflection with a large knob on the probe handle
- Flex to the right and flex to the left with a small knob on the probe handle.

The probe shaft has markings indicating the depth of insertion **(Table 1)**. Various probe positions are used to image the heart, from the upper esophagus to the stomach.

The TEE probe is posterior and closer to the heart than the TTE probe. If the probe is in the upper esophagus, the closest structures are the great vessels. If the probe is in the midesophagus, the closest structure is the left atrium; in the transgastric, it is the left ventricle. The right and left display orientation during TEE is similar to a chest X-ray. Increasing the imaging plane proceeds clockwise. The sector's apex displays structures closest to the TEE probe in TEE.

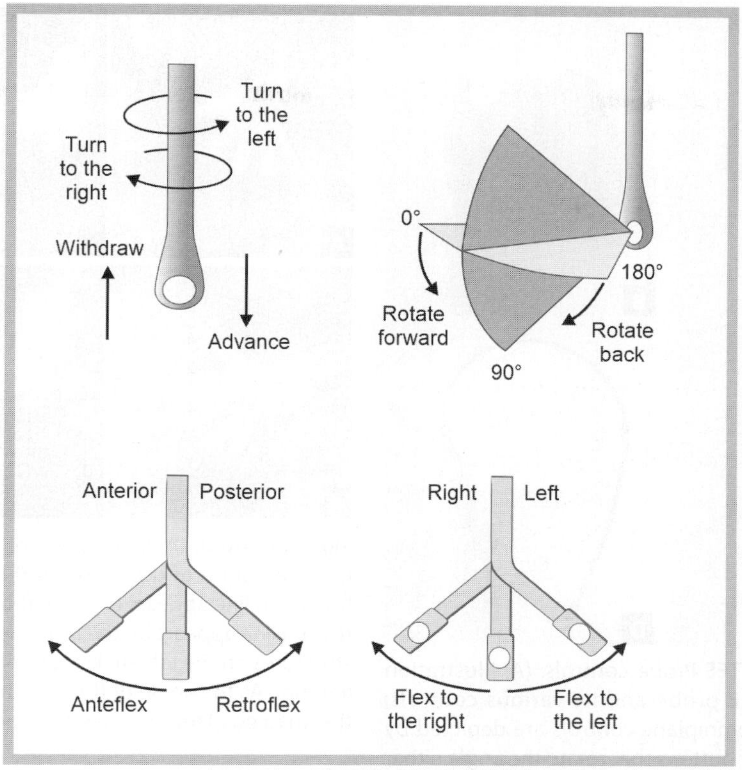


**Fig. 1:** This image depicts the various probe manipulation maneuvers.

So, the apex of the image sector displays posterior structures, and the arc of the sector displays anterior structures.

Currently, the standard probes used in TEE are multiplane. The orientation of the imaging plane can be changed from 0° to 180°. A circular electronic switch in the shaft of the probe can make changes of 1°.

The orientation of the sector at 0° and 90° is shown in **Figures 3A and B**.

**Q2. How long the transesophageal echocardiography probe can be left in the esophagus?**

**Ans.** The continued high-frequency pulsing of the acoustic array within a TEE probe causes its internal temperature to rise. The rise in tip temperature can be transferred to the patient, causing thermal damage or even burning of the esophagus. TEE transducers contain a temperature sensor, called a thermistor, within the tip to sense the temperature (of the tip, not the patient) and disable the ultrasound system if the tip temperature becomes excessively high. The TEE transducers have piezoelectric crystals. If a piezoelectric crystal is heated to its curie point, the domains become disordered, and the crystal becomes completely depolarized. A piezoelectric crystal's curie point or curie temperature is when it loses its piezoelectricity, and its tetragonal crystalline structure changes to a cubic one. Hence, it can function long without depolarization, but only at a temperature below the curie point. Normal ICU temperature will be halfway between 0° and its curie point.

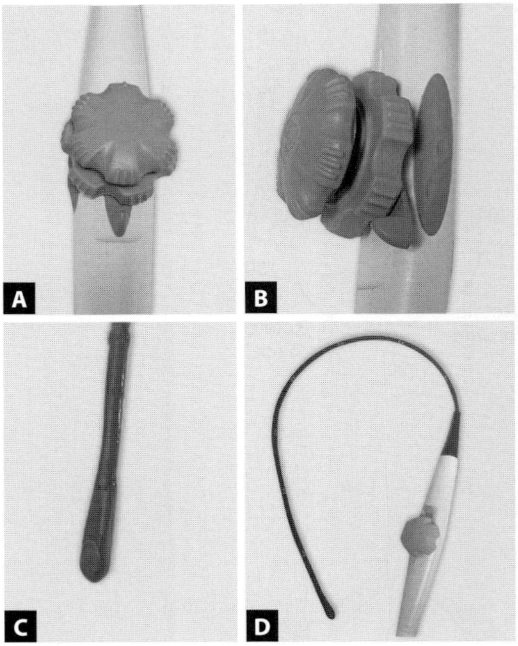

**Figs. 2A to D:** TEE Probe controls: (A) Illustration of a typical TEE probe and its various controls; (B and C) The omniplane controls are depicted by the two circular buttons that rotate the angle either forward or back; (D) Furthermore, the probe can be anteflexed or retroflexed by the large internal control wheel or turned left or right with the small external control wheel.

**TABLE 1:** Appropriate depth of insertion for transesophageal echocardiography (TEE) probe according to view.

| *View* | *Depth of insertion* |
|---|---|
| Upper esophageal view | 25–30 cm |
| Midesophageal view | 30–40 cm |
| Transgastric view | 40–45 cm |

Heat sterilization should not be done for probes as it depolarizes the crystal.

Transesophageal echocardiography transducers have two upper thermal limits: the first is set at 41°C, and the second is 42.5°C. If the temperature reaches 41°C, a warning appears, and if it reaches 42.5°C, the system freezes unconditionally and restarts only if it cools. Similarly, if the temperature reaches 17.5°C, the system freezes unconditionally and restarts only if it rises to 18°C.

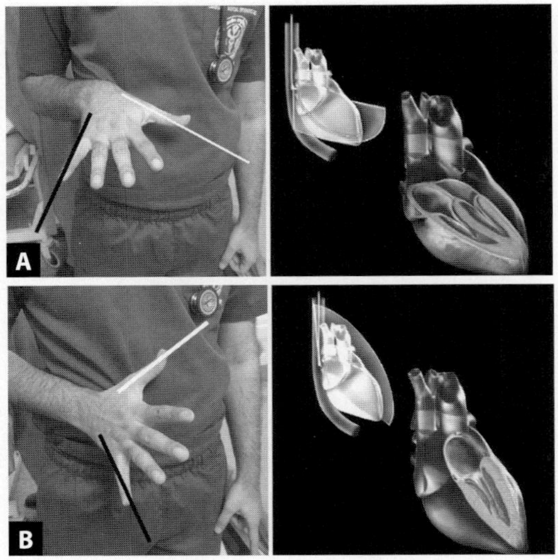

**Figs. 3A and B:** (A) Orientation of the sector at 0°; (B) Orientation of the sector at 90°. At 0° and 90°, the green line appears on the left of the sector, and the red line appears on the right. However, at 0°, the structures on the left are lateral, and at 90°, they are anterior. As the angle of the TEE probe is increased, the imaging plane changes in a clockwise direction.

Important TEE views with associated Doppler measurements required for image acquisition and interpretation competence **(Table 2)**.[4]

## APPLICATIONS OF TRANSESOPHAGEAL ECHOCARDIOGRAPHY IN THE INTENSIVE CARE UNIT

- *Hemodynamic assessment and evaluation **(Table 3)***: TEE enables functional hemodynamic monitoring along with systemic blood pressure, central venous pressure, and biomarkers of tissue perfusion.

**TABLE 2:** Transesophageal echocardiography (TEE) views along with Doppler measurements required for image acquisition and interpretation competence.

| *TEE view name* | *How to obtain the view* | *Information obtained from the view* |
|---|---|---|
| Midesophageal four-chamber view **(Figs. 4A and B)** | • *Transducer angle:* 0–10°<br>• *Level:* Midesophagus (30–35 cm from incisors) | • Assessment of left ventricle (LV) size and function<br>• Evaluation of LV contractility (anterolateral and inferoseptal walls) and presence of regional wall motion abnormality (RWMA)<br>• Estimation of volume status<br>• Right ventricle (RV) to LV cavity size ratio (RV dysfunction/ventricular interdependence)<br>• RV-free wall contractility<br>• Detection of pericardial effusion/tamponade physiology<br>• Assessment of left atrial (LA) and right atrial (RA) size<br>• Mitral valve (MV) and tricuspid valve (TV) two-dimensional, color flow, and Doppler assessment |
| Midesophageal two-chamber view **(Figs. 5A and B)** | • *Transducer angle:* 80–100°<br>• *Level:* Midesophagus | • *RWMA:* Left anterior descending (LAD) territory (anterior wall and right of screen), right coronary artery (RCA) (inferior wall and left of screen)<br>• Visualization of the left atrial appendage for LA clot detection |
| Midesophageal long-axis (LAX) view **(Figs. 6A and B)** | • *Transducer angle:* 120–140°<br>• *Level:* Midesophagus | • Assessment of LV size and function<br>• RWMA in the anteroseptal and inferolateral walls and apex of LV<br>• Gross valvular abnormalities (MV and AV) via two-dimensional and color flow assessment<br>• Detection of systolic anterior motion (SAM) in hypertrophic obstructive cardiomyopathy (HOCM) with left ventricular outflow tract (LVOT) obstruction<br>• Aortic root and ascending aortic pathology assessment<br>• Measurement of LVOT for calculating cardiac output (CO) and aortic valve area (AVA)<br>• Position of mechanical circulatory support devices (e.g., percutaneous temporary LV assist device)<br>• Ascending aorta (Ao) assessment |
| Midesophageal bicaval **(Figs. 7A and B)** and modified bicaval views **(Figs. 8A and B)** | • *Transducer angle:* 90–110°<br>• *Level:* Midesophagus<br>• *Maneuver:* Probe turned to the right | • RA pathology assessment<br>• Superior vena cava (SVC) and IVC assessment<br>• Intra-atrial septum assessment for atrial septal defect (ASD) or patent foramen ovale (PFO)<br>• Detection of thrombus, tumor, or mass in RA, paradoxical thrombus, or tumors/clots from IVC<br>• Guidance for placement and confirmation of central venous catheters and extracorporeal membrane oxygenation (ECMO) cannula |

*Contd...*

*Contd...*

| ***TEE view name*** | ***How to obtain the view*** | ***Information obtained from the view*** |
|---|---|---|
| Midesophageal aortic valve LAX view **(Figs. 9A and B)** | • *Transducer angle:* 120–140°<br>• *Level:* Midesophagus<br>• *Maneuver:* From ME LAX, withdraw + anteflexion | • Assessment of AV pathology (stenosis, regurgitation, infective endocarditis, tumor, Lambl's excrescences, and aortic dissection)<br>• Evaluation of ascending aortic aneurysm or dissection<br>• Prosthetic AV evaluation<br>• Detection of subaortic or supra-aortic membrane/stenosis<br>• LVOT and aortic annulus measurements |
| Midesophageal aortic valve short-axis (SAX) view **(Figs. 10A and B)** | • *Transducer angle:* 30–45°<br>• *Level:* Midesophagus<br>• *Maneuver:* Slight anteflexion | • AV pathology (bicuspid AV, endocarditis, and stenosis/regurgitation)<br>• Evaluation of tricuspid and pulmonary valves<br>• Detection of ventricular septal defects (VSD) |
| Midesophageal RV inflow–outflow view **(Figs. 11A and B)** | *Transducer angle:* 55–75° | Assessment of pulmonary valve pathology, main PA, and right ventricular outflow tract (RVOT) pathology |
| Transgastric LV SAX mid-papillary view **(Figs. 12A and B)** | • *Transducer angle:* 0–20°<br>• *Level:* Transgastric<br>• *Maneuver:* Advance + anteflexion | • Evaluation of cardiac function, LV hypertrophy, and volume status<br>• Coronary artery evaluation<br>• RWMA assessment<br>• Fractional area change (FAC) calculation for LV systolic function assessment<br>• Interventricular septum position for RV-LV interdependence (detecting RV pressure and/or volume overload)<br>• Detection of pericardial effusion |
| Deep transgastric five-chamber view **(Figs. 13A and B)** | • *Transducer angle:* 0–20°<br>• *Level:* Transgastric<br>• *Maneuver:* Advance, anteflex, and left flex | • AV pathology assessment (stenosis and regurgitation)<br>• Calculation of LVOT-velocity time integral (VTI) for cardiac output and AV area<br>• Shunt fraction calculation across septal defects (Qp)<br>• Confirmation of the position of temporary percutaneous LV assist device |
| Inferior vena cava (IVC)—hepatic vein (HV) view **(Figs. 14A and B)** | • *Transducer angle:* 50–70°<br>• *Level:* Transgastric<br>• *Maneuver:* Right flexion and advance | • IVC collapsibility, distension, and size assessment for volume responsiveness or venous congestion detection<br>• IVC compression assessment<br>• Doppler profile of IVC and hepatic veins to evaluate tricuspid valve function |
| Descending aortic SAX **(Figs. 15A and B)** and LAX views **(Figs. 16A and B)** | • *Transducer angle:* 0–10° and X-plane for perpendicular axis<br>• *Level:* Transgastric to midesophagus | • Detection of aortic aneurysm, dissection, and quantification of aortic atherosclerosis<br>• Guidance for the placement of the intra-aortic balloon pump (IABP) position and guide wire arterial cannula for ECMO |

*Contd...*

*Contd...*

| *TEE view name* | *How to obtain the view* | *Information obtained from the view* |
|---|---|---|
| | • *Maneuver:* Distal aorta on the left of the screen, proximal on the right | • Detection of pleural effusion |
| Ascending aortic SAX view **(Figs. 17A and B)** | • *Transducer angle:* 0–30°<br>• *Level:* Upper esophagus<br>• *Maneuver:* Anteflexion | • Aortic pathology assessment (aortic dissection and dilation)<br>• Pulmonary artery (PA) pathology evaluation (pulmonary embolism, dilated PA in pulmonary hypertension, and PA acceleration time measurement)<br>• Calculation of PA mean and diastolic pressures using Doppler-based hemodynamic calculations<br>• Confirmation of the position of the PA catheter and guidance for the placement of percutaneous right ventricular assist device (RVAD) |

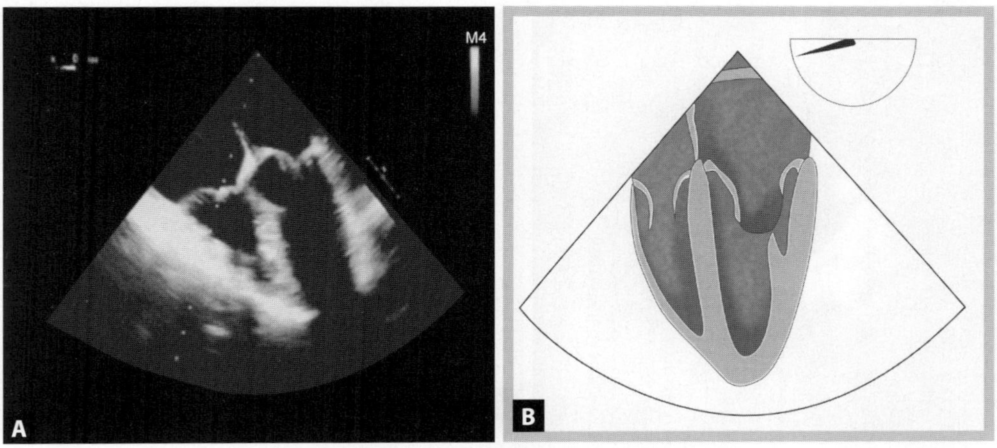


**Figs. 4A and B:** Midesophageal four-chamber view.

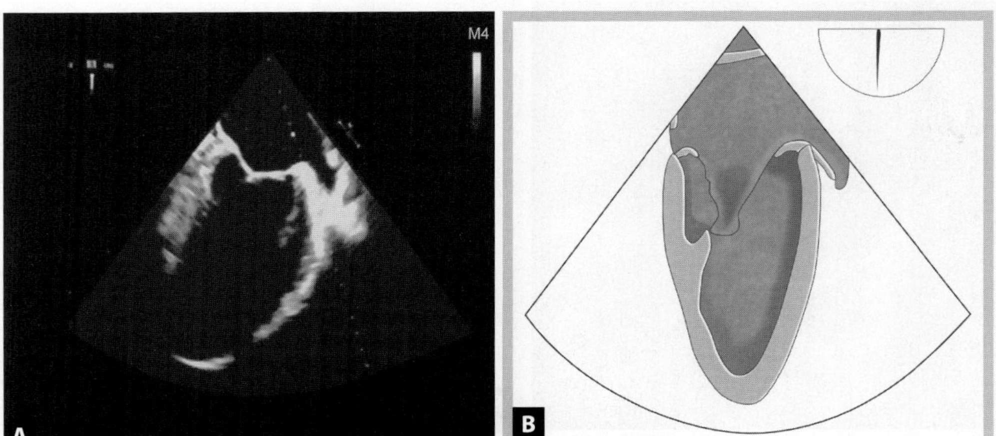


**Figs. 5A and B:** Midesophageal two-chamber view.

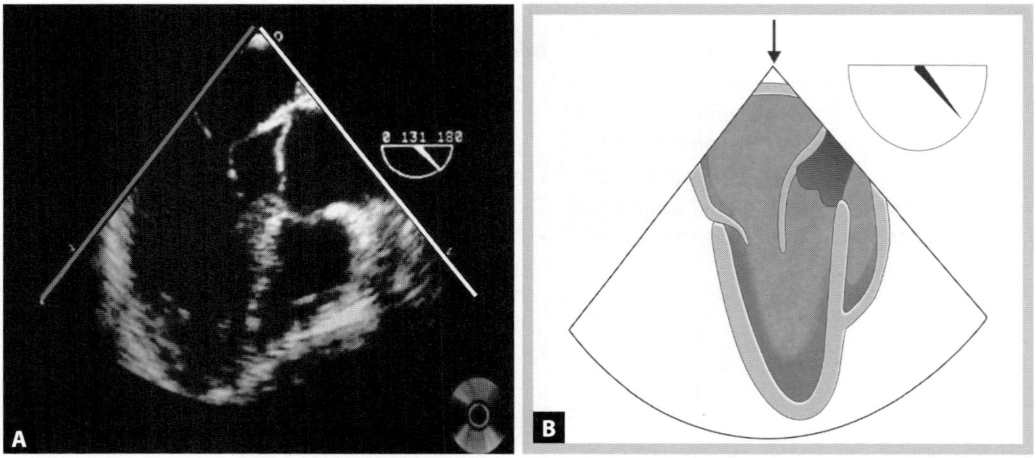


**Figs. 6A and B:** Midesophageal long-axis view.

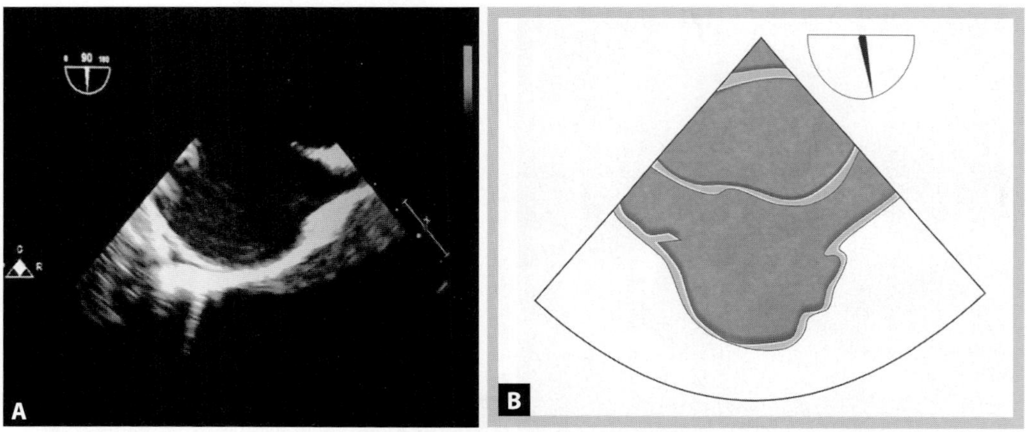


**Figs. 7A and B:** Midesophageal bicaval view.

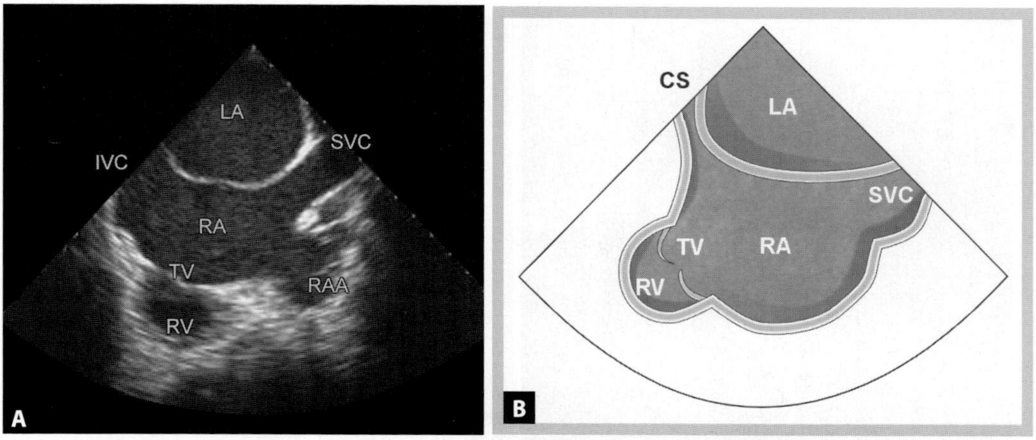


**Figs. 8A and B:** Midesophageal modified bicaval view. (CS: coronary sinus; IVC: inferior vena cava; RA: right atrium; RV: right ventricle; LA: left atrium; SVC: superior vena cava; TV: tricuspid valve)

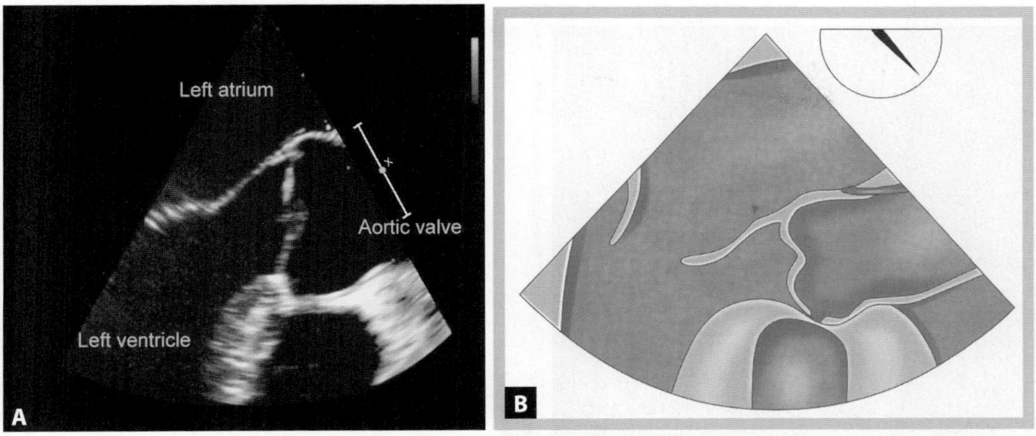


**Figs. 9A and B:** Midesophageal aortic valve long-axis view.

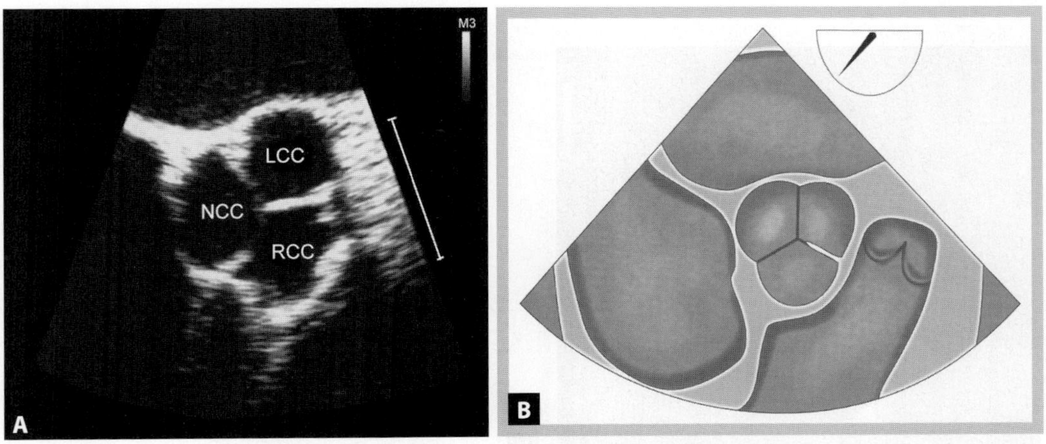


**Figs. 10A and B:** Midesophageal aortic valve short-axis view.
(LCC: left coronary cusp; NCC: Noncoronary cusp; RCC: right coronary cusp)

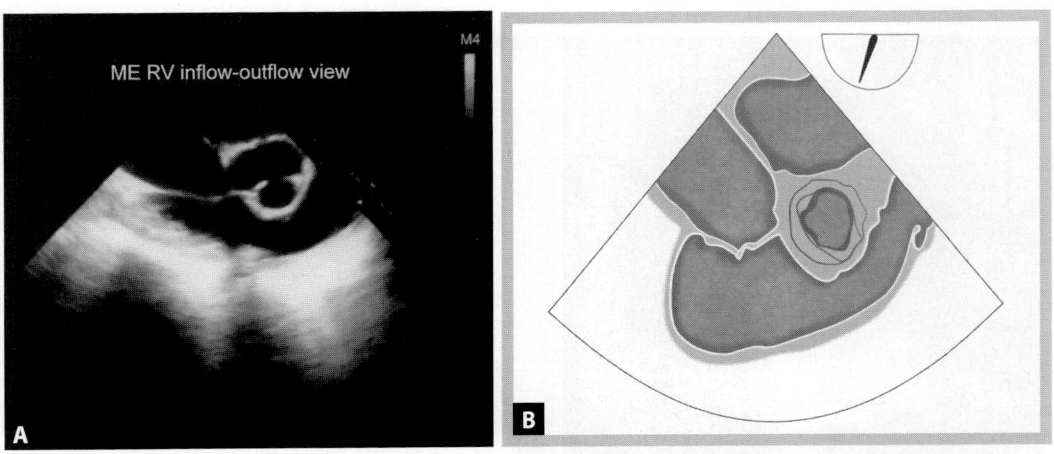


**Figs. 11A and B:** Midesophageal (ME) right ventricle (RV) inflow-outflow view.

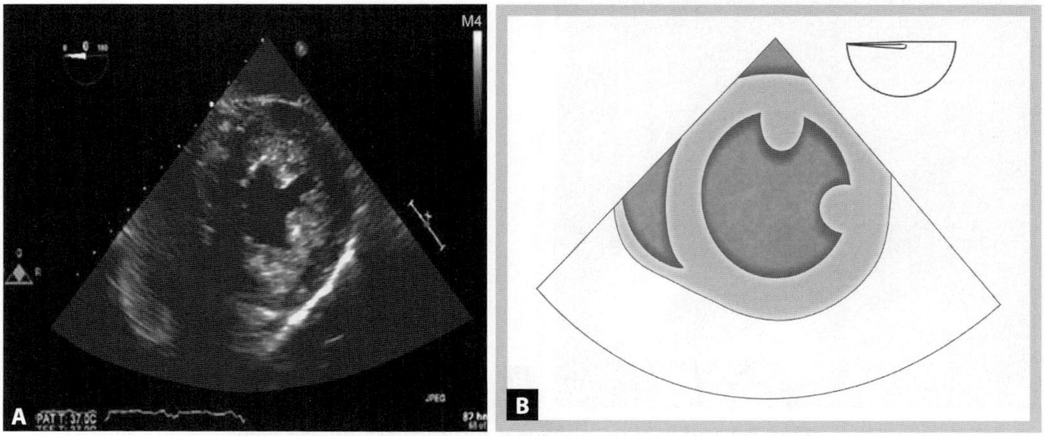


**Figs. 12A and B:** Transgastric left ventricle (LV) short-axis (SAX) mid-papillary view.

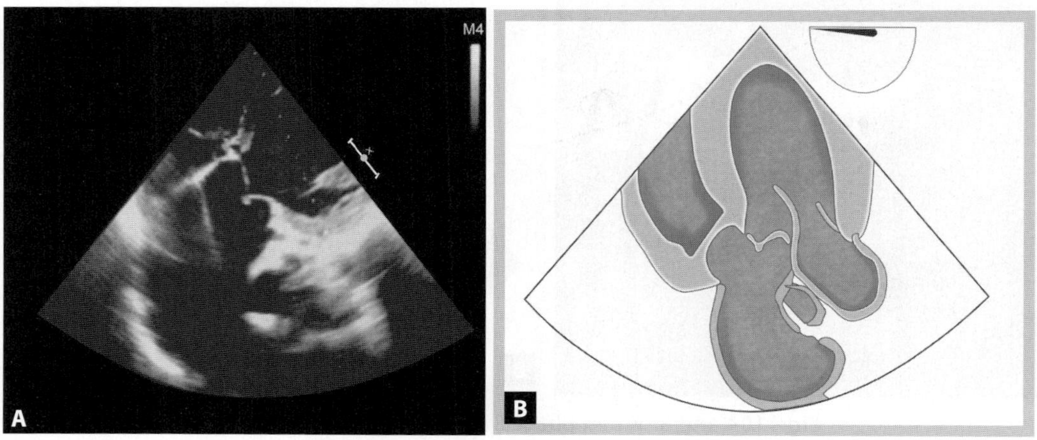


**Figs. 13A and B:** Deep transgastric five-chamber view.

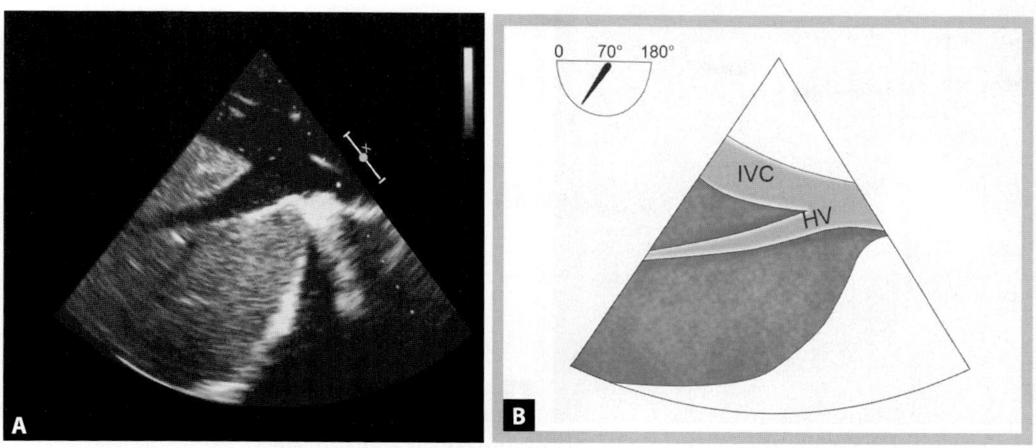


**Figs. 14A and B:** Inferior vena cava-hepatic vein (IVC-HV) view.

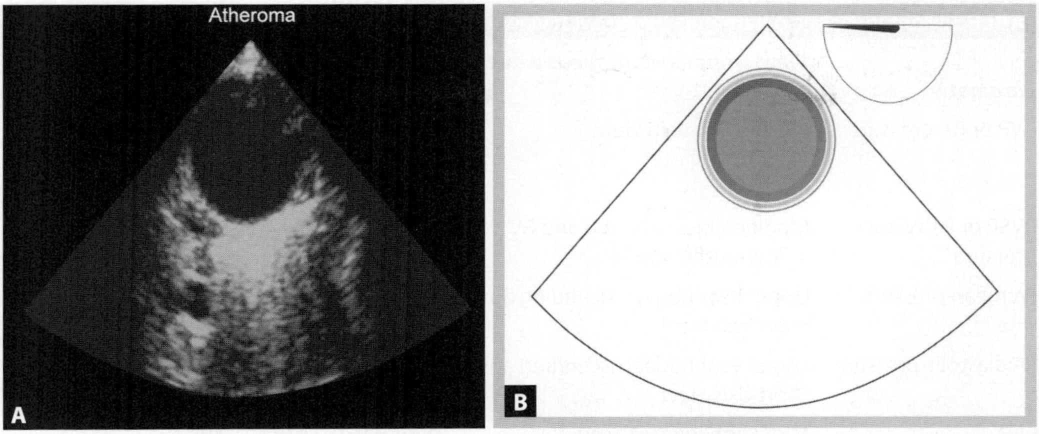


**Figs. 15A and B:** Descending aorta short-axis (SAX) view.

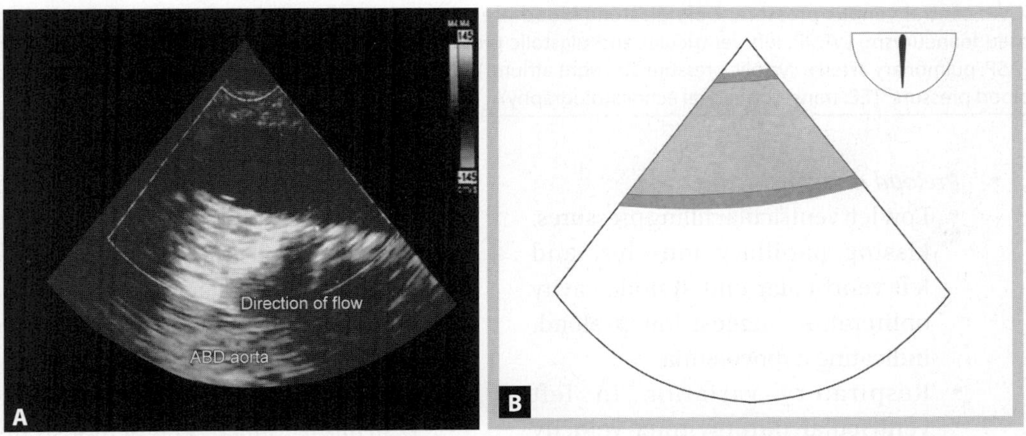


**Figs. 16A and B:** Descending aorta long-axis (LAX) view (ABD: abdominal).

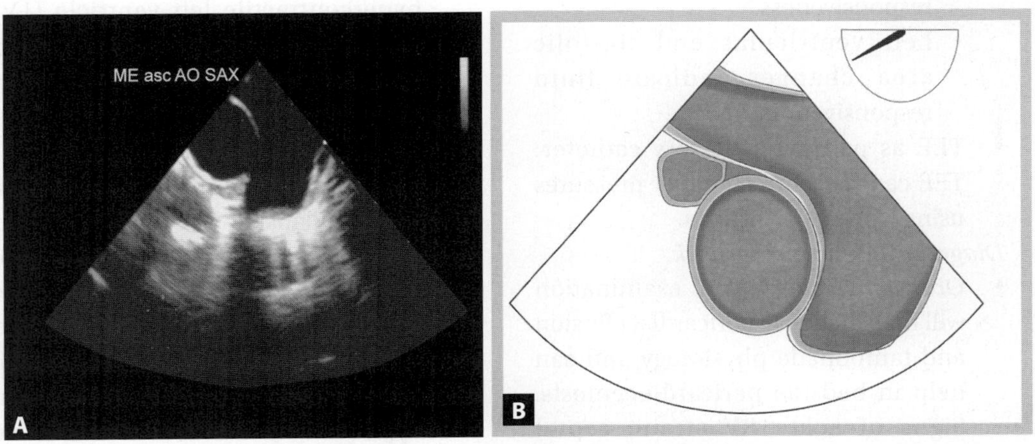


**Figs. 17A and B:** Ascending aorta short-axis (SAX) view.

**TABLE 3:** Hemodynamic parameters on TEE with view and relevant equations.

| *Parameter* | *View, Doppler continuous wave in all views* | *Equation* |
|---|---|---|
| CVP or RA pressure | IVC-hepatic vein view | IVC collapsibility index = (IVC maximum diameter – IVC minimum diameter)/IVC maximum diameter × 100 |
| RVSP or PA systolic pressure | Modified bicaval views and RV inflow-outflow view | RVSP or PASP = $4\ (V_{peak}\ TR)^2 + RAP$ |
| PA mean pressure | Upper esophageal ascending aortic short-axis view | PASP = $4\ (V_{peak}\ PR)^2 + RAP$ |
| PA diastolic pressure | Upper esophageal ascending aortic short-axis view | PADP = $4\ (V_{end\text{-}diastolic}\ PR)^2 + RAP$ |
| LAP | Midesophageal 4C view, midesophageal long-axis view | LAP = $SBP - 4\ (V_{peak}\ MR)^2$ |
| LVEDP | Deep transgastric 5C view | LVEDP = $DBP - 4\ (V_{end\text{-}diastolic}\ AR)^2$ |

(CVP: central venous pressure; DBP: diastolic blood pressure IVC: inferior vena cava; LAP: lumbar artery pseudoaneurysm; LVEDP: left ventricular end-diastolic pressure; PADP: pulmonary artery diastolic pressure; PASP: pulmonary arterial systolic pressure; RA: right atrium; RVSP: right ventricular systolic pressure; SBP: systolic blood pressure; TEE: transesophageal echocardiography)

- *Preload assessment:*
    - Low left ventricular filling pressures, kissing papillary muscles, and left ventricular end-systolic cavity obliteration suggest low preload, indicating hypovolemia.
    - Respiratory variation in left ventricular outflow tract velocity time integral (LVOT VTI) indicates stroke volume variation and fluid responsiveness.
    - Left ventricular end-diastolic area changes indicate fluid responsiveness.
- TEE as pulmonary artery catheter: TEE can measure chamber pressures using Doppler principles.

▪ *Diagnose the etiology of shock:*
- *Obstructive shock:* TEE examination will help diagnose pericardial effusion and tamponade physiology and can help in bedside pericardiocentesis. Signs of acute RV strain, septal deviation to the left, and evidence of RV overload point toward a pulmonary embolism, causing obstructive shock. TEE helps in the diagnosis of left-sided heart lesions, causing obstructive shock, such as critical aortic valve stenosis and coarctation of the aorta.
- *Distributive shock:* TEE demonstrates a collapsible inferior vena cava (IVC), superior vena cava (SVC), hypercontractile left ventricle (LV) with a preserved or higher ejection fraction. Left ventricular outflow tract velocity time integral (LVOT-VTI) shows respiratory variations.
- *Hypovolemic shock:* TEE shows a small, collapsible IVC with decreased LV end-diastolic area (LVEDA), reduced LVOT-VTI, and low cardiac output. TEE enables qualitative and quantitative assessment of preload, which helps differentiate between hypovolemic shock and distributive

shock. In both conditions, the end-diastolic diameter will be decreased with hyperdynamic LV. LVEDA measurement helps differentiate between both, in which LVEDA is normal in distributive shock and reduced with hypovolemic shock.

- *Cardiogenic shock:* TEE can demonstrate reduced ejection fraction, reduced LVOT-VTI, dilated IVC, ischemia causing regional wall motion abnormality (RWMA), gross valvular abnormalities, or infective endocarditis. TEE can demonstrate LV dysfunction, RV dysfunction, or biventricular dysfunction.

- *In cardiopulmonary resuscitation (CPR):* During cardiac arrest, TEE plays a crucial role by providing real-time heart imaging, allowing for an assessment of cardiac function and identification of potential reversible causes of the arrest. It helps minimize the duration of pulse checks and guides resuscitative efforts more effectively. TEE offers immediate feedback on the effectiveness of CPR and the return of spontaneous circulation. Additionally, it aids in predicting the need for mechanical circulatory support (MCS), facilitates the precise placement of MCS devices **(Table 4)**, prevents complications, and helps assess the response to therapy postplacement, as well as assists in the weaning process from MCS.
- *TEE can help evaluate lungs.*
  - Transesophageal lung ultrasound (TELU) can help visualize the left lung better via the aorta. Posterosuperior segments of the lungs can only be seen with TEE, as the scapula prevents a proper acoustic window. Performing TELU with each TEE examination in the ICU will help better understand the patient.
  - To assess the apical, mid, and basal levels of the lung, begin by visualizing the left subclavian artery, left superior pulmonary vein, and the IVC-RA junction at 0°. Rotate the omniplane to 90° and turn the probe to each side to examine the anterior, mid, and basal segments at each level. This approach allows for visualization of various lung features, including A lines, B lines, air bronchograms, and areas of lung hepatization. Lung consolidation can be observed in these hepatized areas, while air bronchograms, which are hyperechoic foci within consolidated regions, indicate the presence of dynamic or static conditions. A dynamic air bronchogram suggests consolidation, whereas a static air bronchogram indicates atelectasis.
- *TEE can help evaluate the veins:*
  - Standard view on TEE helps analyze SVC, IVC, hepatic vein, coronary sinus, and pulmonary veins.
  - Venous excess ultrasound score, or VExUS, can help guide fluid therapy and prognosticate acute kidney injury (AKI). The score is determined by assessing the IVC, hepatic vein, portal vein, and renal vein.
- *TEE can help evaluate hypoxemia:* Cause of hypoxemia can be diagnosed by evaluating heart, lungs, and pulmonary artery.

Transesophageal echocardiography is a minimally invasive procedure with a low risk of complications. Advanced critical care TEE is performed only on intubated and mechanically ventilated patients; hence, the risks of airway complications are less. The patients are well-sedated and monitored in the ICU environment. Hence, respiratory or cardiovascular compromise risks are minimal

**TABLE 4:** Role of transesophageal echocardiography (TEE) in placing MCS devices.

| ***Device*** | ***Site of cannulation/final position*** | ***TEE view*** |
|---|---|---|
| Intra-aortic balloon pump (IABP) | Femoral artery | Descending thoracic aorta (DTA) short-axis (SAX) and long-axis (LAX) views—guide wire in descending aorta |
| | Axillary artery | Aortic arch SAX and LAX views—guide wire in the aortic arch and the balloon in the DTA |
| | Final position | Rotate the probe counterclockwise at the end of the aortic arch to visualize the left subclavian artery (LSCA)—balloon should be placed 2–3 cm below the LSCA |
| Left ventricular assist device (LVAD) | Femoral cannulation | Descending aorta (DA), SAX, and LAX views Aortic arch SAX and LAX views. Midesophageal (ME) LAX views—guide wire and catheter visualized in the DTA and advanced into the left ventricle (LV) via the ascending aorta (AA) |
| | Axillary cannulation | AA SAX and LAX views. ME four-chamber (4C) view—the guide wire and catheter are visualized in the aortic arch and advanced into the LV via the AA |
| | Final position | Transgastric SAX view—the metal cap at the LVAD inlet appears as a tear-drop shape and should be positioned 3.5–4 cm from the aortic valve inside the LV cavity, with the outlet 3 cm from the aortic valve in the proximal AA. LV size and function are assessed before and after deployment |
| Right ventricular assist device (RVAD) | Peripheral cannulation | ME 4C view, RV inflow-outflow view—the wire and cannula are placed in the right atrium, right ventricle (RV), and main pulmonary artery (PA) |
| | Final position | AA SAX and LAX views for distal tip positioning—the cannula enters from the superior vena cava (SVC) and/or inferior vena cava (IVC), with the distal tip in the main PA trunk |
| Veno-arterial extracorporeal membrane oxygenation (ECMO) | *Peripheral cannulation:*<br>• Femoral artery<br>• Femoral vein<br>• Axillary artery<br>• Internal jugular vein | • DA SAX and LAX views—the cannula is placed in the DTA<br>• ME LAX view—the cannula is placed in the IVC/right atrium (RA)<br>• AA SAX and LAX views—the cannula is placed in the aortic arch<br>• ME 4C view—the cannula is placed in the SVC/RA |
| | *Central cannulation:*<br>• Venous cannula<br>• Arterial cannula | • ME-RV inflow-outflow view—placed in the RA or IVC and SVC<br>• ME bicaval view—placed in the aortic arch |
| Venovenous ECMO | Drainage return | ME 4C view, RV inflow-outflow view, ME bicaval view, transgastric IVC—hepatic vein view—the cannula is placed in the FV |

when intensivists in the ICU perform TEE. The major risks of advanced critical care TEE are related to mechanical injury from probe insertion and manipulation in the esophagus. Minor oropharyngeal injury is uncommon and is of limited clinical concern. Major injury to the hypopharynx, esophagus, or stomach, even though uncommon, can cause severe clinical consequences, requiring surgical interventions or even death. Hence, appropriate patient selection is important.

## UPPER GASTROINTESTINAL BLEEDING AFTER TRANSESOPHAGEAL ECHOCARDIOGRAPHY

The overall major bleeding rate of the intraoperative TEE is very low (0.0–0.8%).[5] Upper gastrointestinal bleeding (UGIB) following TEE is managed with endoscopic thermal ablation or clipping of bleeding vessels if conservative measures fail.

## ESOPHAGEAL PERFORATION AFTER TRANSESOPHAGEAL ECHOCARDIOGRAPHY

Esophageal perforation (EP) is one of the most severe complications following TEE, with a reported incidence between 0.03% and 0.09%.[6] The major cause of TEE-induced esophageal rupture may be explained by the prolonged, continuous pressure of the TEE probe on the esophageal mucosa and the possible low blood circulation in the esophagus due to critical illness. A prompt diagnosis and initiating an effective treatment on time are crucial for the patient's survival. A history of multiple attempts to insert the TEE probe along with subcutaneous emphysema, voice changes, and systemic inflammatory response syndrome (SIRS) should raise a clinical suspicion of esophageal perforation. Primary repair is the modality of choice when dealing with esophageal perforations, especially when diagnosed during the first 24 hours.

## TRANSESOPHAGEAL ECHOCARDIOGRAPHY IN COAGULOPATHIC PATIENTS

Coagulopathy and thrombocytopenia are considered relative contraindications for the performance of TEE according to ASE guidelines.[5] Kitkungvan et al. evaluated the safety of TEE in patients with cancer with platelet counts <100,000/mL and found a complication rate of only 0.3%.[7] Nowak-Machen et al. examined TEE's safety in critically ill patients undergoing extracorporeal membrane oxygenation (ECMO) support with an average activated partial thromboplastin time (aPTT) of 60 seconds. The only complication seen in their population was minor oropharyngeal bleeding (2.3%).[8]

Transesophageal echocardiography in the ICU has emerged as a pivotal diagnostic and monitoring tool, offering real-time, detailed imaging of cardiac structures and function. Its utility in critically ill patients lies in its ability to provide a comprehensive assessment of complex cardiac conditions that are often challenging to diagnose with TTE, especially in the presence of mechanical ventilation or other factors that impede optimal imaging. TEE's enhanced visualization capabilities aid in accurately evaluating valvular pathologies, intracardiac thrombi, endocarditis, and hemodynamic status, facilitating timely and precise therapeutic interventions. As a result, its integration into ICU protocols significantly enhances patient management, contributing to improved outcomes through targeted treatment strategies based on precise diagnostic information.

## REFERENCES


1. Porter TR, Abdelmoneim S, Belcik JT, McCulloch ML, Mulvagh SL, Olson JJ, et al. Guidelines for the cardiac sonographer in the performance of contrast echocardiography: a focused update from the American Society of Echocardiography. J Am Soc Echocardiogr. 2014;27(8):797-810.
2. Si X, Ma J, Cao DY, Xu HL, Zuo LY, Chen MY, et al. Transesophageal echocardiography instead or in addition to transthoracic echocardiography in evaluating haemodynamic problems in intubated critically ill patients. Ann Transl Med. 2020;8(12):785.
3. Charron C, Vignon P, Prat G, Tonnelier A, Aegerter P, Boles JM, et al. Number of supervised studies required to reach competence in advanced critical care transesophageal echocardiography. Intensive Care Med. 2013;39(6):1019-24.
4. Shanewise JS, Cheung AT, Aronson S, Stewart WJ, Weiss RL, Mark JB, et al. ASE/SCA guidelines for performing a comprehensive intraoperative multiplane transesophageal echocardiography examination: recommendations of the American Society of Echocardiography Council for Intraoperative Echocardiography and the Society of Cardiovascular Anesthesiologists Task Force for Certification in Perioperative Transesophageal Echocardiography. Anesth Analg. 1999;89(4):870-84.
5. Hahn RT, Abraham T, Adams MS, Bruce CJ, Glas KE, Lang RM, et al. Guidelines for performing a comprehensive transesophageal echocardiographic examination: recommendations from the American Society of Echocardiography and the Society of Cardiovascular Anesthesiologists. J Am Soc Echocardiogr. 2013;26(9):921-64.
6. Agha RA, Borrelli MR, Farwana R, Koshy K, Fowler AJ, Orgill DP, et al. The SCARE 2018 statement: Updating consensus Surgical CAse REport (SCARE) guidelines. Int J Surg. 2018;60:132-6.
7. Kitkungvan D, Kalluru D, Lunagariya A, Sanchez L, Yusuf SW, Hassan S, et al. Safety of Transesophageal Echocardiography in Patients with Thrombocytopenia. J Am Soc Echocardiogr. 2019;32(8):1010-5.
8. Nowak-Machen M, Schmid E, Schlensak C, Consferent C, Haeberle HA, Rosenberger P, et al. Safety of transesophageal echocardiography during extracorporeal life support. Perfusion. 2016;31(8):634-9.

CHAPTER 35

# Self Assessment in Critical Care Echocardiography

*Rakupathy S, Gourav Mittal, Puneet Khanna*

## SECTION A: ULTRASOUND PHYSICS

**Q1. The relationship between frequency (f), wavelength (λ), and velocity (c) of ultrasound waves:**

a. Velocity varies inversely with wavelength and frequency
b. Velocity varies directly with wavelength and frequency
c. Frequency and velocity vary inversely with wavelength
d. Frequency and velocity vary directly with wavelength

**Q2. The loss of ultrasound energy can be due to:**

a. Scattering
b. Acoustic impedance
c. Reflection and refraction
d. All of the above

**Q3. How to improve brightness at deeper structures?**

a. Time gain compensation (TGC)
b. Focal point adjustment
c. Low-frequency probe
d. All of the above

**Q4. All are true about pulse wave (PW) Doppler, *except*:**

a. PW doppler emits short bursts of ultrasound waves and receives returning echoes from a particular depth within the heart
b. Blood flow velocity can be measured by the Doppler shift principle
c. PW Doppler measures high velocities across the valves
d. The angle of PW Doppler impacts the measurement

**Q5. Bernoulli equation assumes all, *except*:**

a. Pulsatile blood flow
b. Laminar blood flow
c. Density of blood is constant
d. Blood flow resistance is zero

**Q6. Which of the following is a primary advantage of continuous wave (CW) Doppler ultrasound over PW Doppler?**

a. Higher resolution in deep tissues
b. Ability to measure high-velocity blood flow without aliasing
c. Better spatial resolution
d. ENHANCED imaging of small structures

**Q7. True about pulse repetition frequency (PRF) is:**

a. PRF and $v_{max}$ are inversely proportional
b. Deeper structures require low PRF
c. Increasing the PRF relative to the target depth decreases aliasing
d. Low PRF improves the visualization of high-velocity flows

**Q8. Aliasing can be corrected by:**

a. Increasing velocity scale
b. Low-frequency probe and low PRF
c. Baseline adjustment
d. All of the above

**Q9. Advantages of phased array probes all, *except*:**

a. Piezoelectric crystals are arranged in a rectangular grid, and each of them can be controlled independently
b. Beam steering and focusing electronically allows precise measurement at deeper structures
c. Both axial and lateral resolution are better
d. Inferior to curvilinear probe for resolution of deeper structures

**Q10. Relationship between probe frequency and penetration**

a. High-frequency probes have longer near-field
b. The angle of divergence increases with high frequency
c. Near field increases with decreasing frequency
d. Low-frequency probe has low angle of divergence

**Q11. All of the following are limitations of M-mode, *except*:**

a. Provides one-dimensional information
b. Measurement of moving objects
c. Tissue characteristics are poorly defined
d. Cannot provide blood flow information

**Q12. The incorrect statement about color flow Doppler is:**

a. Provides the spatial resolution between the structure and blood flow
b. Cannot measure blood flow velocities
c. Aliasing artifacts can be overcome by color Doppler
d. Uses multiple PW Doppler samples over an area represented by different colors

**Q13. Regarding angle of ultrasound beam**

a. Doppler shift is proportional to the tangent of the angle between the ultrasound beam and the direction of blood cells
b. Higher the angle, the better the estimate
c. Doppler shift is significantly affected when the angle exceeds >20°
d. None of the above

**Q14. What is the depth of penetration of the 3.5 MHz phased array probe?**

a. 4–8 cm
b. 5–10 cm
c. 6–12 cm
d. 9–18 cm

**Q15. Tissue Doppler imaging (TDI) measures:**

a. Blood flow velocity
b. Both systolic and diastolic function
c. It could not be used for tissues other than the heart.
d. None of the above

**Q16. What is the approximate speed at which sound travels through human tissues?**

a. About 1,540 m/s
b. About 1,540 km/s
c. About 1,540 cm/s
d. About 1,540 m/s

**Q17. Which factor contributes to an increase in the frame rate during ultrasound imaging?**

a. Increasing the depth of imaging
b. Decreasing the sector angle
c. Increasing line density
d. Adding color Doppler to B-mode imaging

**Q18. Which characteristic of a reflected ultrasound wave is most critical for generating a two-dimensional (2D) image?**

a. Pulse repetition period (PRP)
b. Period
c. Amplitude
d. Pulse duration

**Q19. Which of the following is not affected by increasing the imaging depth?**

a. PRF
b. PRP
c. Pulse duration
d. Duty factor

**Q20. 2D ultrasound images are produced due to which phenomenon when ultrasound waves interact with tissue?**

a. Specular reflection
b. Backscatter
c. Refraction

**Q21. Under which condition is ultrasound attenuation greater as it travels through tissue?**

a. Greater depth
b. In blood
c. Lower transducer frequency
d. In bone > in air

**Q22. Which adjustment will increase the frame rate in ultrasound imaging?**

a. Increase transmit power (TP)
b. Increase transmit frequency (TF)
c. Decrease sector angle
d. Increase imaging depth

**Q23. Lateral resolution in ultrasound imaging improves by:**

a. Decreasing transmit frequency
b. Decreasing power
c. Beam focusing
d. Reducing transducer diameter

**Q24. Which adjustment can improve axial resolution in ultrasound imaging?**

a. Reduce beam diameter
b. Beam focusing
c. Reduce gain
d. Increase transmit frequency

**Q25. What does the duty factor refer to in ultrasound imaging?**

a. Damping material physical properties
b. Transducer range of frequencies
c. Power generation by the transducer
d. Fraction of time the transducer is emitting ultrasound

**Q26. The duty factor increases with the following:**

a. Gain increase
b. Pulse duration increase
c. Decreasing PRF
d. Dynamic range decreased

**Q27. What is the Nyquist limit at a PRF of 1,000 Hz?**

a. 500 Hz
b. Cannot calculate
c. 2,000 Hz
d. 1,000 Hz

**Q28. How can the Nyquist limit be increased?**

a. With PRF increase
b. With PRF decrease
c. None of above

**Q29. The Nyquist limit can also be increased by:**

a. With an increase in transducer frequency
b. With a reduction in transducer frequency
c. Filter reduction
d. None of the above

**Q30. Aliasing in Doppler ultrasound is reduced by:**

a. Reduction in depth
b. With an increase in the PRF
c. Transducer frequency reduction
d. Switching to CW Doppler
e. All of the above

**Q31. If the ultrasound scan image is dark throughout, how do you troubleshoot?**

a. By output power increase
b. By receiver gain increase
c. Switch to higher frequency transducer
d. Receivers gain reduction

**Q32. Flow resistance depends most strongly on:**

a. Vessel length
b. Vessel radius
c. Blood viscosity
d. All of the above

**Q33. Which of the following is represented in real-time on a color Doppler display?**

a. Doppler spectrum
b. Flow direction
c. Gray-scale anatomy
d. b and c
e. All of the above

**Q34. For obtaining one line of color Doppler, how many pulses are required?**

a. One
b. 10,000
c. 10
d. 100

**Q35. The Bernoulli equation is a classic example of:**

a. Law of conservation of momentum
b. Law of conservation of energy
c. Law of conservation of mass
d. None of the above

**Q36. The continuity equation is the best example of:**

a. Conservation of mass
b. Conservation of momentum
c. Conservation of energy
d. None of the above

**Q37. The color flow jet area of mitral regurgitation (MR) depends upon:**

a. Amount of regurgitation alone
b. Driving pressure and the regurgitant volume
c. Presence of aortic regurgitation (AR)
d. Degree of mitral stenosis (MS)

**Q38. The PRF is influenced by:**

a. The ultrasound source
b. Medium of transmission
c. a and b
d. Neither

**Q39. Reducing the transducer footprint will impact:**

a. Lateral resolution
b. Temporal resolution
c. Axial resolution
d. None of the above

**Q40. Increasing the transmit power will lead to:**

a. Sensitivity decrease
b. Lateral resolution increase
c. Penetration increase
d. None of the above

## Answers and Explanations

1. **Ans. b**
The velocity of an ultrasound wave is directly proportional to wavelength and frequency.
2. **Ans. d**
As ultrasound waves cross two different interfaces, some of it is reflected, deflected (refraction), scattered, and attenuated (acoustic impedance).
3. **Ans. d**
Gain increases the brightness at the cost of background noise. TGC is a series of sliding controls for gain adjustment. Low-frequency (higher wavelength) probes have better penetration for deeper structures. The focal point can be shifted to deeper structures to increase the visualization.
4. **Ans. c**
Pulsed wave Doppler measures blood flow velocities by using the Doppler principle. It emits short pulses of ultrasound waves and measures blood flow velocities directed toward a particular depth (sampling gate). The angle of the beam impacts measurement that higher the angle, the underestimation of velocities will occur. It cannot measure high-velocity flows across heart valves.
5. **Ans. a**
The assumptions made by Simplified Bernoulli's equation are that blood flow is nonpulsatile, laminar, zero resistance, and the density of blood is constant.

6. **Ans. b**

Continuous wave Doppler can measure high-velocity blood flow because it continuously transmits and receives ultrasound waves, bypassing the limitations of PRF and avoiding aliasing, a common issue with PW Doppler.

7. **Ans. b**

Pulse repetition frequency is defined as the number of ultrasound pulses emitted by the transducer in a given period of time. It is inversely proportional to the maximum depth that can be effectively imaged and directly proportional to the flow velocity of fast-moving objects. Deeper structures require more time for echoes to return, so a lower PRF is necessary to avoid missing echoes from these deeper tissues. A higher PRF is beneficial for capturing fast-moving blood flow. However, if the PRF is too high for the depth being examined, aliasing artifacts may occur.

8. **Ans. d**

Aliasing artifact is due to the inability of the sampling gate to measure the velocity of target objects, resulting in flow reversal in returning echoes. Low PRF and low-frequency probes allow measurement at deeper structures, whereas the velocity scale can be adjusted according to the desired depth and velocity of objects being measured.

9. **Ans. d**

Piezoelectric crystals in phased array probes are arranged in rectangular grids with individual elements, each capable of generating ultrasound beams. Beam steering and focusing can be electronically controlled by adjusting the timing and intensity of stimulation. It can produce a greater resolution of deeper structures by enhancing both axial and lateral resolution compared to curvilinear probes, which is best for near-surface organs in the abdomen.

10. **Ans. a**

The near field is the initial columnar portion of the beam, and the far field is the late diverging segment of the beam. As frequency increases, the near field lengthens, and the angle of divergence decreases and, resulting in better resolution.

11. **Ans. b**

M-mode provides information about timing and movement along a single line in one dimension. PW and color Doppler are needed for blood flow measurement, and B-mode provides detailed tissue characteristics.

12. **Ans. c**

Color Doppler, a form of PW Doppler, provides instantaneous distribution of flow across structures, depicted as a mixture of red and blue colors. It is a semi-quantitative technique, and aliasing occurs when the velocity exceeds the Nyquist limit.

13. **Ans. c**

Doppler shift is proportional to the cosine of the angle between the ultrasound beam and blood cells. When the beam is parallel to blood cells (angle is zero; cosine 0 = 1), it provides the best estimate of velocity. In clinical practice, angles <15° are not affected by Doppler shift.

14. **Ans. d**

Wavelength

= velocity of sound in blood/frequency

= 1,540,000 (mm/s)/350,000 (Hz)

= 0.44 mm

Depth of penetration
= 200–400 × wavelength
= 200–400 × (0.44 mm)
= 9–18 cm

15. **Ans. b**

Tissue Doppler measures the movement of tissues, a form of PWD. It can measure both systolic ($S_m$) and diastolic (e') function of LV. Recently, other tissue functions have also been evaluated by TDI (e.g., diaphragm). It cannot measure blood flow velocities.

16. **Ans. a**

The speed of sound in human tissues, particularly in soft tissues, is approximately 1,540 m/s. This value is crucial for accurate imaging in ultrasound as it affects the calculation of distances and the formation of images.

17. **Ans. b**

Reducing the sector angle decreases the number of scan lines needed for each frame, which allows the ultrasound machine to refresh the image more quickly. This increases the frame rate, enhancing temporal resolution and providing smoother motion imaging.

18. **Ans. c**

The amplitude of the reflected ultrasound wave is the primary factor that influences the brightness of the pixels in a 2D ultrasound image. Variations in amplitude correspond to different tissue densities and interfaces, allowing for the detailed visualization of structures within the body.

19. **Ans. c**

Increasing depth affects the pulse repetition period (the time between pulses), PRF (the number of pulses per second), and duty factor (the percentage of time the transducer is emitting sound). However, pulse duration (the time for one pulse) is determined by the transducer and remains constant, regardless of depth.

20. **Ans. b**

Two-dimensional images are primarily created by backscatter, where the ultrasound waves are scattered in many directions upon hitting tissue interfaces. This scattering provides the detailed information necessary to form an image.

21. **Ans. a**

Attenuation increases with depth as the ultrasound waves lose more energy the further they travel. Higher frequency transducers also experience more attenuation, and bone attenuates ultrasound much more than soft tissue or air.

22. **Ans. c**

Reducing the sector angle lowers the number of scan lines per frame, which in turn increases the frame rate. Increasing depth or transmit frequency usually results in a lower frame rate, while increasing transmit power does not have a direct impact on the frame rate.

23. **Ans. c**

The lateral resolution, which is the ability to distinguish two points perpendicular to the ultrasound beam, improves with beam focusing, as it narrows the beam width. Decreasing transducer diameter and reducing transmit frequency generally worsen lateral resolution, while reducing power does not directly affect resolution.

24. **Ans. d**

Axial resolution, which refers to the ability to distinguish two points along the path of the ultrasound beam, improves with higher transmit frequency as it shortens the wavelength, leading to better detail. Reducing beam diameter and focusing the beam primarily enhances lateral resolution, while gain adjustment affects image brightness but does not influence resolution.

25. **Ans. d**
The duty factor is the fraction or percentage of time that the ultrasound transducer is actively emitting sound waves. It indicates the proportion of time spent transmitting sound waves compared to the time spent listening to echoes.

26. **Ans. b**
The duty factor increases with longer pulse duration, as the transducer spends more time emitting sound during each cycle. Increasing gain or changing dynamic range does not affect the duty factor; while, decreasing PRF typically increases the listening time, not the duty factor.

27. **Ans. a**
The Nyquist limit is half of the PRF. At a PRF of 1,000 Hz, the Nyquist limit is 500 Hz, which is the highest Doppler frequency that can be accurately measured without aliasing.

28. **Ans. a**
The Nyquist limit can be increased by increasing the PRF. A higher PRF raises the Nyquist limit, allowing for the accurate measurement of higher Doppler frequencies without aliasing.

29. **Ans. d**
The Nyquist limit is not directly affected by the transducer frequency or the filter settings. It is primarily dependent on the PRF. Therefore, none of the options listed directly increases the Nyquist limit.

30. **Ans. e**
Aliasing can be reduced by decreasing the imaging depth (which increases the PRF), increasing the PRF, lowering the transducer frequency, or using CW Doppler, as it is not subject to aliasing.

31. **Ans. b**
The first step to brighten a dark ultrasound image is to increase the receiver gain, which amplifies the received signal and enhances image brightness. Increasing output power is a secondary option, but increasing gain is typically faster and safer.

32. **Ans. b**
According to Poiseuille's law, flow resistance is primarily influenced by the vessel radius. A small change in radius can greatly affect resistance, as it is inversely proportional to the fourth power of the radius. While vessel length and blood viscosity also impact resistance, their effect is less significant compared to the radius.

33. **Ans. d**
Color Doppler provides real-time grey-scale anatomy alongside the direction and speed of blood flow. However, the Doppler spectrum, which shows detailed flow velocity information, is not usually displayed in real-time on the color Doppler screen.

34. **Ans. c**
Usually, about 10 pulses are necessary to gather one line of color Doppler information. This allows for precise evaluation of flow characteristics and reduces the impact of noise.

35. **Ans. b**
The Bernoulli equation is based on the principle of conservation of energy. It describes the relationship between pressure, velocity, and height

in a flowing fluid, demonstrating that the total mechanical energy remains conserved throughout the flow.

36. **Ans. a**

The continuity equation is derived from the law of conservation of mass, which states that the mass flow rate must remain constant across different cross-sections of a pipe. This implies that the product of cross-sectional area and velocity must remain constant.

37. **Ans. b**

The color flow jet area of MR is influenced by both the driving pressure across the valve and the volume of regurgitant blood. A higher driving pressure and greater regurgitant volume led to a larger jet area.

38. **Ans. c**

The PRF is determined by both the ultrasound system settings (source) and the characteristics of the medium through which the ultrasound waves travel. The speed of sound in the medium affects the rate at which echoes return, thereby influencing the PRF.

39. **Ans. a**

Reducing the transducer footprint typically affects lateral resolution because it changes the width of the ultrasound beam. A smaller footprint can make it harder to focus the beam, reducing lateral resolution. Axial resolution and temporal resolution are not directly impacted by the footprint size.

40. **Ans. c**

Increasing transmits power boosts the intensity of the ultrasound waves, allowing them to penetrate deeper into the tissue, thus enhancing the imaging of deeper structures. It does not directly affect lateral resolution or sensitivity.

## SECTION B: CRITICAL CARE ECHOCARDIOGRAPHY

**Q41. Critical care echocardiography involves:**

a. Done by cardiologist
b. Done by an intensivist and interpreted by a cardiologist
c. Inadequate for patient monitoring
d. Involves both transthoracic echocardiogram (TTE) and transesophageal echocardiogram (TEE)

**Q42. TTE image quality depends on:**

a. Patient's position
b. Body contour
c. Experience of intensivist
d. All of the above

**Q43. All of the following are used to identify artifacts, *except*:**

a. Findings to be rechecked in all possible views
b. Color flow with appropriate settings
c. TGC and depth modification
d. Under the guidance of a cardiologist

**Q44. TTE is preferred in:**

a. Evaluation of left atrial appendage (LAA)
b. Evaluation of prosthetic valves
c. Evaluation of left ventricular (LV) thrombus
d. Patent foramen ovale

**Q45. The minimum number of echocardiographic studies required for advanced training**

a. 100
b. 200
c. 300
d. 500

**Q46. All of the following are appropriate indications for TEE, *except*:**

a. Management of atrial fibrillation
b. Diagnosing infective endocarditis
c. Evaluation of aortic pathology
d. Fluid resuscitation in cardiogenic shock

**Q47. How to achieve a right ventricular (RV) inflow view?**

a. Patient in left lateral position
b. Parasternal longitudinal view
c. Tilting the probe toward the left shoulder with the ultrasound beam focusing downward
d. All of the above

**Q48. In the A3C view, the following structure is not seen:**

a. LA
b. Left ventricular outflow tract (LVOT)
c. LV
d. Right ventricular outflow tract (RVOT)

**Q49. In the apical two-chamber view (A2C) view, which of the following structure is not seen:**

a. Left atrium (LA)
b. LV
c. Interventricular septum
d. Right atrium (RA)

**Q50. In the subcostal view, which of the following structures is not seen?**

a. LA
b. RV
c. Interventricular septum
d. Aortic valve (AV)

**Q51. The suprasternal view is used to visualize:**

a. LA
b. Descending thoracic aorta
c. Mitral valve
d. Right ventricle

**Q52. Pleural and pericardial effusion in parasternal-long axis (PLAX) view can be differentiated by:**

a. Echogenicity
b. Descending thoracic aorta
c. Pleural line
d. Vertebra

**Q53. How to visualize LAA?**

a. In apical four-chamber view (A4C), tilting the probe anteriorly with patient in left lateral position
b. In PLAX view, probe tilted toward left shoulder
c. Need TEE always
d. Using suprasternal view

**Q54. Rocking maneuver is best described by:**

a. The transducer changes orientation either toward or away from the orientation marker
b. The transducer moves in different planes
c. The transducer moves perpendicular to the orientation marker
d. None of the above

**Q55. What is the optimal Doppler gate?**

a. Smaller the Doppler gate, the better the resolution
b. Optimal depth with high PRF
c. Size should be at least two-thirds size of the vessel in interrogation
d. All of the above

## Answers and Explanations

41. **Ans. d**
Critical care echocardiography is usually done and interpreted by an intensivist. It is adequate for diagnosing and monitoring therapeutic interventions in the intensive care unit (ICU). It also includes TEE for certain situations where TTE is nondiagnostic.

42. **Ans. d**
The image quality of TTE depends on the patient's position, size, and skill of the operator.

43. **Ans. d**
The image has to be reviewed in all possible views. It is better to use gain modification and appropriate color flow to delineate cardiac structures.

44. **Ans. c**
Apart from LV thrombus, all other options mentioned need TEE for complete evaluation.
45. **Ans. c**
According to the American Society of Echocardiography (ASE) and Society of Cardiovascular Anesthesiologists (SCA) guidelines, 300 examinations are required for advanced training.
46. **Ans. d**
Fluid resuscitation in cardiogenic shock does not need TEE unless TTE is nondiagnostic. Rest all other options will be better managed with TEE.
47. **Ans. d**
RV inflow view is achieved by tilting the probe toward the left shoulder in PLAX and the ultrasound beam directed downward with a patient in the left lateral position. RA and RV with tricuspid valve is best visualized in this view.
48. **Ans. d**
The right ventricular outflow tract is not seen in the A3C view. LA, LVOT, AV, and anterior septum and posterolateral segments of LV are best visualized in this view.
49. **Ans. d**
Right atrium; is not seen in the A2C view. It is mainly used to see LA, LV and mitral valve.
50. **Ans. d**
Aortic valve is not completely evaluated by the subcostal view but both ventricles and atria are visualized, especially when there is difficulty in image acquisition in critically ill patients.
51. **Ans. b**
The aortic arch and descending thoracic aorta are visualized in this view to rule out aortic dissection and coarctation of the aorta.
52. **Ans. b**
The hypoechoic area above the descending thoracic aorta (circular structure in cross-section) is usually pericardial effusion.
53. **Ans. a**
Transesophageal echocardiogram best evaluates LAA, but sometimes TTE can also visualize LAA by tilting the echo probe anteriorly in A4C view.
54. **Ans. a**
Rocking—side to side along the long axis of the probe
Tilting—side to side along the short axis of the probe
Rotation—clockwise or counterclockwise along a central axis of the probe
55. **Ans. d**
The optimal Doppler gate is the minimum gate size with a location at a desired level (e.g., at the center of the vessel), and the angle of insonation is zero. PRF should be high enough to avoid aliasing.

## SECTION C: ECHOCARDIOGRAPHY IN RIGHT HEART DYSFUNCTION

**Q56. Right ventricular systolic pressure (RVSP) increases with all of the following, *except*:**
a. Age
b. Sex
c. Body mass index (BMI)
d. Diastolic dysfunction

**Q57. Assumptions in RVSP measurement could be:**
a. Normal RA pressure
b. Detectable tricuspid regurgitation (TR) jet
c. Least possible Doppler angle
d. All of the above

**Q58. All of the following are false, *except*:**

a. Absence of TR jet excludes pulmonary hypertension (PHT)
b. RVSP underestimates RV pressure in right heart failure (RHF)
c. The higher the Doppler angle, the better the estimate
d. None of the above

**Q59. Mean pulmonary artery pressure (mPAP) is:**

a. One-half of pulmonary arterial systolic pressure (PASP)
b. One-quarter of PASP
c. Two-thirds of PASP
d. Could not be calculated from PASP

**Q60. True about the eccentricity index is:**

a. Ratio of the axis perpendicular to the septum (D1) to the axis parallel to the septum (D2)
b. Value <1.1 indicates RV dysfunction
c. Measured in PLAX view
d. Eccentricity only in diastole suggests volume overload

**Q61. Additional echocardiographic signs of PHT is/are:**

a. RVOT Doppler midsystolic notching
b. RA area at end-systole
c. High pulmonary regurgitant velocity
d. All of the above

**Q62. The hemodynamic classification of PHT is based on:**

a. PASP, pulmonary capillary wedge pressure (PCWP), and pulmonary vascular resistance (PVR)
b. Pulmonary artery diastolic pressure (PADP), PCWP, and PVR
c. mPAP, PCWP, and PVR
d. RVSP, PCWP, and PVR

**Q63. Limitation of echocardiography to find the etiology of PHT is:**

a. PHT due to left heart disease could not be diagnosed
b. Could not differentiate between class I, III, IV of PHT
c. Mean pulmonary pressures calculated from RVSP have a poor correlation with actual values
d. All of the above

**Q64. PHT due to lung disease is classified as:**

a. Precapillary PHT
b. Post capillary PHT
c. Combined
d. None of the above

**Q65. Pulmonary artery:**

a. Dilates only in pressure overload
b. Diameter >25 mm is a sign of PHT
c. Measured in A4C view
d. PA diameter could not be used for estimation of PHT

**Q66. Predictors of severity and prognosis of PHT:**

a. Tricuspid annular plane systolic excursion (TAPSE)
b. RV free wall longitudinal strain
c. Pericardial effusion
d. All of the above

**Q67. Identify the correct statement about RV systolic function.**

a. Longitudinal shortening contributes more than radial fibers in RV systole
b. S′ measures global systolic RV function
c. Modified Simpsons biplane technique is commonly used for measurement
d. None of the above

**Q68. Regarding TAPSE:**

a. Measure of global RV systolic function
b. Not depend on RV afterload
c. A value more than 17 mm reliably rules out RV dysfunction all the time
d. None of the above

**Q69. What is false about McConnell sign?**

a. Hyperkinetic RV-free wall
b. Absence of McConnell sign rules out pulmonary embolism
c. Specific for pulmonary embolism
d. All of the above

**Q70. Echocardiographic parameters to differentiate between acute and chronic PHT all, *except*:**

a. RA size
b. RV-free wall thickness
c. Pulmonary artery acceleration time
d. All of the above

**Q71. The 60/60 sign is characterized by:**

a. TR jet gradient >60 mm Hg and PAT >60 milliseconds
b. TR jet gradient >60 mm Hg and PAT <60 milliseconds
c. TR jet gradient <60 mm Hg and PAT >60 milliseconds
d. TR jet gradient <60 mm Hg and PAT <60 milliseconds

**Q72. A 30-year-old female patient with a history of cesarean section 3 days back presented to the ICU with tachycardia, hypoxemia, and hypotension. The best management option is:**

a. Low D-Dimer value cannot rule out pulmonary embolism in the setting of pregnancy
b. Computed tomography pulmonary angiogram (CTPA) is the preferred investigation at this time
c. Echocardiography with N-terminal prohormone of brain natriuretic peptide (NTpro-BNP) gives reliable information
d. None of the above

**Q73. The following parameters will affect the accuracy of TRVmax in the estimation of RVSP:**

a. Severe TR
b. Pulmonary stenosis
c. High RA pressures
d. All of the above

**Q74. RV inflow view:**

a. Can assess TR jet reliably
b. Modification of PSAX
c. RA at the top of RV in this view
d. None of the above

**Q75. Pulmonary artery acceleration time:**

a. Reliably estimates PHT in RHF
b. Accuracy is operator dependent
c. Highly specific for pulmonary embolism
d. None

**Q76. Calculation of RVSP from TR velocity signal is an example of:**

a. Conservation of mass
b. Conservation of energy
c. Conservation of momentum
d. None

**Q77. Pulmonary artery dilatation is seen in all of the following conditions, *except*:**

a. Atrial septal defect (ASD)
b. Valvular pulmonary stenosis
c. Pulmonary arterial hypertension (PAH)
d. Infundibular pulmonary stenosis

## Answers and Explanations

56. **Ans. b**
Right ventricular systolic pressure increases with increasing age, body weight, and diastolic dysfunction.

57. **Ans. d**
Presence of a detectable TR jet, with Doppler angle of insonation at 0° and normal RA pressures quantified by inferior vena cava (IVC) measurements. Other assumptions such as negligible RVOT obstruction and laminar flow through the tricuspid valve.

58. **Ans. b**
The absence of a TR jet does not rule out PHT in 30% of individuals. The higher

the angle, the worse the estimate. RVSP underestimates RV pressure in RHF.

59. **Ans. c**
Pulmonary artery systolic pressure and mPAP have a good correlation ($r = 0.9$). mPAP = 0.66 × PASP.

60. **Ans. d**
The eccentricity index is the ratio of parallel to the septum D2/perpendicular to the septum D1. The value >1.1 is abnormal and indicates RV dysfunction. It is measured in PSAX view at the level of papillary muscles. Eccentricity in diastole indicates volume overload, and in systole, it indicates pressure overload.

61. **Ans. d**
Additional signs of PHT are:
- Ventricles—RV > LV and eccentricity index >1.1
- Pulmonary artery—RVOT acceleration time <105 milliseconds, early diastolic pulmonary regurgitation velocity >2.2 m/s, mean PA diameter >25 mm
- IVC >2.1 cm with <50% collapsing, RA area >18 $cm^2$

62. **Ans. c**
According to the sixth International Symposium on PAH 2018, hemodynamic classification is based on mPAP, PVR, and PCWP. mPAP >20 mm Hg and pre- and postcapillary PAH is based on PVR and PCWP.

63. **Ans. b**
Mean PAP has a good correlation with PASP and PAH due to left heart disease, which can be diagnosed with echocardiography. Precapillary PAH is the basis for classes I, III, and IV and cannot be differentiated.

64. **Ans. a**
Pulmonary arterial hypertension due to lung disease is precapillary PAH, and PAH due to heart disease is postcapillary PAH. If chronic heart disease with change in pulmonary vasculature leads to combined pre and postcapillary PAH

65. **Ans. b**
Pulmonary artery diameter measurement is an additional sign of PAH. The value >25 mm is abnormal and measured in the PSAX view. PA is dilated in both pressure and volume overload.

66. **Ans. d**
Predictors of severity and prognosis of PAH are:
- Pericardial effusion
- RV dimensions
- TAPSE and S'
- TR jet velocity
- Eccentricity index
- RA area and RV fractional area change (FAC)

67. **Ans. a**
Longitudinal shortening contributes 75% of RV systole. S' indicates regional RV contractile function. The modified Simpson biplane method is used for left ventricular ejection fraction (LVEF) estimation.

68. **Ans. d**
Tricuspid annular plane systolic excursion measures regional RV function, and low TAPSE values do not rule out RV dysfunction. TAPSE is load-dependent.

69. **Ans. d**
McConell's sign is characterized by hypokinesia of the RV-free wall and normal apical contractility. It is highly specific for acute pulmonary embolism but has low sensitivity.

70. **Ans. d**

| | ***Acute pulmonary hypertension*** | ***Chronic pulmonary hypertension*** |
|---|---|---|
| RA size | Equal to LA | Graeter than LA |
| RV-free wall thickness | <5 mm | >5 mm |
| Pulmonary acceleration time | <60 milliseconds | <105 milliseconds |
| TR jet pressure gradient | <45 mm Hg | >45 mm Hg |

(LA: left atrium; RA: right atrium; RV: right ventricle; TR: tricuspid regurgitation)

71. **Ans. d**
The 60/60 sign is characterized by TR jet velocity <60 mm Hg and pulmonary artery acceleration time <60 milliseconds. It is highly specific for acute pulmonary embolism but has low sensitivity.
72. **Ans. c**
Given the clinical condition, the probable diagnosis will be acute pulmonary embolism. D-dimer has a negative predictive value of 0.98 and can be used to rule out pulmonary embolism with low clinical probability. Here, the patient is having hypotension; bedside echocardiography with NTpro-BNP will give reliable information. CTPA is the gold standard for diagnosing PE, but it cannot be done when the patient is unstable.
73. **Ans. d**
Right atrium pressure, TR jet velocity, and RVOT obstruction are the factors that affect RVSP measurement.
74. **Ans. a**
RV inflow view is a modification of the PLAX view by tilting the probe toward the left shoulder, directing the beam downward. It is used to assess the TR jet velocity.
75. **Ans. b**
Pulmonary artery acceleration time has a poor correlation with RVSP, especially in patients with RHF. A study conducted on 234 critically ill cardiothoracic patients showed no significant correlation in the setting of RHF (*p* 0.27). It is operator-dependent. It has a specificity of around 94%. A low PAT is also present in RV infarction, chronic obstructive pulmonary disease (COPD), and pulmonary stenosis.
76. **Ans. b**
Valvular pulmonary stenosis does not typically cause dilatation of the pulmonary artery. Instead, it causes poststenotic dilatation. Conditions such as ASD, infundibular pulmonary stenosis, and PHT are associated with pulmonary artery dilatation.
77. **Ans. b**
Valvular pulmonary stenosis does not typically cause dilatation of the pulmonary artery. Instead, it causes post-stenotic dilatation. Conditions such as ASD, infundibular pulmonary stenosis, and PHT are associated with pulmonary artery dilatation.

## SECTION D: ECHOCARDIOGRAPHY IN LV DYSFUNCTION

**Q78. LVEF is best measured by:**

a. Eyeballing method
b. Fractional shortening
c. End-point septal separation (EPSS)
d. Modified Simpson's biplane disc method

**Q79. All of the following are limitations in the estimation of LV systolic function in critically ill patients, *except*:**

a. Overestimation of LVEF
b. Poor image quality in one-third of the patients
c. Eyeballing LV contractility with secondary MR can be used reliably
d. M-mode needs to be placed perpendicular to the cardiac structures, which is difficult in most of critically ill patients

**Q80. Limitations of Simpson's technique for EF evaluation all, *except*:**

a. Assumption that LV is ellipsoid
b. Reproducibility
c. Operator dependent
d. Load independent

**Q81. True about LV contractility all, *except*:**

a. Longitudinal shortening
b. Oblique shortening
c. Circumferential shortening
d. Radial shortening

**Q82. Regarding EPSS:**

a. Movement of the mitral valve toward the interventricular septum (IVS) can be measured at the moment
b. A form of PW doppler
c. Load independent measure
d. A value >10 mm rules out LV dysfunction

**Q83. FAC:**

a. FAC is a direct estimate of LVEF
b. Measured in both PLAX and PSAX views
c. FAC (%) = (LVESA – LVEDA)/LVEDA × 100
d. Normal range is 52–72% (using Teichholz formula)

**Q84. False about the technical aspects of measuring LVEF using Simpson's method**

a. A4C and A3C are the two views used for biplane measurement
b. Papillary muscles to be excluded
c. Mitral valve hinge at the base of both sides to be connected
d. Usually, the tracing has to be parallel to the epicardium in case of poor image quality

**Q85. Identify the wrong match:**

a. A4C – Simpson's method
b. A4C – FAC
c. PSAX – FAC
d. PLAX – EPSS

**Q86. When are the LV mass index and relative wall thickness high?**

a. Concentric hypertrophy
b. Eccentric hypertrophy
c. Concentric remodeling
d. Normal

**Q87. Incorrect regarding myocardial strain:**

a. Measure of myocardial deformation
b. Strain = $(L_0 - L_1)/L1$
c. More the negative value, the better the contractility
d. Measure of global LV function

**Q88. False statement about Global longitudinal strain (GLS) is:**

a. Longitudinal strain is calculated from A2C, A3C, and A4C views
b. Circumferential and radial strains are obtained from PLAX view
c. Six segments, each at the levels of mid, apical, and basal segments, are measured
d. Average of all the segments gives GLS (–18 to –25%)

**Q89. All are advantages of myocardial speckle tracking, *except*:**

a. Not angle dependent
b. Provides objective measures in the way of bull's plot
c. Values are standardized and validated
d. Ischemic areas at risk (subclinical) can also be detected

**Q90. Correct statement about S′ peak mitral annular descend velocity (PMADV):**

a. Correlates with global LV function with good accuracy
b. Measured by TDI
c. A single lateral mitral annular S′ value >5.4 cm/s has EF >50%
d. All of the above

**Q91. During a TTE to assess LV dimensions, which of the following is the *least* important view for accurate measurement?**

a. PLAX
b. A4C
c. A2C
d. Short axis view at the level of the papillary muscles

**Q92. Which of the following findings on echocardiography is the LEAST suggestive of left ventricular hypertrophy (LVH)?**

a. Increased wall thickness of the left ventricle
b. Impaired relaxation of the left ventricle
c. Dilation of the LA
d. Normal LVEF

**Q93. Which phase of electrocardiogram (ECG) corresponds to left ventricular internal dimension end-diastole (LVIDd) and LVIDs?**

a. At or before the peak of R wave – LVIDd and end of T wave – LVIDs
b. At or before peak of R wave – LVIDs and end of T wave – LVIDd
c. P wave – LVIDd and R wave – LVIDs
d. ECG could not be used for echo measurement

**Q94. All of the following are criteria for diastolic dysfunction, *except*:**

a. LA volume index is >34 mL/m$^2$
b. TR velocity is >2.8 m/s
c. Average E/e′ is >14
d. LVH >10 mm

**Q95. Following is/are the causes of diastolic dysfunction:**

a. Coronary artery disease (CAD)
b. Hypertrophic cardiomyopathy
c. Obesity
d. All of the above

**Q96. Which of the following findings on PW Doppler echocardiography is *most* suggestive of E-wave diastolic dysfunction?**

a. A wave peak velocity greater than E wave peak velocity (A > E)
b. E wave peak velocity greater than A wave peak velocity (E > A) with normal deceleration time
c. Normal E and A wave peak velocities with prolonged deceleration time
d. Both A and E wave velocities are significantly reduced

**Q97. How will the echocardiography guide fluid administration in a patient with diastolic dysfunction?**

a. E > A with prolonged isovolumic relaxation time (IVRT) changes to E < A with shortened IVRT → left atrial pressure (LAP) pressure is increasing
b. E < A with prolonged IVRT changes to E > A with shortened IVRT → LAP pressure is increasing
c. E > A with prolonged IVRT changes to E > A with shortened IVRT → LAP pressure is decreasing
d. LAP pressure estimation cannot be used for fluid status optimization

**Q98. Noninvasive indices of LV relaxation:**

a. IVRT
b. Mitral annulus e′
c. Strain rate during early diastole ($SR_E$)
d. All of the above

**Q99. Limitations of PW Doppler in diastolic dysfunction assessment:**

a. Presence of atrial fibrillation
b. Presence of mitral valve disease

c. Presence of basal and segmental wall abnormalities
d. All of the above

**Q100. E/e′ interpretation for worsening diastolic dysfunction and increasing LAP:**

a. E increases and e′ decreases progressively
b. Both E and e′ decreases
c. Both E and e′ increases
d. E decreases and e′ increases progressively

**Q101. How to differentiate cardiogenic and noncardiogenic pulmonary edema by echocardiography?**

a. LV systolic and diastolic dysfunction with dilated IVC and lung ultrasound showing anterior B-lines and smooth pleural lines suggestive of cardiogenic pulmonary edema
b. LV systolic or diastolic dysfunction with collapsing IVC and lung ultrasound showing anterior B-lines and smooth pleural lines suggestive of noncardiogenic pulmonary edema
c. Normal LV function with diffuse B-lines suggestive of cardiogenic pulmonary edema
d. Could not be differentiated by echocardiography

**Q102. Commonly used strategies for weaning from mechanical ventilation with diastolic dysfunction:**

a. Provided positive pressure support postextubation
b. Achieve neutral/negative fluid balance (E/e′ < 8)
c. NTpro-BNP guided spontaneous breathing trials
d. All of the above

**Q103. All below represent LV end-systolic circumferential wall stress principal determinants *except*?**

a. LV end-systolic dimension
b. LV end-systolic pressure
c. LV systolic wall thickness
d. LV pressure at mitral valve closure

**Q104. End-systolic wall stress increase will lead to a reduction of all following *except*:**

a. EF
b. Fractional shortening
c. Circumferential shortening velocity
d. LV positive dp/dt

**Q105. An increase in LV end-systolic wall stress corresponds to the following change in LV end-systolic volume?**

a. Increase
b. Decrease
c. No effect

**Q106. The mitral E/A ratio is least affected by:**

a. Modulus of LV chamber stiffness
b. LAP
c. Elastic recoil of LV
d. Cardioversion for atrial fibrillation performed 2 hours ago
e. Pulmonary artery pressure

**Q107. Mitral A-wave amplitude reduction least effected by is:**

a. Recent cardioversion
b. Myopathic LA
c. An acute rise in left ventricular end-diastolic pressure (LVEDP)
d. Severe AS with mild LV hypertrophy and normal LVEF

**Q108. A high E/A ratio can occur both in high LA pressure and atrial mechanical failure. Among the following, which factor will not help in differentiating the above?**

a. Pulmonary vein S/D time velocity integral ratio
b. Amplitude and duration of AR-wave
c. E-wave deceleration time
d. Mitral annular velocity with TDI

**Q109. An abnormal LV relaxation pattern represents:**

a. Mean LA pressure of 10 mm Hg and LVEDP of 22 mm Hg
b. Mean LA pressure of 10 mm Hg and LVEDP of 12 mm Hg
c. Mean LA pressure of 22 mm Hg and LVEDP of 10 mm Hg
d. Mean LA pressure of 28 mm Hg and LVEDP of 30 mm Hg
e. Mean LA pressure of 28 mm Hg and LVEDP of 40 mm Hg

## Answers and Explanations

78. **Ans. d**
Modified Simpson's biplane method is the gold standard for the estimation of LVEF. It measures end-systolic and end-diastolic volume. LVEF = (EDV – ESV)/ EDV × 100.

79. **Ans. c**
The estimation of LVEF in critically ill patients has certain limitations, such as achieving a good echo window, hyperdynamic circulation with overestimation, and M-mode has to be applied perpendicular to the LV cavity in PLAX view while calculating FAC. Eyeballing has been shown to predict LVEF reliably in all critically ill patients, comparable with modified Simpson's technique.

80. **Ans. d**
Limitations of Simpson's method for LVEF estimation are:
- Assumption that LV cavity is ellipsoid
- Reproducibility depends on achieving the same plane for EDV and ESV measurement
- Depends on the skill and experience of the operator

81. **Ans. b**
Left ventricular contractility is in three-dimensional plane (twisting and shortening)
- Longitudinal shortening
- Circumferential shortening
- Radial shortening

82. **Ans. a**
End Point Septal Separation assesses LVEF in PLAX view using M-mode echocardiography. A value <7 mm indicates normal LVEF, 7–10 mm → equivocal, and >10 mm indicates poor LVEF.

83. **Ans. b**
Fractional area change is an alternate way of assessing LV contractility and is not a direct estimate of LVEF since it does not use geometric assumptions such as EF estimation. A value >35% indicates good LV contractility. FAC% = (LVESA – LVEDA)/LVEDA × 100. It can be assessed in both PLAX and PSAX views.

84. **Ans. a**
Apical A4C and A2C are used for Simpson's biplane method to estimate LVEF. For accurate measurement, papillary muscles are to be excluded, and the mitral valve hinge at the base of both sides is to be connected. When tracing the endocardial border, always follow the epicardial border.

85. **Ans. b**

| *A4C* | *Simpson's method* |
|---|---|
| PLAX | FAC |
| PSAX | FAC |
| PLAX | EPSS |

86. **Ans. a**

| | *LV mass index <115* | *LV mass index >115* |
|---|---|---|
| Relative wall thickness >0.42 | Concentric remodeling | Concentric hypertrophy |
| Relative wall thickness <0.42 | Normal | Eccentric hypertrophy |

87. **Ans. b**

Myocardial deformation is measured by strain, which is the ratio of change in myocardial fiber length to baseline length. Strain = $(L_1-L_0)/L_0 \times 100$. It is a measure of global LV function. GLS value –18% to –25% (more negative value indicates better LV contractility).

88. **Ans. b**

Longitudinal strain is calculated from A2C, A3C, and A4C views. Circumferential and radial strains are obtained from the PSAX view. Six segments, each at the level of apical, mid, and basal segments, are measured, and an average of all the segments gives the GLS value (normal –185 to –25%).

89. **Ans. c**

In speckle tracking, the system measures unique acoustic patterns within the myocardium called speckles. These speckles can be tracked over time, and speckle displacement can be used to calculate tissue velocity and strain. It is an objective measure and not angle-dependent (not based on the Doppler principle). The advantage is the detection of subclinical areas of myocardial ischemia at risk.

90. **Ans. d**

Peak mitral annular descend velocity S′ has a good correlation with LVEF estimation ($r$ = 0.85) measured by tissue Doppler in A4C view. A value >5.4 cm/s indicates LVEF of >50% with 88% sensitivity and 97% specificity.

91. **Ans. d**

The three most important views for LV dimension measurement by TTE are:

1. PLAX view
2. A4C
3. A2C

These three views combined provide the necessary information to calculate key LV dimensions such as left ventricular end-diastolic diameter (LVEDD) and left ventricular end-systolic diameter (LVESD), which are then used to derive other parameters, such as ejection fraction (EF).

92. **Ans. d**

Common echo findings suggestive of LVH include:

- LVH—increased wall thickness of the left ventricle
- Impaired relaxation of the left ventricle-diastolic dysfunction
- Dilation of the LA
- LVEF normal/slightly increased

93. **Ans. a**

At or before peak of R wave – LVIDd and end of T wave – LVIDs

94. **Ans. d**

Criteria for diastolic dysfunction: ≥2 variables are present

1. LA volume index is >34 mL/m$^2$
2. TR velocity is >2.8 m/s
3. E/e′ is >14
4. Septal e′ velocity <7 and lateral e′ velocity <10

95. **Ans. d**

Causes of diastolic dysfunction:

- Hypertension
- Diabetes
- Obesity
- Restrictive cardiomyopathy
- CAD
- Infiltrative and storage disorders

96. **Ans. a**

In a healthy heart, the mitral valve filling pattern on PW Doppler echo typically shows a dominant E wave, representing early filling during diastole due to atrial contraction. The A wave, representing passive filling after atrial contraction, is usually smaller than the E wave (E > A). E-wave diastolic dysfunction refers to a condition where the E-wave velocity is impaired or reduced. This can be caused by various factors affecting the ventricle's ability to relax and fill properly during diastole.

- Option (a) describes the most characteristic finding: An A wave exceeding the E wave in peak velocity (A > E) is a strong indicator of E-wave diastolic dysfunction. This reversal in the normal pattern suggests that passive filling (A wave) is stronger than active filling (E wave), which can occur when the ventricle is stiff and has difficulty relaxing.
- Option (b) describes normal filling: An E wave greater than the A wave (E > A) with a normal deceleration time is indicative of normal diastolic function.
- Option (c) can be abnormal but not most suggestive: Prolonged deceleration time of the E wave can be a sign of diastolic dysfunction, but it is not the most specific finding for E-wave dysfunction alone. It can also occur in other conditions.
- Option (d) is not specific to E-wave dysfunction: Reduced A and E wave velocities can occur in various conditions, not just E-wave dysfunction specifically.

Therefore, an A wave exceeding the E wave in peak velocity (A > E) is the most suggestive finding of E-wave diastolic dysfunction on PW Doppler echocardiography.

97. **Ans. a**

If a patient with impaired relaxation (grade 1 diastolic dysfunction) is given fluids, there is worsening of pulmonary edema (high LAP) and grade 2 diastolic dysfunction (pseudonormal pattern), it is better to stop giving fluids and start diuretics.

98. **Ans. d**

Following are the noninvasive measures of diastolic dysfunction
- IVRT
- Mitral annulus e'
- Strain rate during early diastole ($SR_E$) and isovolumic relaxation ($SR_{IVR}$)

99. **Ans. d**

Limitations of PW Doppler in diastolic dysfunction
- Atrial fibrillation
- Mitral valve disease
- Regional wall motion abnormalities
- Conduction abnormalities

100. **Ans. a**

E/e' interpretation for worsening diastolic dysfunction and increasing LAP.

Progressive increase in E wave velocity and decrease in e'.

101. **Ans. a**

To differentiate cardiogenic and noncardiogenic pulmonary edema by echocardiography.

Left ventricular systolic and diastolic dysfunction with dilated IVC and lung ultrasound showing anterior B-lines and smooth pleural lines suggestive of cardiogenic pulmonary edema

Anterior B-lines with irregular pleural lines (shredding) with or without LV dysfunction is suggestive of noncardiogenic pulmonary edema

102. **Ans. d**

Preexisting cardiac dysfunction patients are at risk of weaning failure. The best strategy to prevent weaning-induced diastolic dysfunction is to achieve neutral or negative fluid balance by optimal diuresis (deresuscitation phase) and monitoring the weaning process with NTproBNP values (more accurate to rule out than to rule in postextubation respiratory distress) and providing positive pressure support postextubation in high-risk patients.

103. **Ans. d**

LV end-systolic circumferential wall stress is determined by the LV end-systolic dimension, end-systolic pressure, and systolic wall thickness. The pressure at mitral valve closure is not a determinant.

104. **Ans. d**

Increased LV end-systolic wall stress negatively impacts EF, fractional shortening, and the velocity of circumferential shortening but does not directly affect LV positive dp/dt, which is a measure of contractility.

105. **Ans. a**

An increase in LV end-systolic wall stress typically leads to an increase in LV end-systolic volume, as the higher wall stress reduces the efficiency of ventricular contraction.

106. **Ans. e**

The mitral E/A ratio is influenced by factors such as the tau (relaxation time constant), LV chamber stiffness, LAP, and LV elastic recoil. Pulmonary artery pressure is the least likely to directly affect the E/A ratio.

107. **Ans. d**

Severe aortic stenosis with mild LVH and a normal LVEF is unlikely to significantly reduce the A-wave amplitude. However, conditions such as recent cardioversion, a myopathic LA, and an acute increase in LVEDP can all contribute to a decrease in A-wave amplitude.

108. **Ans. b**

The amplitude and duration of the AR-wave are less useful in distinguishing high LA pressure from atrial mechanical failure compared to other parameters such as E-wave deceleration time, pulmonary vein S/D ratio, and mitral annular velocity.

109. **Ans. e**

An abnormal LV relaxation pattern is typically linked to elevated LAP (mean LA pressure) and increased LVEDP.

## SECTION E: ECHOCARDIOGRAPHY IN ACUTE CORONARY SYNDROME

**Q110. Akinesia is defined as:**

a. <10% of LV thickening
b. <50% of LV thickening
c. No LV thickening from baseline
d. <30% of LV thickening

**Q111. The number of segments to be seen for complete examination of regional wall motion abnormalities (RWMA)**

a. 5
b. 8
c. 15
d. 17

**Q112. All of the following are the causes of RWMA, *except*:**

a. Stroke
b. Stress cardiomyopathy
c. Chronic kidney disease (CKD)
d. All of the above

**Q113. Basal septal hypokinesia is seen in infarction due to:**

a. Left anterior descending artery
b. Left circumflex artery
c. Right coronary artery (RCA)
d. Left obtuse marginal artery

**Q114. The advantage of echocardiography over ECG and troponin is/are:**

a. Early detection of RWMA
b. Mechanical complications can be diagnosed
c. Can be used to rule out other differentials
d. All of the above

**Q115. In PSAX view, apical RWMA is seen due to infarction of:**

a. LAD
b. LCX
c. RCA
d. Left obtuse marginal artery

**Q116. The anteroseptal wall can be visualized in:**

a. A2C view
b. A3C view
c. A4C view
d. PLAX view

**Q117. Inferoseptal wall is best visualized in:**

a. A2C view
b. A3C view
c. A4C view
d. PLAX view

**Q118. The following are the mechanical complications of ACS, *except*?**

a. MR due to papillary muscle rupture
b. VSR
c. Pericardial effusion
d. Severely reduced LVEF

**Q119. Which myocardial segment most commonly has false-positive wall motion abnormalities on TTE?**

a. Posterior basal wall
b. Anterior septum
c. Lateral wall
d. Apex

## Answers and Explanations

110. **Ans. a**
Hypokinesia <50% from baseline
Akinesia <10% from baseline

111. **Ans. d**
According to ASE (2016), 17 segments have to be examined for RWMA detection.

112. **Ans. d**
Causes for RWMA:
- Stroke
- Stress cardiomyopathy
- CKD

113. **Ans. a**
Basal septum is supplied by RCA.

114. **Ans. d**
Troponin rises usually after 2–3 hours in myocardial infarction. Echocardiography can be useful to detect RWMA in these situations. The other advantage is echo can be used to rule out other diagnoses such as pulmonary embolism, and respiratory causes such as pneumothorax, etc. Mechanical complications such as ventricular septal rupture, and papillary muscle rupture lead to acute MR, tamponade, etc., are detected

115. **Ans. a**
Left anterior descending artery supplies the apical segment. Sometimes contributed by the left circumflex artery

116. **Ans. b**

117. **Ans. c**

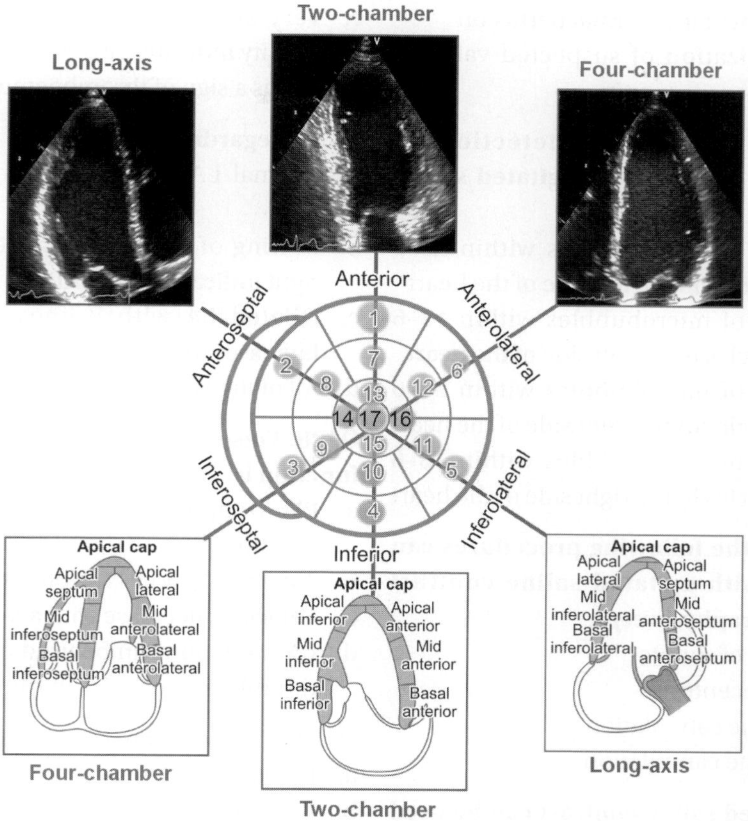


*Source:* Lang RM, Badano LP, Mor-Avi V, Afilalo J, Armstrong A, Ernande L, et al. Recommendations for cardiac chamber quantification by echocardiography in adults: an update from the American Society of Echocardiography and the European Association of Cardiovascular Imaging. J Am Soc Echocardiogr. 2015;28(1):1-39.e14.

118. **Ans. c**

119. **Ans. a**

Most commonly seen in the posterior basal wall due to factors such as imaging artifacts and the presence of adjacent structures.

## SECTION F: HEART VALVES, TAMPONADE, AND EFFUSION

**Q120. A 52-year-old woman with heart failure is undergoing echocardiography. Which of the following findings would be MOST suggestive of poor ventriculoarterial (VA) coupling?**

a. Aortic peak velocity (Ao peak) greater than mitral E wave peak velocity (E)
b. Aortic peak velocity (Ao peak) equal to mitral E wave peak velocity (E)
c. Aortic peak velocity (Ao peak) less than mitral E wave peak velocity (E) with normal pulsatility
d. Prolonged deceleration time of the Mitral E wave

**121. Which of the following is the LEAST likely application of bubble contrast echocardiography?**

a. Detection of intracardiac shunts
b. Evaluation of LV endocardial border definition

c. Assessment of myocardial perfusion
d. Characterization of suspected valvular vegetations

**Q122. The criteria for detection of intracardiac shunts using agitated saline contrast:**
a. Presence of microbubbles within ≤3–6 cardiac cycles in the left side of the heart
b. Presence of microbubbles within ≥3–6 cardiac cycles in the left side of the heart
c. Presence of microbubbles within ≤3–6 cardiac cycles in the right side of the heart
d. Presence of microbubbles within ≥3–6 cardiac cycles in the right side of the heart

**Q123. All of the following procedures can be guided with agitated saline contrast echocardiography, *except*:**
a. Detection of shunts
b. Pericardiocentesis
c. Central line cannulation
d. Arterial line cannulation

**Q124. Agitated saline contrast can be used in the following:**
a. LV thrombus
b. Cardiac tumor
c. TR jet visualization
d. All of the above

**Q125. Use of echocardiography in extra-corporeal membrane oxygenation (ECMO) patients:**
a. Assessment of overdistension
b. Estimation of filling pressures
c. Detection of thrombi
d. All of the above

**Q126. All of the following are true, *except*:**
a. LAA is a multilobed, trabeculated structure in the posterolateral aspect of LA
b. TTE can be used to detect LAA thrombus and spontaneous echo contrast (SEC) with good accuracy
c. Very slow swirling pattern with echo density indicates severe grading of SEC
d. SEC is a sign of thromboembolic risk

**Q127. Regarding LAP:**
a. Normal LA size does not rule out high LAP
b. Bowing of the interatrial septum to the right indicates high LAP
c. Dilated LA with B-lines in the lungs increases the likelihood of high LAP
d. All of the above

**Q128. False statement regarding the LAA function is:**
a. PW Doppler velocities can assess LAA function
b. A normal flow has a triphasic wave pattern
c. Velocities decrease with age
d. LAA function can be used to quantify the thromboembolic risk in AF

**Q129. RV dimensions can be measured at:**
a. RV base diameter
b. RV mid diameter
c. RV length
d. All of the above

**Q130. Cardiac tamponade can be diagnosed by:**
a. Diastolic collapse of RA and RV
b. Dilated IVC
c. Variation in mitral/tricuspid flow
d. All of the above

**Q131. Large pericardial effusion is defined as:**
a. End systolic separation of chambers from pericardium
b. Echo-free space throughout the cardiac cycle, surrounding heart >20 mm
c. End diastolic separation of chambers from pericardium
d. Echo-free space throughout the cardiac cycle, surrounding heart >40 mm

**Q132. Ascites can be differentiated from pericardial effusion by:**

a. Falciform ligament
b. Coronary ligament
c. Ligamentum venosum
d. Could not be differentiated

**Q133. Doppler features of tamponade include all, *except*:**

a. Exaggerated inspiratory decrease in mitral inflow velocity
b. Exaggerated inspiratory increase in tricuspid inflow velocity
c. Exaggerated inspiratory decrease in tricuspid inflow velocity
d. Flow variability during each phase of respiration in mitral inflow has to be calculated

**Q134. The diagnostic criteria for tamponade with the highest accuracy:**

a. Duration of diastolic collapse of RA as ratio on the cardiac cycle length >0.34
b. Swinging heart with large pericardial effusion
c. No respiratory variation in IVC and dilated IVC
d. Respiratory changes of MV and tTV inflow Doppler velocities

**Q135. Regarding RA diastolic collapse:**

a. Best seen in PLAX view
b. Occurs in early diastole near T wave of ECG
c. Usually presents after hemodynamic instability
d. Duration of collapse more than one-third of a cardiac cycle has 100% specificity

**Q136. Cardiac tamponade can be differentiated from constrictive pericarditis by all of the following, *except*:**

a. Higher diastolic velocities in pericarditis and reduced diastolic velocities in tamponade
b. Mitral inflow E wave is higher for pericarditis and A wave is predominant in tamponade
c. Mitral inflow A wave is higher for pericarditis and E wave is predominant in tamponade
d. After drainage, an echo will return to baseline in tamponade whereas high RA pressures in pericarditis

**Q137. All of the following are echocardiographic criteria for pericarditis, *except*:**

a. Usually not associated with effusion
b. Pericardial thickening >2 mm
c. Exaggerated RV LV interdependence
d. Collapsing IVC

**Q138. Diagnostic criteria for tamponade:**

a. Fixed and dilated IVC
b. Interventricular interdependence
c. Hepatic vein diastolic flow reversal during expiration
d. All of the above

**Q139. Echocardiographic features of infective endocarditis:**

a. Oscillating intracardiac mass
b. Valvular dehiscence
c. Paravalvular leak/abscess
d. All of the above

**Q140. The severity of MS is determined by:**

a. Mitral valve area by planimetry
b. Mean valvular pressure gradient
c. PHT
d. None of the above

**Q141. Severe MS is characterized by:**

a. Mitral valve area <1.5 cm$^2$
b. Pressure half time ≥150 milliseconds
c. PASP >30 mm Hg
d. All of the above

**Q142. All of the following are quantitative parameters of MR, *except*:**

a. Vena contracta width
b. Regurgitant volume

c. Regurgitant fraction
d. Effective regurgitant orifice area

**Q143. Severe MR is characterized by all *except*:**
a. Central jet MR >40% LA
b. Vena contracta ≥0.7 cm
c. Regurgitant volume ≥60 mL
d. All of the above

**Q144. What is the relation between severity of AR and pressure halftime?**
a. Higher the PHT, severe the AR
b. Lower the PHT, milder the AR
c. Higher the PHT, milder the AR
d. Lower the PHT, severe the AR

**Q145. Echocardiographic criteria for aortic stenosis:**
a. Aortic jet velocity
b. Pressure gradient
c. AV area
d. All of the above

**Q146. Pressure half-time is:**
a. Qualitative
b. Quantitative
c. Semi quantitative
d. Structural

**Q147. The proximal isovelocity surface area (PISA) method for determining the area of a regurgitant orifice is based on which scientific principle?**
a. Conservation of mass
b. Conservation of energy
c. Conservation of momentum
d. Jet momentum analysis

**Q148. Simplified Bernoulli equation for determining the pressure gradient not suitable in?**
a. Determining the peak instantaneous gradient across a nonobstructed MV
b. Determining the peak gradient across a severely stenotic AV
c. Determining the mean gradient across a severely stenotic AV
d. Determining the mean gradient across a stenotic TV

**Q149. The size of the regurgitant jet for a given regurgitant volume reduced in all, *except*:**
a. Heart rate (HR) increase
b. Sector angle increase
c. Imaging depth increase
d. Blood pressure (BP) increase

**Q150. A bicuspid AV is usually associated with:**
a. ASD
b. Coarctation of the aorta
c. Coronary anomalies
d. None of the above

**Q151. All of the following can have dilated coronary sinus *except*?**
a. Right atrial hypertension
b. Persistent left superior vena cava (LSVC)
c. Coronary A–V fistula
d. Unroofed coronary sinus
e. Azygos continuity of IVC

**Q152. In a person with suspected paravalvular (mechanical) MR, which view best reveals MR jet?**
a. PLAX
b. A4C
c. A2C
d. Apical long axis view

**Q153. Rheumatic MS most common location of leaflet thickening and calcification?**
a. More at the tip
b. Uniform throughout the leaflets
c. More at the base

**Q154. Where is leaflet calcification, most pronounced in degenerative MS?**
a. More at the tip

b. More at the base
c. Uniform throughout the leaflets

**Q155. Which of the following represents the predominant mechanism behind chronic ischemic MR?**
a. Mitral leaflet closure reduction
b. Papillary muscle dysfunction
c. Rupture of chordae tendineae
d. Rupture of papillary muscle

**Q156. Which of the following will not help in differentiating a LA myxoma from a LA thrombus?**
a. Transpulmonary contrast agent enhancement
b. Color flow imaging showing blood vessels
c. Attachment to the atrial septum
d. Similar mass in LV with normal LV function

**Q157. What is the most common location of a LA thrombus?**
a. LAA b. LA body
c. Atrial septum d. Atrial roof

**Q158. Mitral leaflet total surface area accounts for what percentage of the mitral annular area.**
a. 300% b. 175%
c. 150% d. 50%

**Q159. Compared to the anterior mitral leaflet (AML), the posterior mitral leaflet (PML) is:**
a. Shorter
b. Longer
c. The same length as the anterior leaflet
d. Of variable length

**Q160. Mitral annulus major diameter is best imaged from which view?**
a. Apical 2C view
b. Apical long-axis view
c. Apical 5C view
d. PLAX

**Q161. Which of the following is not associated with bicuspid AV:**
a. Aortic root disease
b. Coarctation of the aorta
c. Aortic stenosis or regurgitation
d. VSD

**Q162. What is the usual cause of aortic stenosis in a 50-year-old individual?**
a. Unicuspid AV b. Bicuspid AV
c. Calcific d. RHD

**Q163. Acute AR signs include:**
a. Normal left ventricle size
b. Hyperdynamic LV function
c. Premature mitral valve closure
d. a, b, and c
e. None

**Q164. Which of the following will not lead to an increase in intrapericardial pressure?**
a. Cardiac tamponade
b. Acute massive PE
c. Acute traumatic rupture of TV causing acute TR
d. Acute RV infarct
e. Severe AS with normal LV function

**Q165. A patient with a prosthetic mitral valve with a mean diastolic gradient of 10 mm Hg at an HR of 70 beats/min and a pressure half-time of 200 milliseconds represents?**
a. Severe MR
b. Prosthetic mitral valve stenosis
c. Severe anemia with high output failure
d. Normal prosthetic valve

**Q166. The appearance of saline contrast after five beats from RA to LA in a patient with cirrhosis of the liver is suggestive of:**
a. Normal physiology
b. Portopulmonary syndrome
c. Patent foramen ovale
d. Hepatopulmonary syndrome

## Answers and Explanations

120. **Ans. c**

Ventriculoarterial coupling refers to the interaction between the contraction of the left ventricle and the ejection of blood into the aorta. Normal VA coupling: In a healthy heart, the aortic peak velocity (Ao peak) is typically slightly greater than or equal to the Mitral E wave peak velocity (E). This reflects the efficient transfer of energy from the contracting ventricle to the blood ejected into the aorta. Poor VA coupling: When VA coupling is impaired, the ventricle might not be transferring energy effectively to the blood. This can be reflected by a lower Ao peak velocity compared to the Mitral E wave velocity (E) with normal pulsatility (waveform appearance) of the aortic flow. Overall, a Doppler finding of Ao peak velocity less than Mitral E wave peak velocity (E) with normal pulsatility is the most suggestive of poor VA coupling in this scenario.

121. **Ans. b**

Bubble contrast echocardiography is a technique that uses an agitated saline solution containing microbubbles to enhance the ultrasound signal. Microbubbles do not normally pass through healthy heart valves, but they can appear in the opposite chamber if a shunt is present. In areas with poor blood flow, the microbubbles remain intact for a longer duration, allowing identification of perfusion defects. Microbubbles can adhere to these vegetations, making them more easily visualized with echo and aiding in their characterization.

122. **Ans. a**

Agitated saline contrast (microbubbles) introduced into the right heart will pass through the defects to the left side and can be used to differentiate intracardiac and intrapulmonary shunts. The presence of agitated saline contrast within three to six cardiac cycles in the left heart is considered positive for the presence of the intracardiac shunt.

123. **Ans. d**

Procedures guided by agitated saline contrast are:

- Detection of shunts
- Intensifying TR jet when there is difficult
- Echo guided pericardiocentesis
- Central venous catheter (CVC) insertion
- Delineate right heart masses

124. **Ans. d**

As explained in the previous answer.

125. **Ans. d**

Role of echocardiography in ECMO.
During initiation—the cannula position
Maintenance—LV assessment, estimation of filling pressures, and LV venting
Complications—tamponade, valvular diseases, detection of thrombus, or SEC

126. **Ans. b**

The LAA is a multilobed, trabeculated structure situated on the posterolateral side of the LA. Reduced contractility of the LAA can lead to blood stasis and the development of SEC. SEC is graded based on the swirling pattern and echogenicity. A very low swirling pattern with an echo-dense appearance indicates severe grading (grade #3) of SEC, which typically requires anticoagulation.

127. **Ans. d**

A dilated LA with an LA volume index (LAVI) ≥34 mL/m$^2$ should raise suspicion for elevated LAP. However, a normal LA size does not rule out elevated LAP. Bowing of the interventricular septum (IVS) toward the right ventricle (RV) is indicative of high LAP.

128. **Ans. b**

Pulse wave Doppler velocities can assess LAA function, and it gradually decreases with age. It can be used to quantify the thromboembolic risk in AF. In normal sinus rhythm, a quadriphasic flow pattern is seen.

129. **Ans. d**

Two common sites for measuring RV dimensions are the basal distance (at the tricuspid annulus) and the mid-RV measurement (in the middle segment of the RV). The length of the right ventricle is less commonly used for assessment.

130. **Ans. d**

Cardiac tamponade is confirmed by:

- Echo-free space
- Diastolic collapse of RA and RV
- Dilated IVC
- Variation in mitral and tricuspid inflow

131. **Ans. b**

Pericardial effusion:

| | |
|---|---|
| Small | Echo-free space throughout the cardiac cycle, surrounding heart, <10 mm |
| Medium | 10–20 mm |
| Large | >20 mm |

132. **Ans. a**

Falciform ligament is used to differentiate ascites from pericardial effusion.

133. **Ans. c**

- Exaggerated inspiratory decrease in mitral inflow velocity
- Exaggerated inspiratory increase in tricuspid inflow velocity
- Flow variability during each phase of respiration in mitral inflow has to be calculated.

134. **Ans. a**

| ***Parameters*** | ***Sensitivity*** | ***Specificity*** |
|---|---|---|
| Duration of diastolic collapse of RA as ratio on the cardiac cycle length >0.34 | 90% | 100% |
| Swinging heart with large pericardial effusion | NA | NA |
| Dilated IVC with no respiratory variation | 97% | 40% |
| Respiratory phasic variation in MV and TV inflow Doppler velocities | NA | NA |

(RA: right atrium; IV: inferior vena cava)

135. **Ans. d**

Cardiac tamponade is best visualized in a subcostal/A4C view. It occurs in late diastole near the R wave of ECG and usually presents before hemodynamic instability. Duration of the collapse of more than one-third of the cardiac cycle has 100% specificity and 94% sensitivity.

136. **Ans. c**

Higher diastolic forward flow velocities in effusive constrictive pericarditis and markedly reduced diastolic velocities in tamponade. Mitral inflow E wave is higher for pericarditis, and A wave is predominant in tamponade. After drainage, the echo will return to baseline in tamponade, whereas high RA pressures in pericarditis.

137. **Ans. d**

In constrictive pericarditis, pericardial thickening >2 mm is present in 80% of patients and is usually not associated with effusion. Exaggerated RV LV interdependence such as respiratory septal movement, >25% variation in mitral E velocity, >40% variation in tricuspid E velocity, hepatic vein diastolic flow reversal, and dilated IVC.

138. **Ans. d**
As explained in the previous answer.

139. **Ans. d**
Echocardiographic features of infective endocarditis include vegetation, abscess, and new dehiscence of a prosthetic valve. Echocardiography evaluates the number, size, shape, location, echogenicity, and mobility of vegetations, making it a valuable tool for predicting embolic risk.

140. **Ans. a**
Mitral valve area by planimetry method determines the severity of MS. Mean valvular pressure gradient determines the prognosis.

141. **Ans. d**
Mitral valve area ≤1.5 $cm^2$ (≤1 $cm^2$—very severe MS)
Pressure half time ≥150 milliseconds (≥220 milliseconds—very severe MS)
PASP >30 mm Hg.

142. **Ans. a**
Echocardiographic assessment of MR:

| *Qualitative* | *Semiquantitative* | *Quantitative* | *Structural* |
|---|---|---|---|
| Mitral valve morphology | Vena contracta width | Effective regurgitant orifice area EROA (PISA) | Left ventricle |
| Color flow jet area | Pulmonary vein flow | Regurgitant volume | Left atrium |
| Flow convergence | Mitral inflow | Regurgitant fraction | |
| Continuous wave Doppler jet | TVI mitral/TVI aortic | | |

(EROA: effective regurgitant orifice area; MR: mitral stenosis; PISA: proximal isovelocity surface area; TVI: transvalvular impedance)

143. **Ans. d**
ECHO findings of Severe MR:
- Central MR jet covering >40% of the LA
- Vena contracta measurement >0.7 cm
- Regurgitant volume exceeding 60 mL
- Regurgitant fraction >50%
- Effective regurgitant orifice >0.4 $cm^2$

144. **Ans. d**
Pressure half time is the time required for the pressure gradient to decrease to its half of baseline value. In severe AR, the gradient falls rapidly and, so the pressure half time will be lower.

145. **Ans. d**
Echocardiographic criteria for aortic stenosis:
- AV area
- Aortic jet velocity
- Mean pressure gradient

146. **Ans. c**
Pressure half time is a semiquantitative measure used for quantifying regurgitant lesions.

147. **Ans. a**
The PISA method uses the principle of conservation of mass, which states that the mass flow rate must be constant across any cross-section of the flow. By analyzing the flow convergence region, the regurgitant flow rate can be calculated, leading to the determination of the regurgitant orifice area.

148. **Ans. a**
The simplified Bernoulli equation is typically used to estimate pressure gradients in situations where flow

acceleration and deceleration occur, such as across stenotic or narrowed valves. It is not applicable for calculating the peak instantaneous gradient across a nonobstructed mitral valve, as there is no significant pressure drop or flow acceleration in this situation.

149. **Ans. d**
Increasing HR, sector angle, or imaging depth can all reduce the apparent size of the jet due to various technical and physiological reasons. However, increasing BP typically does not reduce the jet size and might even make it more prominent.

150. **Ans. b**
A bicuspid AV is frequently associated with coarctation of the aorta. Although it can be linked to coronary anomalies, coarctation is the more common and direct association.

151. **Ans. e**
Azygos continuity of the IVC typically does not lead to dilation of the coronary sinus. However, conditions such as right atrial hypertension, a persistent LSVC, coronary arteriovenous fistula, and an unroofed coronary sinus can all result in coronary sinus dilation.

152. **Ans. b**
The A4C is the best position to visualize the MR jet as it provides a comprehensive view of the LA and mitral valve from which regurgitation jets can be assessed.

153. **Ans. a**
In rheumatic MS, thickening and calcification of the mitral valve leaflets typically occur more at the tips, leading to fusion and restricted motion.

154. **Ans. b**
In degenerative MS, calcification tends to be more pronounced at the base of the leaflets near the annulus.

155. **Ans. a**
Chronic ischemic MR primarily results from restricted closure of the mitral leaflets due to remodeling and displacement of the papillary muscles.

156. **Ans. d**
Left atrial myxomas often enhance with contrast agents, have blood vessels visible on color flow imaging, and are typically attached to the atrial septum. A similar mass in the left ventricle is not a distinguishing characteristic.

157. **Ans. a**
The LAA is the most common location for thrombus formation in the LA, especially in conditions like atrial fibrillation.

158. **Ans. c**
The total surface area of the mitral leaflets is generally around 150% of the mitral annular area, allowing for sufficient coaptation and effective valve function.

159. **Ans. a**
The posterior mitral leaflet (PML) is typically shorter than the AML but has a broader base.

160. **Ans. b**
The apical long-axis view provides the best imaging of the major diameter of the mitral annulus.

161. **Ans. d**
While bicuspid AV is associated with aortic root disease, coarctation of the aorta, and aortic stenosis or regurgitation, it is not typically associated with ventricular septal defects.

162. **Ans. b**
In individuals around 50 years old, a bicuspid AV is a common cause of aortic stenosis due to congenital valve deformity leading to early calcification and stenosis.

163. **Ans. d**

Acute AR can cause premature mitral valve closure due to elevated LVEDP, hyperdynamic LV function due to the acute volume overload, and initially normal LV size before dilation occurs.

164. **Ans. e**

Severe aortic stenosis with normal LV function does not increase intrapericardial pressure. However, conditions such as cardiac tamponade, acute massive pulmonary embolism, acute traumatic rupture of the tricuspid valve, and acute RV infarction can lead to an increase in intrapericardial pressure.

165. **Ans. b**

A mean diastolic gradient of 10 mm Hg and a pressure half-time of 200 milliseconds suggest prosthetic mitral valve stenosis.

166. **Ans. c**

The delayed appearance of contrast in the LA compared to the RA is suggestive of a patent foramen ovale, allowing shunting of contrast between the atria.

## SECTION G: TRANSESOPHAGEAL ECHOCARDIOGRAPHY

**Q167. All of the following are absolute contraindications of TEE, *except*:**

a. Perforated viscus
b. Esophageal stricture
c. Active peptic ulcer disease
d. Restriction of neck mobility

**Q168. All of the following are common TEE views, *except*:**

a. Midesophageal view
b. Transgastric view
c. Deep gastric view
d. Suprasternal view

**Q169. Indications for TEE are:**

a. Evaluation of LAA
b. Evaluation of prosthetic valve
c. Critically ill patients, where TTE is nondiagnostic, and TEE findings will alter management.
d. All of the above

**Q170. The number of TEE examinations for basic training as per ASE is:**

a. 300 b. 250
c. 50 d. 100

**Q171. General indications of TEE are:**

a. Intraoperative TEE
b. Guidance for transcatheter procedure
c. To diagnose infective endocarditis with high pretest probability
d. All of the above

**Q172. The LAA evaluation by TEE includes:**

a. Visualization of LAA in multiple beam axis
b. Color-flow filling defect in LAA
c. Pulsed wave (PW) Doppler emptying velocities >0.4 m/s
d. All of the above

**Q173. The anteflex/retroflex of the TEE probe is done by manipulation of:**

a. Small wheel
b. Big wheel
c. Multibeam omniplane control
d. None of the above

**Q174. The long-axis view in TEE is obtained by:**

a. Midesophageal view with angle at 0°
b. Midesophageal view with angle at 130°
c. Transgastric view
d. Midesophageal view with angle at 90°

**Q175. The short-axis view in TEE is obtained by:**

a. Transgastric view with anteflexion
b. Midesophageal view with angle at 130°

c. Transgastric view with retroflexion
d. Midesophageal view with angle at 90°

**Q176. The standard four-chamber view in TEE is obtained by:**
a. Midesophageal view
b. Transgastric view
c. Bicaval view
d. None of the above

**Q177. The common complication of TEE probe insertion is:**
a. Bleeding
b. Swallowing difficulty
c. Esophageal injury
d. Dental injury

**Q178. A 55-year-old male presents with sudden onset tearing chest pain radiating to the back. Which of the following findings on echocardiogram is representative of an aortic dissection?**
a. Normal AV function
b. Thickened aortic wall with a double-lumen sign
c. Enlarged left ventricle
d. Mitral valve regurgitation

**Q179. A 60-year-old male with prior no comorbidities presented with acute onset chest pain with no radiation, with blurred vision episode. There was a difference in upper limbs BP readings (right 50/30 mm Hg, left 140/78 mm Hg) with no right radial pulse. ECG showed LVH, TTE showed BAV and severe AR, and there is an intimal flap extending toward the aortic arch in a suprasternal window. The diagnosis is:**
a. Cardiac tamponade
b. Hypertrophic cardiomyopathy
c. Aortic aneurysm
d. Aortic dissection

**Q180. Which of the following is not associated with an increased risk of aortic dissection?**
a. Pregnancy
b. Bicuspid AV
c. Marfan's syndrome
d. MS

**Q181. Weaning failure from CPB during CABG TEE performed. Fresh findings include an akinetic inferior wall with 3+ MR originating at the medial commissure, and the inferior wall looked excessively bright. Likely diagnosis?**
a. Air embolism into RCA
b. Volume overload
c. Excessively high BP
d. RCA graft thrombosis
e. Poor myocardial preservation

## Answers and Explanations

167. **Ans. d**

Following are the absolute contraindications of TEE:
- Perforated viscus
- Esophageal tumor
- Esophageal diverticulum
- Esophageal perforation and laceration
- Esophageal stricture
- Active upper GI bleed
- ASE/SCA recommendations

168. **Ans. d**

There are 28 views examined by TEE. Common TEE views are midesophageal, transgastric, deep gastric, and aorta views.

169. **Ans. d**
- Evaluation of LAA
- Evaluation of prosthetic valve
- Critically ill patients, where TTE is nondiagnostic, and TEE findings will alter management.

- Guidance for transcatheter procedures

170. **Ans. a**

Basic training includes:
- Total examinations (TTE/TEE): 150
- TEE examinations: 50
- ASE/SCA recommendations

171. **Ans. d**
- Evaluation of the aorta and the LAA
- Evaluation of prosthetic heart valves
- Examination of paravalvular abscesses
- Intraoperative TEE
- Guidance of transcatheter procedures
- Critically ill patients, where TTE is nondiagnostic, and TEE findings will alter management.

172. **Ans. d**

The LAA evaluation includes:
- Visualization of LAA in multiple beam axis
- Color-flow filling defect in LAA
- PW Doppler emptying velocities >0.4 m/s

173. **Ans. b**

Transesophageal echocardiogram probe controls:
- Small wheel—flex to the right/flex to the left
- Big wheel—anteflex/retroflex
- Omniplane axis—rotate forward/rotate backward

174. **Ans. b**
175. **Ans. a**
176. **Ans. a**

| | |
|---|---|
| A4C | Midesophageal view with angle @0° |
| A2C | Midesophageal view with angle @90° |
| LAX | Midesophageal view with angle @130° |
| SAX | Transgastric view with anteflexion |

(A2C: apical two-chamber; A4C: apical four-chamber; LAX: long axis; SAX: short axis; TEE: transesophageal echocardiogram)

177. **Ans. b**
- *Bleeding:* <0.01%
- *Dysphagia:* 1.8%
- *Esophageal injury*: <0.01%
- *Dental injury*: <0.1%

(*Source*: Hahn RT, Abraham T, Adams MS, Bruce CJ, Glas KE, Lang RM, et al. Guidelines for performing a comprehensive transesophageal echocardiographic examination: recommendations from the American Society of Echocardiography and the Society of Cardiovascular Anesthesiologists. J Am Soc Echocardiogr. 2013;26(9):921-64.)

178. **Ans. b**

Aortic dissection is a life-threatening condition in which a tear forms in the inner layer of the aorta, allowing blood to flow between the layers. A thickened aortic wall with a double-lumen sign is a characteristic finding on echocardiography in aortic dissection. This appears as two distinct channels within the aorta on the ultrasound image.

179. **Ans. d**

Aortic dissection is diagnosed by sudden onset acute chest pain sometimes radiating to back pain. ECG shows LVH, echocardiography shows normal LV contractility, bicuspid AV and AR. Suprasternal window shows intimal flap in the aorta extending to the aortic arch. Clinically, there will be difference in BP reading in upper limbs and absence of pulse in the right radial artery.

180. **Ans. d**

Mitral stenosis is not associated with an increased risk of aortic dissection. Conditions such as Marfan's syndrome, bicuspid AV, and pregnancy can increase the risk of aortic dissection.

181. **Ans. e**

The appearance of an akinetic inferior wall, bright appearance, and new onset of severe MR post-CABG suggests poor myocardial preservation.

## SECTION H: ECHOCARDIOGRAPHY IN FLUID RESPONSIVENESS AND SHOCK

**Q182. Heart-lung interactions are best described by:**

a. Pulsus paradoxus
b. Exaggerated pulsus paradoxus
c. Reverse pulsus paradoxus
d. None of the above

**Q183. During passive leg raising (PLR) test, LVOT VTI is repeated at:**

a. 1 minute
b. 10 minutes
c. 5 minutes
d. No specific timeline

**Q184. The diagnostic accuracy of IVC distensibility index is:**

a. Poor
b. Good
c. Outstanding
d. Unable to discriminate

**Q185. All of the following conditions have limitations in LVOT VTI measurement, *except*:**

a. MR
b. AS
c. AFib
d. Low tidal volume ventilation

**Q186. The specificity of PLR is:**

a. 50%
b. 60%
c. 80%
d. 90%

**Q187. Limitations of heart-lung interaction-based dynamic indices are all, *except*:**

a. Spontaneous ventilation
b. Atrial fibrillation
c. RHF
d. Prone position

**Q188. In obese patients and abdominal surgical patients, does measurement of IVC variability through transhepatic window reliable?**

a. Yes
b. No

**Q189. What is minifluid challenge?**

a. 100 mL in 1 minute
b. 100 mL in 5 minutes
c. 250 mL in 5 minutes
d. 250 mL in 10 minutes

**Q190. The vein not studied in venous excess ultrasound score (VEXUS) is:**

a. Renal
b. Hepatic
c. Portal
d. Jugular

**Q191. Identify the incorrect match regarding pulse pressure variation limitation:**

a. Arrythmia—false negative
b. Low tidal volume ventilation—false negative
c. Spontaneous breathing—false positive
d. Increased abdominal pressure—false positive

**Q192. What is the correlation between cardiac output from LVOT VTI and invasive cardiac output measurement?**

a. Good correlation
b. Poor correlation
c. Moderate correlation
d. Cannot be compared

**Q193. Passive leg raising is not reliable in:**

a. Noninvasive ventilation (NIV) patients
b. COPD patients
c. Obese patients
d. All of the above

**Q194. What is the correlation between IVC diameter and RAP?**

a. Strong positive correlation
b. Moderate correlation
c. Inversely related
d. Not related at all

**Q195. A 43-year-old male presented to ICU with BP of 79/45 mm Hg [mean arterial pressure (MAP) of 55 mm Hg] and HR of 130 beats/min. His central venous pressure (CVP) was 5 mm Hg, and LVOT VTI was 23 cm/s and LVOT diameter was 2 cm. What is the systemic vascular resistance (SVR) of this patient?**

a. 500
b. 1,000
c. 1,500
d. 1,800

**Q196. Identify the incorrect statement regarding aortic root diameter:**

a. Independent predictor of aortic dissection
b. Measured in PLAX view
c. Extend from right coronary sinus to the opposite sinus of Valsalva
d. Measured in suprasternal view

**Q197. Two-point compression ultrasound can be used to rule out deep venous thrombosis in emergency settings. State true or false.**

a. True
b. False

**Q198. Calculate cardiac output with the following information: LVOT velocity of 1 m/s, TVI of 25 cm, LVOT diameter of 2 cm, aortic transvalvular velocity of 1.5 m/s, and HR of 70 beats/min?**

a. 6.3 L/min
b. 4.5 L/min
c. 5.5 L/min
d. Insufficient data

**Q199. Which of the following will not lead to increased respirophasic variations in transvalvular flows?**

a. A large RV infarct
b. Cardiac tamponade
c. Constrictive pericarditis
d. Status asthmaticus
e. Hypovolemic shock

**Q200. Calculate AV area with continuity equation for the patient in question 198, LVOT diameter was 2 cm and the LVOT velocity by pulse Doppler was 1 m/s.**

a. 0.2 $cm^2$
b. 0.3 $cm^2$
c. 0.5 $cm^2$
d. 0.8 $cm^2$

## Answers and Explanations

182. **Ans. c**

Heart-lung interactions are characterized by an inspiratory rise in arterial systolic and diastolic pressures, related to an inspiratory increase in LV stroke output secondary to positive pressure ventilation.

183. **Ans. a**

During passive leg raising (PLR), when the patient's position changes from semirecumbent at 45° to head-down with the legs elevated at 45°, there is autotransfusion of blood from the lower limbs into the circulation. The LVOT velocity-time integral (VTI) should be measured at baseline and then repeated at 1-minute interval after the position change to assess the change in cardiac output from baseline.

184. **Ans. b**

Meta-analyses of 31 studies on the IVC variability index showed a sensitivity of 0.75 and a specificity of 0.83. The area under the receiver operating characteristics (ROCs) curve was 0.86.

185. **Ans. d**

Limitations of LVOT VTI measurement are:

- AV disease
- MR
- Angle dependence
- Doppler gate at LVOT position
- Arrhythmia

186. **Ans. d**

The passive leg raise test has specificity of 90% to detect fluid responsiveness.

187. **Ans. d**

Limitations of dynamic indices of fluid responsiveness are:

- Spontaneous ventilation
- Arrhythmia
- Low tidal volume ventilation
- RHF

188. **Ans. a**

In obese and abdominal surgical patients with poor subcostal window (bowel gas), transhepatic IVC can be assessed for fluid responsiveness with good accuracy [area under the receiver operating characteristic curve (AU-ROC 0.88)], especially when there is high degree of respiratory variation.

189. **Ans. a**

- *Fluid challenge:* 250 mL crystalloids transfused over 15–20 minutes to detect a change in cardiac output of 15% from baseline
- *Minifluid challenge:* 100 mL crystalloid transfusion over 1 minute

Advantage is that with minifluid challenge, the risk of edema is less but the limitation is that the change in cardiac output is too small to detect fluid responsiveness.

190. **Ans. d**

- Venous excess ultrasound score—ultrasound imaging of the systemic veins such as IVC, portal vein, hepatic vein, and renal vein to assess for venous congestion in septic AKI patients for deresuscitation
- If IVC >2 cm, then subsequently other veins are examined for congestion.

191. **Ans. a**

| ***Parameters*** | ***False positive*** | ***False negative*** |
|---|---|---|
| Arrhythmia | ++ | |
| Low tidal volume ventilation | | ++ |
| Spontaneous breathing | ++ | ++ |
| Increased abdominal pressure | ++ | |

192. **Ans. c**

Measurement of cardiac output by LVOT VTI has many limitations (described in answer 128). It has moderate correlation ($r = 0.66$) in literature when compared to invasive cardiac output measurements.

193. **Ans. d**

Passive leg raise test to assess fluid responsiveness is not reliable in hypovolemic patients, obese, raised intra-abdominal pressure, and COPD patients.

194. **Ans. b**

There is a moderate correlation between IVC diameter and RAP ($r = 0.56–0.63$) but there is a strong correlation between IVC variability and RAP ($r = 0.72$)

195. **Ans. a**

SV = 3.14 × LVOT VTI × LVOT $r^2$

SV = 3.14 × 23 × 1

SV = 72 mL

C0 = SV × HR= 72 × 130 = 9,360 mL/min

SVR = (MAP – CVP)/C0 × 80

SVR = (55 × 5)/9.36 × 80

SVR = 430 dyne.s.$cm^{-5}$

196. **Ans. d**

Aortic root dilatation associated with severe AR is an independent risk factor for aortic dissection. It is measured in PLAX view extending from right coronary sinus to sinus of Valsalva.

197. **Ans. d**

Two-point compression ultrasound is usually done to rule out deep vein thrombosis (DVT) in critically ill patients. It examines common femoral vein bifurcation and popliteal vein bifurcation for venous compression and previous studies showed that it is comparable to the radiologist whole limb ultrasound to rule out DVT. However, the later studies showed that 5–10% of false negative in the emergency settings.

198. **Ans. a**

$SV = 3.14 \times \text{LVOT VTI} \times \text{LVOT } r^2$

$SV = 3.14 \times 25 \times 1$

SV = 78.5 mL

$CO = SV \times HR$

$CO = 78.5 \times 70$

CO = 5,495 mL/min

199. **Ans. e**

Hypovolemic shock typically does not cause increased respirophasic variations in transvalvular flows. However, conditions such as status asthmaticus, constrictive pericarditis, cardiac tamponade, and a large RV infarct can lead to these variations, as they affect intrathoracic pressures and ventricular interdependence.

200. **Ans. d**

Using the continuity equation, the calculated AV area based on the LVOT diameter and velocity is 0.8 $cm^2$.

# Index

Page numbers followed by *b* refer to box, *f* refer to figure, *fc* refer to flowchart, and *t* refer to table.

## Q



## R

## U



## V



## W



## Z